THE WOMAN PATIENT

Volume 3
Aggression, Adaptations,
and Psychotherapy

WOMEN IN CONTEXT: Development and Stresses

THE WOMAN PATIENT

Volume 1: Sexual and Reproductive Aspects of Women's Health Care
Edited by Malkah T. Notman and Carol C. Nadelson

Volume 2: Concepts of Femininity and the Life Cycle
Edited by Carol C. Nadelson and Malkah T. Notman

Volume 3: Aggression, Adaptations, and Psychotherapy
Edited by Malkah T. Notman and Carol C. Nadelson

BECOMING FEMALE: PERSPECTIVES ON DEVELOPMENT

Edited by Claire B. Kopp

WOMEN'S SEXUAL DEVELOPMENT: EXPLORATIONS OF INNER SPACE

Edited by Martha Kirkpatrick

WOMEN'S SEXUAL EXPERIENCE: EXPLORATIONS OF THE DARK CONTINENT

Edited by Martha Kirkpatrick

THE WOMAN PATIENT

Volume 3
Aggression, Adaptations, and Psychotherapy

EDITED BY

MALKAH T. NOTMAN, M.D.
AND
CAROL C. NADELSON, M.D.

Tufts University School of Medicine
Boston, Massachusetts

PLENUM PRESS · NEW YORK AND LONDON

Library of Congress Cataloging in Publication Data

Main entry under title:

Aggression, adaptations, and psychotherapy.
  (The woman patient; v. 3) (Women in context)
  Bibliography: p.
  Includes index.
  1. Aggressiveness (Psychology). 2. Women—Mental health. 3. Women—Crimes
against. 4. Psychotherapist and patient. I. Notman, Malkah T. II. Nadelson, Carol C. III.
Series. IV. Series: Women in context. [DNLM: 1. Delivery of health care. 2. Genital
diseases, Female. 3. Women. WP 100.3 W872 1978]
RC451.4.W6A37   616.89′0088042   82-5325
ISBN 0-306-40859-7   AACR2

©1982 Plenum Press, New York
A Division of Plenum Publishing Corporation
233 Spring Street, New York, N.Y. 10013

Printed in the United States of America

Contributors

E. P. Benedek, M.D. • Clinical Professor of Psychiatry, University of Michigan Medical Center; Director of Research and Training, Center for Forensic Psychiatry, Ann Arbor, Michigan

Karen A. Cohen • Program Coordinator for Health Education, Capital Area Community Health Plan, Albany, New York

G. A. Farley • Private practice, Ann Arbor, Michigan

Susan M. Fisher, M.D. • Lecturer, Department of Psychiatry, University of Chicago School of Medicine, Chicago, Illinois

Rochelle Friedman, M.D. • Psychiatrist, Massachusetts Institute of Technology, Cambridge, Massachusetts; Clinical Associate in Psychiatry, Massachusetts General Hospital, and Clinical Instructor in Psychiatry, Harvard University School of Medicine, Boston, Massachusetts.

Abraham Genack, M.D., Ph.D. • Department of Psychiatry, Harvard Medical School and Mount Auburn Hospital, Boston; Medical Director, Metropolitan Beaverbrook Mental Health and Retardation Center, Watertown, Massachusetts

Stuart T. Hauser, M.D., Ph.D. • Associate Professor of Psychiatry, Harvard Medical School, Boston, Massachusetts

Astrid Nøklebye Heiberg, M.D. • Associate Professor, Psychiatric Institute, University of Oslo, and Deputy Minister of Health, Norway

Berit Helöe, D.D.S. • Department of Oral Surgery and Oral Medicine, University of Oslo, Norway

Elaine (Hilberman) Carmen, M.D. • Associate Professor, Department of Psychiatry, University of North Carolina School of Medicine, Chapel Hill, North Carolina

Irving Hurwitz, Ph.D. • Associate Professor, School of Education, Boston College, Chestnut Hill; Consultant Division of Child Psychiatry, New England Medical Center, Boston, Massachusetts

Lewis A. Kirshner, M.D. ● Assistant Professor of Psychiatry, Harvard Medical School, Boston; Harvard Community Health Plan, Wellesley, Massachusetts

Gerald L. Klerman, M.D. ● Professor of Psychiatry, Harvard Medical School and Director, Stanley Cobb Psychiatric Research Laboratories, Massachusetts General Hospital, Boston, Massachusetts

Harriet E. Lerner, Ph.D. ● Staff Psychologist, The Menninger Foundation, Topeka, Kansas

Don R. Lipsitt ● Associate Professor of Psychiatry, Harvard Medical School and Mount Auburn Hospital, Cambridge, Massachusetts

Mirjam Mathe, M.D. ● Assistant Clinical Professor of Psychiatry, Albert Einstein College of Medicine; Clinical Director, Outpatient Child Psychiatry, Soundview Throgs Neck Mental Health Center, New York

Barbara S. McCrady, Ph.D. ● Butler Hospital, Brown University, Providence, Rhode Island

Jean Baker Miller, M.D. ● Clinical Professor of Psychiatry, Boston University Medical School, Boston; Director, Stone Center for Developmental Studies and Services, Wellesley, Massachusetts

Carol C. Nadelson, M.D. ● Professor and Vice-chairman, Director of Training and Education, Department of Psychiatry, Tufts University School of Medicine-New England Medical Center Hospital, Boston, Massachusetts

Theodore Nadelson, M.D. ● Clinical Professor of Psychiatry, Tufts University School of Medicine; Chief of Psychiatry, Boston Veterans Administration Medical Center, Boston, Massachusetts

Malkah T. Notman, M.D. ● Clinical Professor, Department of Psychiatry, Tufts University School of Medicine-New England Medical Center Hospital, Director, Women's Resource Center, and Director of Psychotherapy, Boston, Massachusetts

Cynthia R. Pfeffer, M.D. ● Assistant Professor of Psychiatry, Cornell University Medical College; Chief, Child Inpatient Unit, The New York Hospital-Cornell Medical Center, Westchester Division, White Plains, New York

Nancy Rudes, M.S.W. ● Private practice, New York

Earle Silber, M.D. ● Supervising and Training analyst, Washington Psychoanalytic Institute, Washington, D.C.

Veronica Tisza ● Lecturer, Department of Psychiatry, Harvard Medical School; Consultant, Department of Child Psychiatry, Massachusetts General Hospital, Boston, Massachusetts

Myrna M. Weissman, Ph.D. ● Professor of Psychiatry and Epidemiology; Director, Depression Research Unit, Yale University School of Medicine, Department of Psychiatry; Connecticut Mental Health Center, New Haven, Connecticut

Joan J. Zilbach, M.D. ● Associate Clinical Professor of Psychiatry, Tufts University School of Medicine; Lecturer, Harvard Medical School; Senior Psychiatrist and Co-director, Family Therapy and Research Program, Judge Baker Guidance Center, Boston, Massachusetts

Preface

This volume continues some of the issues raised in Volume 2 and focuses more closely on therapeutic intervention. The theoretical discussion of aggression provides a background for the presentation of patterns of aggression and violence affecting women, as well as possible connections between physical and emotional symptoms and indirect expressions of aggression. The section on aggression against and by women is an extension of some of the content of *The Woman Patient*, Volume 1 (e.g., the chapter on rape). Theoretical and clinical views that are not often linked in this fashion are included here because we are interested in understanding the development of a self-concept that incorporates the constructive aspects of "aggression" as well as an understanding of violence. In this context, loss, abandonment, delinquency, and child and adolescent suicide are also extensions of these issues.

The chapters that follow address aspects of symptom formation and concepts of illness. There is, as yet, no definitive explanation for why women experience certain illness patterns more or less than men. Current considerations have been reviewed, but these do not answer. They are a beginning on which we must build. It is apparent that any discussion of these subjects better elucidates the complexity if it includes an intermingling of general problems with concrete symptoms. Those specific problems that are usually thought of as psychological such as depression, and behaviors (such as substance abuse) provide a focus for understanding wider issues.

In the section on psychotherapy, the relationship between the woman patient and her therapist in analytic therapy is discussed generally as well as specifically with regard to women's relationships to their families.

As in the previous volumes in this series, we hope to raise questions and stimulate thought rather than to provide any kind of definitive answers to many of the questions raised.

We would like to thank all of the contributing authors for their hard work, patience, and tolerance during the process of writing and rewriting; our families for their support; and our editor, Hilary Evans, for her continual enthusiasm and help.

CAROL C. NADELSON
MALKAH T. NOTMAN

Boston, Massachusetts

Contents

PART I

Aspects of Aggression and Violence

Chapter 1

Social Change and Psychotherapeutic Implications

CAROL C. NADELSON AND MALKAH T. NOTMAN

Psychotherapists see women who are successful in many areas, but who are in conflict about their aspirations and activities. Since therapists are influenced by the same cultural, familial, and intrapsychic factors as their patients, they may find their objectivity clouded by their own values and attitudes, so that it may be difficult for them to examine with their patients the conflicts presented:

> An important example that is now being brought most forcefully to our attention has to do with the radical transformation currently taking place in the conceptualization of the position of women in our society, the rapidly changing reality of being a woman in today's world. I submit that many of our familiar usages and the comfortably established assumptions underlying them, concerning such psychoanalytically salient conceptions in our understandings of the psychology of women, as our notions of passive and active, of "normal masochism," and of so-called feminine and masculine attributes and behaviors, must necessarily be profoundly affected by the changing meanings enforced by the changing realities of the new woman's world. To not be aware of or be unable or unwilling to accommodate to a social reality that has been so profoundly transformed within our generation is to unnecessarily and perhaps irreparably burden the delicate balance of transferences and countertransferences on which the progressive resolutions of our therapeutic analytic task depend. If the analyst and analysand have profoundly different visions of this reality—of the "proper" or normal role of women in society—an analytic impass may readily ensue in which, the structure of the relationship being "tilted"

CAROL C. NADELSON, M.D. ● Professor and Vice Chairman, Department of Psychiatry, Tufts University School of Medicine; Director of Training and Education, Department of Psychiatry, Tufts-New England Medical Center Hospital, Boston, Massachusetts. MALKAH T. NOTMAN, M.D. ● Clinical Professor of Psychiatry, Tufts University School of Medicine; Chief of Psychiatry, Boston Veterans Administration Medical Center, Boston, Massachusetts.

(Greenacre) the way it is, the patient is the more usually bent into pseu-
docompliances with analytic interpretive pressures, though it can oppo-
sitely take the course of active withdrawals by the patient of major seg-
ments of psychic functioning from the analytic arena.[1]

The ability to differentiate what is "mentally healthy" from subjective personal values is critical. At the same time, an important and
often subtle distinction must be made between psychopathology and
a nonconformist choice. Interpreting as "sick" any behavior that is
primarily deviant is a well-known fallacy; however, missing the psychopathology deriving from important intrapsychic conflict also does
the patient a disservice.

Concepts of what is "healthy," as well as of what is "appropriate," "rational," or "acceptable," are difficult to define, and they
vary with different groups and with the historical context. In most
cases, "objective" criteria are not available. In 1970, the Brovermans
and their associates demonstrated that therapists' concepts about what
behaviors and attitudes are considered mentally healthy are affected
by sex-role stereotypes.[2] While many changes have occurred in the
decade since this report, and the sex-role stereotype of therapists' assessments of their patients may not be as pervasive, values and expectations always enter into therapeutic decisions to some extent.

Recent social changes have led to greater support for women's
pursuit of serious career commitments, and women have been more
motivated to enter and remain in careers. Nevertheless, concerns about
achievement and its effects on "femininity" remain prominent problems for many women in spite of, or perhaps because of, social pressure in this direction.

In this volume, we consider many issues that are important to
those seeking to understand the impact of social changes on women.
This is not an encyclopedic volume, and not all the important topics
are included. In this chapter, we provide an introductory overview of
some of the theoretical and clinical issues that concern women and
their therapists.

An important aspect of any discussion of the psychology of women
is the role of biology and reproduction. Although they clearly do not
constitute a woman's sole source of identity, women's lives are, in
fact, more influenced by their biological and particularly their reproductive timetable than are men's lives. All women are concerned in
one way or another about this reality, at least from the beginning of
adolescence. While men are also concerned about fertility, they do not
organize their life plans around reproduction and its implications in
the same way that women do. Thus, when femininity or female identity is discussed, we must consider biological as well as intrapsychic

and societal issues, such as the development of gender identity and self-esteem.

To begin, we must understand that the term *femininity* has many meanings. Hypotheses about femininity and feminine development have derived in the past from within a phallocentric culture where this perspective influenced both observations and understanding of human development. The last decade, however, has produced an enormous volume of new research in the psychology of women, and major reconsiderations of psychoanalytic thinking, as well as of other formulations about women's development.

Gender identity has been described as the "knowledge and awareness, conscious or unconscious that one belongs to one sex and not the other."[3] There is increasing evidence that gender identity is established by 18 months of age.[3,4,5,6] An aspect of this process not fully addressed by Freud and early theorists is the implications of its occurrence in the context of a child's interaction with his or her parents and other significant people.[7,8]

While there is some evidence that different skills and characteristics may exist in girls and boys from birth, it has been difficult to definitively establish many of these as innate because the powerful influences of culture begin to have an impact in early infancy. Observations of infants and children emphasize the important role of learning and language development in the child's concept of his or her gender identity. In many subtle ways, parents treat girls and boys differently from early infancy.[9] Therefore, an important component of the development of gender identity is the way in which children are perceived in their relationships to their peers and to adults at an early age. These object relations, in turn, both determine and are influenced by the child's evolving identity.

Arguments and disagreements about biological versus cultural factors are far from being resolved. It has become clear that human potential and adaptability are enormous. Despite the restrictions or the facilitation of biological conditions or the environment, the capacity to override what appears to be biologically determined exists. The work of Stoller and of Money and Ehrhardt exemplifies this point.[3,4] They have demonstrated that gender identity may vary from chromosomal sex, and that the sex of rearing is, in fact, a prime determinant of gender identity. Although recent work by Imperato-McGinley has raised questions about this view, it is nonetheless clear that environmental influences, including the expectations of parents and of society, are important.[10]

The argument that the historical evolution of roles and values has occurred as a response to basic human biological and developmental determinants has also been used to justify sex-role differences. The oversimplification inherent in this view has been well stated by the Rapoports, who said,

> In the human sciences the arguments that a given pattern is the statistical mode, that all through history the pattern has been modal, that primitive tribes show it, and that animals show it, are used daily to support assertions about the limitations of human nature. Because men have tended to be economic providers and women have cared for infants, it is argued that babies need their mothers and that men need to be the breadwinners. Because the nuclear family has been in recent times the basic form of social organization, it is assumed that it is the form best adapted to modern society. Because more men are ambitious and committed to work in contemporary society than are women, it is argued that this is the way men and women basically are.[11]

Thus, formulating conclusions about biological determinants on the basis of manifest behavior is similar to saying that because humans have never been propelled more than 30 miles per hour, it is contrary to human nature and should not occur. We see this as obviously absurd, yet many objections to social change and innovation, especially regarding sex roles, have been supported by similar arguments.

In the past, the inability to control reproduction effectively was a basic assumption. The very expectation that pregnancy would be an inevitable result of sexuality and that women would be subjected to men's sexual desires reinforced women's sense of helplessness and vulnerability, which supported the concept of feminine masochism as inherent. From this perspective, pregnancy could also be seen as implying inevitable suffering. Current views that regard pregnancy as a normal experience, although with stressful components, in the context of the assumption of reproductive choice provide a different perspective.

The procreative function of women has been seen as central to feminine identity. However, not all women actually become mothers, and for those who do, the experience differs. Most women feel some ambivalence. For some women, motherhood is an exciting and rewarding prospect, a fulfillment of creative potential in a new direction, encompassing warmth and closeness. For others, it is a frightening prospect, a task fraught with many possibilities of failure.[12] The actual expression of procreative wishes is an assertion of one part of feminine potential; the development of an identity as a woman is not necessarily interfered with by the choice to control reproduction. That is, a woman does not actually have to have babies to be "feminine."[7,8]

The woman approaching 30 often considers psychotherapy when

she begins to face the possibility that she may not marry, or if she decides not to marry. Even if she has been ambivalent about marriage, the reality of not marrying, or of not having children, may foster a sense of deviance or even defectiveness and may lower her self-esteem. At the same time, current peer pressure toward not having children may make those women who want children feel out of step with their immediate peers, or this pressure may create difficulties for women in facing their ambivalence or their sadness about giving up that option.

IDENTITY AND SELF-ESTEEM

The development of a stable identity and self-esteem is a particularly complex problem for women in the context of the current expanding options and reproductive choices. For many women, past identifications may not provide sufficient models and resources for current life demands, opportunities, or goals. Traditional definitions of feminine (as opposed to maternal) behavior have become translated into expectations of "appropriate" behavior for women, instead of being seen as merely descriptive of traditional norms. However, women are still conflicted and guilty about participation in what is regarded as "unfeminine," even when such behavior is demanded of them by the new situation in which they find themselves. A good example is aggressive and competitive behavior, which is discussed more fully in Chapter 2.

Women are now entering fields where aggression and competition are more open. At the same time, this necessary assertiveness evokes intrapsychic conflict. This conflict derives, in part, from the unconscious destructive impulses that accompany competition and, in part, from early identifications and communications. In the past, women have tended to assert themselves primarily when assertiveness was also in the service of others. They have been inhibited about pursuing self-actualization or stating openly to themselves and to others that they have particular ambitions and goals. Occupational preferences have generally been for caretaking and service roles. While some of these manifestations are changing, women are also concerned about abandoning what are perceived as feminine values, such as sensitivity and concern for others. Self-esteem may suffer as a result of these conflicts. While maintaining care about the welfare of the people with whom one is involved is certainly desirable, these values may come in conflict with the pursuit of "success" in a culture that places a high priority on work and achievement as measures of success.

Horner's work on "fear of success" described some women's per-

ception of achievement as a threat to their concept of femininity.[13]
While achievement and self-assertion have been understood as leading to competence and self-esteem for women as for men, for women
self-assertion and achievement have been traditionally confined to the
areas that are culturally defined as feminine. Thus, there may be important differences in how identity and self-esteem evolve in men as
opposed to women.

Moreover, defective self-esteem plays a significant role in the
etiology of depression, which occurs more frequently in women than
in men. Weissman and Paykel's data also indicate that depressed
mothers have negative effects on their children.[14] This may be particularly a problem for the feminine identification of daughters. If a
mother sees her own femininity as devalued, her daughter is caught
in a dilemma: to be like her mother is to be devalued; to be like her
father is to be "masculine." It is clear, then, that pathological self-
image can be perpetuated from generation to generation.

There may also be conscious or unconscious guilt about surpass-
ing or abandoning one's mother by attaining occupational success. This
conflict, as well as the difficulty of seeing oneself as an assertive, de-
cisive person, complicates the process of making appropriate decisions
about career goals and options.

The role of both parents in the development of stable sexual identity and self-esteem has been repeatedly discussed in the literature.
The course of development in the increasingly frequent one-parent
family must also be considered. Many authors have emphasized the
importance of the relationship with the father in the development not
only of the boy but also of the girl. Life in other than "traditional"
families must be considered by therapists.

Career Choices and Their Implications

Early in life, choices are frequently made because of idealism, ro-
manticism, faddism, or family pressure, often without adequate appreciation of the complexities and realities inherent in those choices.
The rapid increase in the acceptability of careers and, more recently,
the pressure on women to achieve have precipitated conflict about
making these initial decisions or about following through on the decisions already made. This is particularly true for those young women
whose early developmental experiences have been in the context of a
more traditional orientation. Anxiety may occur when a young woman
attempts to follow either a life course that she believes will meet with
disapproval, particularly by her mother, or one that exceeds her
mother's achievements. This may not be true of her mother's actual

current attitudes, but it represents internalized aspects of her mother, which remain despite social change. While in the past a woman might have been able to avoid the entire dilemma by accepting a "traditional" role, current expectations and pressures, including economic ones, frequently make that option less feasible.

PROBLEMS IN CAREER DEVELOPMENT

Women are often poorly prepared to face certain career demands because they have not conceptualized themselves as functioning in these roles during adolescence or childhood. They may find themselves unable to make long-range plans, and they may unconsciously sabotage the efforts of others to help them. When confronted with the option of assuming responsibility, they may choose jobs that are less interesting and rewarding, or they may deprecate their achievements in order to avoid jeopardizing their relationships with men. At times, they regress and become more dependent, helpless, or childlike, to gain approval and aid from male colleagues. They may experience symptoms of depression, anxiety, marital discord, or work inhibition.

Depression or anxiety can also follow a woman's recognition of her anger or discontent with a situation that she previously accepted. She may continue to see herself as helpless and powerless, or she may retreat out of a fear of losing relationships if she expresses angry feelings. In fact, loss of some relationships may indeed occur.[15] Even "successful" women may struggle with this kind of self-image.

Regressing and avoiding conflict are also ways of diminishing anxiety by preventing the open expression of ambition or self-assertion. Because the awareness and the acknowledgment of their aggression are more threatening to women than to men, even when these are conceptualized in terms of mastery and creativity, the therapist may well encounter resistance to achievement whenever it is perceived as being aggressive, at the same time that success is consciously sought.[15,16]

The need to avoid conflict can lead a woman to structure her life so that certain wishes are not explored or fulfilled. Sometimes a life event serves to prevent a confrontation; for example, an unplanned pregnancy may make it less possible to return to work. At times, conflicts are externalized and projected and/or displaced onto family, bosses, peers, the demands of the work, or the presence of discrimination. These reactions are particularly complex to address in therapy because there may be considerable reality in the woman's perception of the external difficulties. The therapist must be able to differentiate the internal from the external influences and to ally with the patient in her exploration of her conflict about self-assertion, in order to help her to examine the ways in which she may mask her competent self. It is important not simply to share her externalizations, nor simplistically to encourage self-assertion, without a full understanding of the situation.

Some women delay taking major professional steps or making personal decisions, such as moving to a better apartment or buying a car, because they fear that these changes would seem to others to be a commitment to an unmarried state. This delay can also lead to choices that undermine serious and potentially rewarding career commitments, in order to keep relationship possibilities open. These women may then become angry and disappointed when rewards do not materialize, but they may remain inhibited about assuming control of their lives.

Other women adopt life patterns in which they identify with the men in their lives and function as "one of the boys." This approach can be adaptive because it permits the woman to be a strong and competent peer; it also prevents the sexualization of relationships. The cost, however, may be an inability to accept sexual, dependent, or other feelings when they occur. These counterdependent mechanisms are often accompanied by rigidity and can interfere with empathy and rich interpersonal relationships.

The woman who attempts to retain her emphasis on relationships without sacrificing the development of competence and assertiveness has had a difficult time, particularly if she is in a "masculine" field. Although attitudes are changing, women in these positions need support in and help with reality testing.

CAREER AND MARRIAGE

Women who combine marriage and a career may experience role strain at some point.[17] This may occur early in the marriage or at a time when the woman begins to increase her involvement in activities outside her family, if she withdrew from these pursuits when her children were small. Her husband's sense of loss and abandonment, as well as his competitiveness when new interests develop, can cause him to become more demanding or even to regress or withdraw. Children can also experience these changes as losses. The mother's guilt about her absence or about the withdrawal of some of her involvement with her family can lead her to give up her outside interests or can stimulate her to overcompensate at home and to become overly self-sacrificing. At times, she may respond by displacing or projecting her anxiety and by becoming overcritical, intolerant, or unresponsive. She may also externalize and see her family as the major source of her problems, rather than understanding her own conflicted responses to pressure. If children develop problems, guilt and anxiety are often precipitated.[18]

At times, marital or sexual difficulties occur. There has been considerable speculation about the possible increase in male impotence as a result of women's more aggressive behavior and increased sexual demands. While there is currently no good evidence to support this contention, it does reflect men's anxiety about their masculinity when traditional roles shift, with women making greater demands for sexual performance and the assumption of tasks and roles that have been traditionally feminine. Psychological withdrawal, including loss of sexual interest or potency, compensatory and sometimes rigid assertions of masculinity, or other symptomatic behavior, may occur as attempts to restore self-confidence and to diminish anxiety.

The specific problems of the dual-career family must also be considered.[11] Generally, in this relationship pattern, each partner makes plans and sets individual goals that may not be consistent with family demands. Thus, problems in dual-career families frequently arise when children are born, since neither partner anticipates the need for change and compromise. Conflicting demands force confrontations that can produce interpersonal tension.

Returning to work presents another kind of problem. A woman returning to a career may find it difficult to find a place for herself, or to increase her time commitment when she has previously worked part-time. In addition to the conflict experienced around the need to become more assertive and independent, there are real issues concerning available opportunities. Positions suitable to the woman's age and experience may not be available, the demands of a particular field may have changed from the time when she was trained, she may not have the credentials to enter at the level she seeks, and she may find herself working with younger and less-experienced colleagues if she does find a job.

Some women attempt to resolve these tensions by seeking their "own space" and leaving their families. Others avoid the challenge by backing down and refusing positions of authority and responsibility. They may accept a compromise, often with anger, and at times with depression.

As people approach midlife, they reflect on the choices they have made. Those women who have not married or had children may feel they have paid too heavy a price. When underlying anger is mobilized, they may find it difficult to respond appropriately or productively, and they may need help in working through these feelings.

On the other hand, those women who have placed family commitments before their careers may face the loss of their primary source of identity when their children leave or when their childbearing ends. Divorce or the death of a spouse and the children's leaving home may precipitate anxiety, depression, or regressive symptomatology. Although often linked with menopausal changes, it is not menopause itself that produces these symptoms, but the events in one's life and family that accompany this period, particularly role loss, when it is present, and the issues of aging. Women with important and gratifying career investments seem to be less vulnerable to depression in the midlife years, and those who have not had children have generally come to terms with this premenopausally. It is the woman who has heavily invested herself in family roles who responds most strongly to menopausal changes.[19] The empty nest itself is overrated as an inevitable source of depression, although both women and men may miss their children as they set out on their own lives. Women find other roles and activities, and their relationships to their husbands often improve when the day-to-day stresses of caring for children are absent. Often it is the father who responds with depression to the departure of the children he has only recently come to know.

THERAPEUTIC IMPLICATIONS

While many of these are clearly applicable to men as well, we define below some therapeutic issues that particularly affect women.

THERAPY REFERRAL. Specific requests may be made for male or female therapists by patients or by other therapists. Women most often seek female therapists in order to avoid a sexualized or a potentially difficult authoritarian transference; they may also be sought for their "maternal" qualities and for their accessibility as role models. Women seeking a woman therapist often feel that she would be more responsive to wishes for self-actualization or can empathize more easily. The reasons for choosing a therapist, however, may be based on stereotyped or traditional views without regard to the characteristics of the individual therapist.[20] Nevertheless, these preferences are important. The patient's feeling of greater comfort or empathy can facilitate the development of a positive therapeutic alliance, which is critical to successful therapy.

REALITY-BASED FACTORS IN THERAPEUTIC APPROACH. Life phase considerations and situational realities are important in the choice of therapeutic modality or approach. It is obvious that a woman who must decide about continuing or aborting a pregnancy requires a short, focused therapeutic approach at the time of the crisis, rather than long-term therapy. A woman of 40 who has conflicts about becoming pregnant cannot afford several years in psychoanalysis to resolve these, even though other considerations might make psychoanalysis an appropriate treatment to be reconsidered another time. Less obvious but important variables are the other needs, priorities, and emotional resources of the woman at a particular moment. For example, a woman medical student with problems in her relationships with men might potentially be a good candidate for intensive psychotherapy or psychoanalysis, but while she is in medical school, it may be more helpful to suggest a therapeutic experience that is less demanding of time and creates less strain on academic performance.

VALUES, ATTITUDES, AND COUNTERTRANSFERENCE ISSUES. The values and attitudes of the therapist influence clinical formulation, the choice of treatment modality, and even the focus of therapy. The therapist does help the patient to sort out priorities, and he or she formulates as well as chooses what to interpret and when. For example, since social relatedness has generally been seen as more critical for women than for men, a woman who has serious problems in interpersonal relationships but who is successful in other areas of her life may find that her therapist is more concerned with her interpersonal relationships than her career-related problems, regardless of the priority she herself has assigned to this area. An interpersonal emphasis is more likely to occur when the patient is an isolated but occupationally successful woman than when the patient is a man. Work or academic requirements that compete with therapy hours are sometimes more likely to be treated as resistances in women than in men by a therapist who does not take these commitments as seriously in a woman. Some therapists still regard success for women in traditional terms, and non-family areas of life may not be given as high priority or may be seen as postponable. Therapists and patients may limit their exploration of choices because they see career and family involvement as being mutually exclusive or as being too complex for success in both.

Therapists may also find it difficult to appreciate the concerns of women who decide to have children late or who are ambivalent about childbearing. The woman executive who wants to have a baby but who has recently undertaken a very demanding job schedule may need the opportunity to explore why she chose to become so commited at the particular time she did, just as the woman of 40 with an established career who suddenly decides to have a baby and give up the career would do well to understand this decision. Both women may be acting defensively, or they may have important positive reasons for their choices.

The traditionally oriented therapist who finds it difficult to accept aggressive or assertive behavior in women may accept a woman's passive, masochistic stance rather than appreciate that it may also be pathological. On the other hand, the woman may be pressured into competitive activity and a major career commitment that she herself does not choose because the therapist feels this choice is now appropriate for women.

Regressive behavior may be erroneously seen as characterologically primitive when it is a style of presentation or a manifestation of low self-esteem, not necessarily related to major defects in ego functioning. A supportive rather than explorative therapeutic approach may then be recommended by the therapist. Such an approach may not enable the woman to work through her conflicts adequately.

A therapist who does not understand the particular meaning of a specific event for a woman—for example, a miscarriage or a hysterectomy—may focus on the underlying psychodynamics and interpret the woman's behavior in terms of psychosexual developmental levels, not recognizing that the woman may be symptomatic as a result of the trauma she has experienced, rather than because of characterological factors.

Countertransference feelings may cause therapists to overidentify with patients. They may be in awe of women who are effective professionally and may not recognize or attend to the concerns they present. The patient herself may support this perception because it is also important for her to present herself as a strong person, a quality that is important in her professional success and self-concept. Thus, both may collude and leave out significant areas for therapeutic work. This can certainly be true of therapy with men as well; a successful or prominent man may dazzle a therapist. However, "success" in men is more consistent with traditional expectation and so does not appear unusual.

The impact of feminist views has led many patients to be mistrustful of formulations presented in psychoanalytic language because of the implications of terms such as *penis envy*.[21] The psychoanalytically oriented therapist or analyst who dismisses this mistrust and does not understand the patient's concerns will come to a therapeutic impasse. It may be necessary to explain, to avoid jargon, and to specifically reinforce the alliance between individuals, not ideologies. If the patient perceives the therapist as taking a provocative, paternalistic, or authoritarian stance, she may find it difficult or impossible to develop a trusting relationship.

CONCLUSION

In order to work with contemporary women, a therapist must be sensitive to the impact and implications of social changes as well as maintaining sensitivity to individual issues. Problems arise from conflicts between the demands of professional or work adaptation and internalized contradictory expectations deriving from developmental experience. A therapist needs to be aware of the impact of real-life events as well as intrapsychic conflict on symptom formation. Earlier formulations and therapeutic approaches also need to be reconsidered in the light of data from a number of disciplines. It is important to incorporate an understanding of both childhood and adult developmental phases with concepts of femininity as a changing process and with different expressions at different life stages.

In this chapter, we have reviewed some of the implications of recent social changes for psychotherapy. Further chapters address many of these more explicitly, sometimes presenting contradictory views. Some chapters also look more closely at feminine development and particular aspects of women's experience. We hope that this volume will stimulate thought, interest, and further study.

REFERENCES

1. Wallerstein RS: Psychoanalytic perspectives on the problem of reality, *Journal of the American Psychoanalytic Association* 21(1):8–33, 1973.
2. Broverman I, Broverman D, Clarkson F, Rosenkrantz P, Vogel S: Sex role stereotypes and clinical judgments of mental health, *Journal of Consulting and Clinical Psychology* 34:1–7, 1970.
3. Stoller R: *Sex and gender.* New York, Science House, 1968.
4. Money J, Ehrhardt A: *Man and woman, boy and girl.* Baltimore, Johns Hopkins University Press, 1972.
5. Kleeman J, cited in Galenson E: Report of a panel on the psychology of women, *Journal of the American Psychoanalytic Association* 24(1):141–160, 1976.
6. Galenson E, cited in Galenson E: Report of a panel on the psychology of women, *Journal of the American Psychoanalytic Association* 24(1):141–160, 1976.
7. Erikson E: *Childhood and society.* New York, Norton, 1950.
8. Notman M, Nadelson C: Conflicts in identity and self-esteem for women, *McLean Hospital Journal* 2(1):14–23, 1977.
9. Moss HA: Sex, age and state as determinants of mother-infant interaction, *Readings on the psychology of women.* Edited by Bardwick J. New York, Harper & Row, 1972.
10. Imperato-McGinley J, Peterson R, Gautier T, Sturla E: Androgens and the evolution of male gender identity among male pseudohermaphrodites with five alpha reductose deficiency, *New England Journal of Medicine* 300(22):1233–1238, 1979.
11. Rapoport R, Rapoport R: *Dual-career families.* New York, Penguin Books, 1971.
12. Bibring G: Some considerations of the psychological processes in pregnancy, *Psychoanalytic Study of the Child* 14:113, 1959.
13. Horner M: Toward an understanding of achievement-related conflicts in women, *Journal of Social Issues* 28(2):157–175, 1972.

16 CAROL C. NADELSON AND MALKAH T. NOTMAN

14. Weissman M, Paykel E: *The depressed woman*. Chicago, University of Chicago Press, 1974.
15. Miller J, Nadelson C, Notman M, Zilbach J: *Reconsiderations of aggression and self-esteem in women*, Paper presented at International Psychoanalytic Association Meeting, New York, August 4, 1979.
16. Gilligan C: In a different voice: Women's conceptions of self and of morality, *Harvard Educational Review* 47(4):13–36, 1976.
17. Johnson F, Johnson C: Role strain in high commitment career women, *Journal of the Academy of Psychoanalysis* 4(1):13–36, 1976.
18. Notman M, Nadelson C, Bennett M: Achievement conflict in women: Psychotherapeutic considerations, *Psychotherapy and Psychosomatics* 29:203–213, 1978.
19. Bailyn L: Family constraints on women's work, *Annals of the New York Academy of Sciences* 208:82–90, 1973.
20. Nadelson C, Notman M: Psychotherapy supervision: The problem of conflicting values, *American Journal of Psychotherapy* 31(2):275–283, 1977.
21. Baker-Miller J: *Toward a new psychology of women*. New York, Beacon Press, 1976.

Chapter 2

Aggression in Women: Conceptual Issues and Clinical Implications

CAROL C. NADELSON, MALKAH T. NOTMAN,
JEAN BAKER MILLER, AND JOAN ZILBACH

In this chapter, we discuss some aspects of aggression in women, the interrelationship between self-esteem and aggression, and particularly the negative effect that women's recognition of their own aggression has on their self-esteem. We clarify these concepts in the light of the recent increased understanding of early childhood development and the impact of parental and societal attitudes, expectations, and definitions on psychological functioning.

Early psychodynamic hypotheses about femininity and feminine development arose within a phallocentric culture, which imposed a bias on the interpretation of data, and on the understanding of female developmental and intrapsychic processes. Most theoretical constructs about human development and behavior have tacitly assumed the male as a model. This was true also in clinical formulations, despite the preponderance of female psychotherapy patients. In other closely related fields, such as psychology, the experimental data have come

CAROL C. NADELSON, M.D. • Professor and Vice Chairman, Director of Training and Education, Department of Psychiatry, Tufts University School of Medicine-New England Medical Center Hospital, Boston, Massachusetts.   MALKAH T. NOTMAN, M.D. • Clinical Professor of Psychiatry, Tufts University School of Medicine-New England Medical Center Hospital; Director, Women's Resource Center, Boston, Massachusetts.   JEAN BAKER MILLER, M.D. • Clinical Professor of Psychiatry, Boston University Medical School, Boston; Director, Stone Center, Wellesley College, Cambridge, Massachusetts.   JOAN ZILBACH, M.D. • Associate Clinical Professor of Psychiatry, Tufts University School of Medicine; Lecturer, Harvard Medical School; Senior Psychiatrist and Co-director, Family Therapy and Research Program, Judge Baker Guidance Center, Boston, Massachusetts.

largely from male subjects. The female, until recently, has been seen as a variant or deviant, and/or data about women have been excluded since they were said to make interpretation of the results difficult or confusing.[1] Concepts about feminine development, and presumed overall human development, are currently undergoing reexamination in many quarters.

In order to fully explore the relationship between aggression and self-esteem in women, a careful consideration of instinct theory and its derivatives and a review of the theoretical concepts of narcissism and masochism would be necessary. That ambitious task is beyond the scope of this chapter, but some theoretical constructs are referred to here in the process of exploring the main theme of this chapter, that self-esteem in women is diminished by women's recognition in themselves of aggression or of its derivatives, that is, assertion, achievement, competence, and success. The manifestations of this loss of self-esteem are expressed as a sense of worthlessness, failure, and wrongdoing.

AGGRESSION

In an effort to clarify the concept of aggression, Maccoby and Jacklin[2] stated that

> The central theme [of aggression] is the intent of one individual to hurt another. But attempts to hurt may reflect either the desire to hurt for its own sake or the desire to control another person (for other ends) through arousing fear.

This view of aggression as a destructive force concurs in general with Freud's concept.[3,4,5] Other psychologists have held different views on aggression, and other psychoanalysts have altered Freud's basic concept. Thompson,[6] for example, stated:

> Aggression is not necessarily destructive at all. It springs from an innate tendency to grow and master life which seems to be characteristic of all living matter. Only when this life force is obstructed in its development do ingredients of anger, rage or hate become connected with it.

Greenacre[7] believes that aggression can be considered "the expression of the life force of growth" and is thus instinctual. Rochlin[8] focused on the defensive components of aggression when he stated, "when narcissism is threatened we are humiliated, our self-esteem is injured and aggression appears." Buxbaum[9] emphasized both the constructive and the destructive aspects and believed that unmodified aggression is destructive. Thus, in both the psychological and the psychoan-

alytic disciplines, there is no general agreement on the definition of aggression.

We define aggression in this chapter as those actions and impulses toward action and assertion that give expression to the individual's own aims and/or have an effect on others. Thus, aggression may be instinctual or defensive, innate or reactive, constructive or destructive, depending on its form and direction. Individual striving toward autonomous action and self-assertion is included in this definition.

It should also be noted that in some instances, different authors aim at different components within the larger subject of aggression. This chapter attempts to integrate some of the understanding that derives from different fields, while recognizing some of the difficulties that underlie basic concepts.

Traditional psychoanalytic theory states that women's aggression is converted into masochism and accompanying passivity. Freud,[10] Deutsch,[11] and others have stated that the efforts to effect this conversion form the key steps in the development of femininity. There was an implicit assumption that women and men begin life with the same quantity of aggression. Women's lifelong task, then, was to divest themselves of their direct aggression in order to achieve "femininity." Further, Freud[10] and Deutsch[11] believed that masochism was actually an innate characteristic in women. Therefore, when women "achieved" this conversion of direct aggression, they were reaching their biologically appropriate condition.

The inextricable binding of narcissism, passivity, and masochism as the "feminine triad" has been accepted until recently as the cornerstone of the normative development of femininity. Although linked together in some women, they are not necessarily uniquely feminine and may have different developmental origins. Tartakoff[12] and others have found these characteristics present, perhaps in different forms, in both men and women and believe masochism to be potentially pathological in both.

Blum[13] pointed out that a woman cannot carry out the function of "good enough mothering" if she has arrived at a predominantly masochistic resolution of her aggression. The implication of this statement is that women do possess and express aggression and activity, which are acceptable so long as they are expressed in the "feminine" mode of service to others, as in mothering. However passivity comes about in many women, as a result of the struggle to transform aggression, it may go beyond acceptable character style and lead to symptom development. Women who attempt to change their passive, masochistic adaptation often encounter serious internal conflict.

Many observations suggest that women do channel their impulses into making and preserving relationships rather than into direct or self-interested activity. In itself, this is an adaptive and constructive form of development. However, problems arise when relationships substitute for activity and action and thus serve a secondary goal. They can become the means by which a woman can feel some power or effectiveness, and thus the major or almost sole source of her self-esteem. To cite just one of many examples, the loss of important relationships and the consequent lowering of self-esteem are important factors in the development of depression. And depression is more frequent in women.[14]

The critical factor leading to depression may often be not the primary loss but the fact that the relationship itself has served a secondary defensive purpose. In the male, "aggression" or direct action is deemed valuable and acceptable in itself, although it is supposed to be directed into socially approved forms and toward socially approved goals. If a man can succeed in so directing his energies, he has the promise of obtaining relationships (and love). That is, others will approve of and love him for his use of his powers and his success. Thus, "aggression" both is rewarded in itself and leads to relationships. For women, "aggression" is first denied and then, secondarily, is channeled into making relationships.

Early in life, women incorporate the conviction, from their relationship with their parents and others, that their own direct, self-generated, self-directed, and self-interested aggression is unacceptable. This perception is further elaborated with each succeeding stage of development. As the "ego ideal" develops for most women, it contains the image of someone who is not overtly "aggressive." Thus, to acknowledge the existence of aggression is threatening to this ego ideal. The women then sees herself as a failure, inadequate and inferior, and her already low self-esteem is diminished further. This lowering of self-esteem may also contribute to depression.

The ego ideal of being someone who is not "aggressive," however, has important value, since women have been the main caretakers in society. Unbridled aggression or uninhibited self-assertion would be inconsistent with that role. Thus some modification of aggression has an important adaptive function. Several questions follow, however:

1. Do women suffer differentially from an excessive societally induced inhibition of aggression, especially as this inhibition begins early in life?
2. Should the inhibition of aggression, which has considerable social value, be restricted primarily to one sex?

3. Is it inevitably equated with a subservient or subordinate position?
4. Can aggression be appropriately expressed without being a destructive characteristic for women?

Evidence that aggression in women is diverted or modified depressively comes from many sources. Goldings[15] stated that overt aggression appears in latency girls' rhymes and stories, although not necessarily in their behavior. This evidence supports the idea of the early existence and then transformation of aggressive impulses and wishes. Kaplan[16] stated that the early inhibition of aggressive expression "prevents adequate sublimations in a girl and restricts the development of a healthy outlet for the discharge of her aggression." In a description of delinquent girls, Kaplan noted that they are less apt to strike out in anger than boys, but when they do become involved in fights, they "fight primitively" without regard for the very real dangers of injury from bigger, stronger opponents, and they often follow these acts with acts of rage against themselves. Symonds[17] confirmed this observation on the basis of extensive work with the psychological aspects of violence.

Whether aggression as activity and assertion can be separated from aggression as action aimed at the harm or destruction of others is a difficult and unsettled question. For women, however, there seem to be special problems. Aggression as action and assertion is experienced primarily as a destructive force, inevitably carrying the implication of the intent to hurt or destroy another. Thus, when women begin to become aware of the extent of their own aggression in a context where it has not been clear to them before, it is most likely to be experienced as incongruent and inappropriate, and therefore as disorganizing and overwhelming, potentially adding to fear and self-condemnation.

The fall in self-esteem that occurs when a woman believes herself to be "too aggressive" has been mentioned. A further consideration of self-esteem and how it relates to aggression is important.

SELF-ESTEEM

Most original formulations about self-esteem development were derived from pathological situations. These ideas were then expanded to explain normative development. According to classical theory, a child was understood to become able to accept her or his realistic limitations and grandiose fantasies and to restrict the expression of instinctual impulses. These impulses are replaced by ego-syntonic goals and by pleasure in those functions and activities that gain approval and support from parents. This process enhances the sense of both effectiveness and "goodness," which is part of the development of self-esteem.

In the early years, the child "has achieved something of a self-concept through reacting to and internalizing the attitudes of family members to him." [18] Self-esteem is gradually modified by experiences with peers and others and with the mastery of physical processes and control of environment, but the basic link to the parents is critical. The child needs and depends on parental love, help, and approval and, by and large, desires to live up to parental expectations, standards, and values, which are gradually internalized. The state of the parents' self-esteem and self-image is also critical in the development of self-esteem in the child.

While self-esteem is usually constantly modified in response to ongoing realistic experiences, when unconscious conflict exists self-esteem is altered. [19] The mastery of unconscious conflict also leads to a basic sense of self-esteem. [20] Thus, as the child moves further in her or his own development, she or he acquires some of the attributes of the parent and identifies with some aspects of parental self-esteem, as well as parental values and attitudes, although always in her or his own unique combination.

The importance of the maternal ego ideal in the development of the young girl's sense of femininity has become more evident and is supported by these formulations. The maternal ego ideal does not usually contain a component of aggression that is perceived as clearly available and is understood as potentially creative. This conflict can result when activity for one's own gratification rather than for the care and nurturance for others becomes a primary source of self-esteem.

Another source of self-esteem derives from physical experiences, sensations, and gratifications. Thompson [6] has stated: "The acceptance of one's body and all its functions is a basic need in the establishment of self-respect and self-esteem." Easser [19] concurred and pointed to women's difficulty in achieving this bodily ease and pleasure, which she attributed to the problems of internal tensions, difficulties in the identification with the mother, and problems in the separation–individuation process. We would also emphasize the underlying societal constraints against women's using their bodies for their own enjoyment *per se,* rather than for others' pleasure.

In early life, the restriction of a girl's physical activity provides a fundamental base for her awareness of the interdiction against aggression. This restriction on her "physicality" has important implications for the more global restriction of activity and assertiveness. The very young child's notion of her physical activity and sexuality incorporates the early prohibitions against aggression, and she comes to feel that her own impulses, desires, and thrusts toward action are inherently "bad." Examples of restrictions in physical and sexual expression abound in the literature and in clinical experience. The recent focus on physical activity and athletic achievement for girls may produce important changes in this aspect of women's self-concept.

The classical view of the developmental origins of femininity and the need to give up active for passive aims must also be considered in relation to self-esteem. In this conceptualization, the girl turns away from her early positive tie to her mother because of disappointment that she does not have a penis, among other issues. She holds her mother responsible for this "lack." However, an overly concrete view of "penis envy" ignores the highly significant symbolic implications that may be central. For a feeling of strength and potency, the little girl may feel that she needs a penis and that without it, she is weak and vulnerable. One might focus on the question of why a penis is necessary for this strength and why a self-image without it is devalued and perceived as weak.

For a woman whose mother does feel devalued, the struggle for positive self-esteem means some degree of psychic separation from the mother, or even rejection of her. Conflict emerges between the need to give up the mother, the need to be loved by the mother, and the intensity of the tie with the powerful pre-Oedipal mother. Thus, the goals of self-actualization and independence may necessitate rebellion against the mother and may be a necessary psychological reaction against the incorporation of the mother's devalued self-image, not specifically because of her responsibility for the lack of a penis.

Feminine psychology can be conceptualized in another light, built on a positive consideration of feminine development rather than on a focus on deficits. This positive approach involves understanding the development of femininity in terms of uniquely female experiences rather than those that are thought of as substitutes for the absence of male characteristics. Positive forces for women are also derived from identification with their mothers.

Many feminine problems can be understood as attempts in various ways to take care of, undo, deny, or hide this strong inner force, which is at the same time perceived as dangerous and conflictual. The awareness of this strength may itself represent an aspect of a tie with the strong pre-Oedipal mother. It is not to be oversimplified by being confused with the girl's sense of another kind of power, namely, the capacity to have a baby. Instead, this refers to a more basic self-conflict, which does not conceptualize women as incomplete without an object or as seeking fulfillment of their identity exclusively in sexuality or parturition. We concur with Easser[19] and Stoller[21] in the concept of primary femininity as a separate feminine developmental phase with a positive self-evaluation in a conflict-free sphere.

We have referred to fear of aggression, lack of integration, and the constriction of aggressive expression. In the psychoanalysis or psychotherapy of women, the need for a positive mobilization of aggression has often been ignored or missed. Such neglect can be seen as "syntonic" with the societal stereotypes present in both patient and therapist.

In sum, women often experience their aggressive wishes and strivings as evidence of their defectiveness or lack of worth, rather than as a basis for positive self-esteem. Aggression and its derivative activities are therefore experienced by women as a major threat.

The Impact of Differential Responses of Parents

The implications of a model of development that emphasizes the significance of early communication between parents and children have been reinforced by a number of investigators. Further, the evidence that parents have different expectations of male and female infants and, in fact, behave differently toward them is quite convincing. Rubin, Provenzano, and Luria[22] found that there were consistent differences in the reports of parents about the characteristics of their infants, depending on the babies' sex. One-day-old infants were studied. Female infants were seen as significantly softer, finer-featured, smaller, and more inattentive than male infants. These differences were not objectively present according to the researchers' observations and measurements (e.g., weight and length). Their data indicate that gender-role stereotypes exist from birth and that the parents in this study acted on them.

Studies of older infants reveal continued parent–child interactional differences based on gender. In one study, mothers smiled, talked, and vocalized more to females; males were held, stimulated, and aroused.[23] Mothers picked up girls more often when they cried, while boys were allowed to remain crying. Since crying can be an active exercise, and large muscle movements may go on unrestrained if the infant remains crying, the male infant may have a different physical experience than the female infant whose crying is curtailed. There are potential implications in this experience for subsequent development.

Another researcher presented the same 6-month-old infant to 11 mothers who were not told the sex of the baby.[24] A different response was reported, depending on the mother's belief about the baby's gender. When the mothers thought that the infant was a girl, "she" was handed a doll more frequently; when they thought it was a boy, a train was given. The mothers did not recognize that their behaviors differed. They also thought the female was softer and perceived other differences, although the same infant was presented in every instance.

Evidence has accumulated to indicate that gender identity is established by 18 months of age.[20,25] Unlike Freud's original view that it began at the later phallic stage with the child's perception of genital differences between boys and girls, recent data make it clear that this awareness occurs earlier.[3] Among the many influences during this early period of life, bodily sensations, including those in the genitals, are believed to contribute to the development of gender identity. We are stressing a part of this process not fully addressed by Freud and early theorists, namely, that these aspects of development take place in the context of a child's earliest interactions with his or her parents and other significant people, who approach the child with deep-seated feelings (and fears) that vary with the infant's gender. Thus, components of the self-concept of children include

1. The primary and/or innate differences existing between boys and girls.
2. The way in which a child is actually treated by adults and peers.
3. Identifications with parents.

In regard to the first of these, there is evidence that biological differences exist between girls and boys in the development of the nervous system and in hormonal balance. However, the relevance of these differences has been difficult to establish because the influence of culture and the wide range of individual variation are so critical. Further, these factors begin to have an impact so early that it is difficult to draw conclusions about which characteristics and behaviors are, in fact, innate and immutable. According to Maccoby and Jacklin,[2] an exhaustive review of research data and cross-cultural observations "in a wide variety of settings, using a wide variety of behavioral indexes," indicates that males demonstrate more aggressive behavior than females. These authors argued that the basis for this difference is biological. When considering competitiveness and dominance (which we would include in our definition of aggression), the evidence is less clear, especially in childhood. Studies of competitive behavior have generally taken place in contrived situations and do not show consistent sex differences. These authors discussed cultural and socialization factors, minimizing parental influence as an important determinant of the differences in aggressive behavior between the two sexes. Further, they feel that there is little differentiation by the sex of the child in parental behavior.

Block,[26] however, after reviewing all of the studies (200) reported by Maccoby and Jacklin,[2] took issue with their assessment of the data and their conclusions. She pointed to major deficiencies in the evidence, emphasizing the differences between mothers and fathers in their interaction with male and female children, and stressing the importance of these differences as determinants of attitudes and behavior. She also focused attention on differences in children at different ages, noting that the data reviewed by Maccoby and Jacklin were on children who were 6 years old and under. Further, Block[26] stated, the data were analyzed in the aggregate, included disparate observations from both mothers and fathers, and did not take into account the relative paucity of studies of fathers' interaction with female and male children.

Block's data indicate that both mothers and fathers appear to emphasize achievement and competition more for their sons than for their daughters and that both parents place greater emphasis on boys' independence, assumption of personal responsibility, and control of affect. Punishment for misbehavior is more commonly given by parents of males than by parents of females. Fathers are more authoritarian, strict, firm, and physically punitive with sons than with daughters. They are less tolerant of aggression directed toward them by their sons. With regard to daughters, both parents expect "ladylike" behavior and discourage rough-and-tumble games and fighting. There is also a greater emphasis on the restriction of daughters' behavior and closer supervision of their activities.

Block pointed out also that the children themselves perceived clear differences in what was expected and communicated. Sons more than daughters described parents who emphasized competition and the control of affective expression, especially as it related to communications about masculinity. In another paper, Block[27] noted that age-specific socialization practices exist and are related to the developmental level of the child. They are also influenced by the tolerance of society for impulse expression in particular areas. In addition to communication via toys, games, sex-role expectations in the performance of chores, etc., evidence has been presented that elucidates some of the ways in which socialization factors may influence the different handling of aggression by women and men. Thus, Block stressed the importance of measuring aggression at different developmental phases and the several different forms in which aggressive behavior can occur.

Conclusion

In this chapter, we have considered the problem of feminine aggression and particularly its relationship to self-esteem. We have discussed some of the evidence that suggests that the interdiction of feminine aggression occurs early in life. Aggression is subject to different influences in girls than in boys. Its direct expression is restricted and more readily suppressed. Most often, it is transformed into action that is in the service of others, and therefore, it can appear to be almost absent. The fact that women can use their aggression to function so well in serving others, can gain satisfaction from fostering the growth and development of others, and can then shift to feeling worthless if the serving relationship is altered suggests that the aggressive energy nevertheless exists but is available only in another form. The force of the self-destructive and self-blaming manifestations in masochism suggests the power of the aggression that is present. The general understanding of aggression has been linked to its manifestations in men and has not been thoroughly explored as it exists in the woman.

Woman's aggression is shrouded in horror and dread. The terrifying destructive violence exhibited by Medea stands as a male culture's perception of the dangerous and primitive nature of women's aggression, and also of its notions about her vulnerability to narcissistic injury. The responses of Clytemnestra are seen as alien to the nature of women, so she is described as "a woman with a man's will." Benedek and Farley[28] pointed out that our denial of aggression in women results in the assumption that violence in women must derive from mental derangement.

The fear of the powerful life-giving and potential life-destroying woman reaches deep into our psychic roots. It seems likely that this cultural interdiction affects the female as an infant. Thus, she is pushed away from active expression, and it becomes a source of conflict rather than a more straightforward path to growth and development. Her physical activity is diverted and inhibited and forms the basis for more complex inhibitions.

We suggest that these inhibitions are compounded at each developmental stage and form the basis of complex inner psychological barriers that have both limited women's development and created the groundwork for psychological distress.

REFERENCES

1. Gilligan C: Women's place in man's life cycle, *Harvard Educational Review* 49(4):431–446, 1979.
2. Maccoby E, Jacklin E: *Psychology of sex differences.* Stanford, Calif.: Stanford University Press, 1974.
3. Freud S (1905): *Standard edition.* Volume 7. *Three essays on the theory of sexuality.* London, Hogarth Press, pp. 135–243, 1957.

4. Freud S (1920): *Standard edition*. Volume 18. *Beyond the pleasure principle*. London: Hogarth Press, pp. 7–64, 1955.

5. Freud S (1923): *Standard edition*. Volume 19. *The ego and the id*. London: Hogarth Press, pp. 12–59, 1961.

6. Thompson C: On women: Some effects of the derogatory attitude toward female sexuality. In *Psychoanalysis and women*. Edited by Miller J. New York, Brunner/Mazel, pp. 58–69, 1973.

7. Greenacre P: *Emotional growth*, Vol. 1. New York, International Universities Press, 1971.

8. Rochlin G: *Man's aggression: The defense of the self*. Boston, Gambit, 1973.

9. Buxbaum E: *Psychology of women: Latency and early adolescence*. Paper presented to American Psychological Association, 1974.

10. Freud S (1925): *Standard edition*. Volume 19. *Some psychical consequences of the anatomical distinction between the sexes*, 1925a. *Standard Edition*, London, Hogarth Press, pp. 248–258, 1961.

11. Deutsch H: The significance of masochism in the mental life of women, *International Journal of Psycho-analysis 11*:48–60, 1930.

12. Tartakoff H: *Psychoanalytic perspectives on women: Past, present and future*. Paper presented at Radcliffe Institute, Cambridge, Mass., 1972.

13. Blum H: Female psychology, masochism and the ego idea, *Journal of the American Psychoanalytic Association 24*(5):305–351, 1976.

14. Weissman M, Klerman G: Sex differences and the epidemiology of depression, *Archives of General Psychiatry 34*:98–111, 1977.

15. Goldings H: Jump rope rhymes and rhythms of latency development in girls, *Psychoanalytic Study of the Child 29*:431–450. New Haven, Conn.: Yale University Press, 1974.

16. Kaplan E: Manifestations of aggression in latency and pre-adolescent girls, *Psychoanalytic Study of the Child 31*:63–78, 1976.

17. Symonds M: Psychodynamics of aggression in women, *American Journal of Psychoanalysis 36*:195–203, 1976.

18. Mead G: *Mind, self and society*. Chicago: University of Chicago Press, 1934.

19. Easser BR: *Womanhood*. Unpublished manuscript, 1975.

20. Bibring E: The development and problems of the theory of the instincts, *International Journal of Psycho-analysis 22*:102–131, 1941.

21. Stoller R: Primary femininity, *Journal of the American Psychoanalytic Association 25*(4):59–78, 1977.

22. Rubin J, Provenzano F, Luria Z: The eye of the beholder: Parents' views on sex of newborns, *American Journal of Orthopsychiatry 44*(4):512–519, 1974.

23. Moss H: Sex, age and state as determinants of mother-infant interaction, *Merrill Palmer Quarterly of Behavior and Development 13*(1):19–36, 1967.

24. Kagen J, Moss H: *Birth to maturity*. New York, Wiley, 1962.

25. Money J, Ehrhardt A: *Man and woman, boy and girl*. Baltimore, Johns Hopkins University Press, 1972.

26. Block J: Conceptions of sex roles: Some cross-cultural and longitudinal perspectives, *American Psychologist 28*(6):512–526, 1973.

27. Block J: Another look at sex differentiation in the socialization behaviors of mothers and fathers. In *Psychology of women: Future directions of research*. Edited by Sherman JA, Denmark FL. New York: Psychology Dimensions, pp. 29–87, 1978.

28. Benedek E, Farley G: Women and violence. In *The woman patient*, Vol. 3. Edited by Nadelson C, Notman M. New York: Plenum Press, 1982.

Chapter 3

Women and Violence

E. P. Benedek and G. A. Farley

Introduction

The long involvement of women in crime, and particularly in crimes of violence, has fascinated dramatists and other observers of the human condition. In the explorations of the particular tragedy that is seen when a woman becomes involved in violence, playwrights have built on recurring themes that are also reflected in modern theoretical notions about the etiology of female criminality. Aeschylus lays bare, in the play *Agamemnon,* the character of Clytemnestra and the events that bring her to a murder. She is described by the author as a woman of character, "a woman with a man's will." Over the 10 years of her husband's absence, the queen has nurtured an evergrowing hatred of him, springing from his slaying of their daughter because an oracle told him to. Her murderous need for revenge is further exacerbated when her husband returns home from Troy, bringing with him his mistress. The dramatist describes the cunning and care with which Clytemnestra, in the grip of hatred, plans and carries out the murder of her husband while he is helpless in the bath. Much of the power of the play comes from the description of the queen's careful planning of this murder, masked by her deceitful facade as a loving wife rejoicing at her husband's return. Thus, the murder is explained by the author as the result of hatred, lust for power, and deceitfulness.

A different explanation of the tragedy of the violent woman is explored by Euripides in the character of Medea. She is shown by the playwright as a woman in the throes of a monstrous and irrational

E. P. Benedek, M.D. • Department of Psychiatry, University of Michigan Medical Center; Director of Research and Training, Center for Forensic Psychiatry, Ann Arbor, Michigan. G. A. Farley, Ph.D. • Private practice, Ann Arbor, Michigan.

passion in which she slays her children. Again, the character of this woman is portrayed as a strong one, marked by power and pride. Early in the play, Medea is revealed, by the author, to nurture bitterness about being a woman. Passages reflect on her evaluation of her own true strength. However, unlike Clytemnestra, who glories in the murder that she has committed, an ambivalent Medea is shown. Her maternal feelings for her children are graphically displayed at war with her need for vengeance on her errant husband. Alternately, she is overwhelmed by the forces within her, which are described by the dramatist as much stronger than rationality or will. It is this inexorable inner psychological force that leads her to the insanity of the murder. The power and drama of this work evolve from the dramatist's exploration of the strength of the internal forces that lead to violence.

The dramatic themes of pride, manliness, deceit, and insanity have repeatedly emerged in even more recent responses to female violence. The possible association of such violence with mental illness was clearly exhibited in the media coverage of such events as Leslie Van Houten's involvement in the Manson murders, Sara Jane Moore's assault on President Ford, and Patricia Hearst's alleged involvement in an armed robbery. Indeed, the general public, when confronted with women who have exhibited violent behavior, frequently assume that it must be the result of mental derangement. The general cultural stereotypes about the behavior of women encourage such a position. It is the purpose of this discussion to explore the nature of violence in women and its relationship to mental illness, where such a relationship exists. We review here the literature on female criminality in general, and violence in particular. It must be borne in mind at the outset that while extensive literature exists addressing male criminality, careful theoretical and research attention have only quite recently been focused on the role of women in crime. This lack of attention is even more noticeable when one considers the special issues of female violence. Much of the literature from the turn of the century is speculative or theoretical in nature, and only more recently has any systematic research investigation of female criminality been undertaken.

THEORIES OF FEMALE CRIMINALITY

Before turning to the special issue of women and violence, it is useful to review the literature that bears on the general etiology of female criminality. Many of the theoretical explanations given for female crime in general have been used to explain more violent behavior in women. This theoretical literature concerning the fundamental basis of women's involvement in crime displays three major themes: bi-

ological causality, the primacy of social roles, and/or the influence of
socioeconomic factors. These three themes recur not only in the theoretical discussion of female crime but in the research literature as well,
and they intertwine through all discussions of women and crime.

At the turn of the century, Lombroso[1] offered what was one of
the earliest biological explanations of criminality, having constructed
a developmental hierarchy of "superiority" involving racial and sexual
variables. Lombroso felt that this hierarchy ranged from the most highly
developed (white males) to the most primitive (nonwhite females). He
explained all crime as a result of inborn atavistic traits reflecting primitiveness of development. He postulated that women, children, and
savages shared many of these traits because of their primitiveness of
development. He noted, in particular, that women were deficient in
"moral sense." He proceeded to explain women's lesser involvement
in criminal behavior as the result of lower intelligence. However,
Lombroso alleged that women given over to crime shared more traits
with men than women whose behavior was more law abiding. While
this rather simplistic somatic theory of criminality has, in general, long
been discredited, it appears to have had an enduring impact on theories of *female* criminality. Klein indicated that more recent theories, in
varying degrees, "rely on those sexual etiologies based on implicit assumptions about physiological and psychological nature of women that
are explicit in Lombroso's work."[2]

A second theoretician who focused on the biological explanation
of female crime was Sigmund Freud. In the *New Introductory Lectures,*[3]
he discussed the psychology of women. While noting that there was,
in fact, considerable variation because of both cultural and social
learning, he alleged that women, because of constitutional differences,
were less aggressive, less defiant, more dependent, and more docile
than men. In examining the psychological development of women,
Freud commented on the apparent weakness of the superego in women.
He presented the development of the superego as emerging with the
resolution of the Oedipal conflict. Theoretically, this internal representation of the moral demands of society derives its power from castration anxiety. In Freud's view, when the fear of castration disappeared,
the primary motives supporting the ultimate development of the superego also disappeared. He viewed women as remaining "in the oedipal situation for an indefinite period . . . the formation of the superego must suffer in these circumstances. It cannot attain the strength
and independence which gives it cultural importance."[3] As a result of
this "deficit," women were seen as lacking in sense of justice, dem-
onstrating a weak moral sense and having less impulse control. Although Freud did not directly relate the superego weakness to female

criminality, it was implied that women were somewhat more inclined toward amorality because of anatomical differences. Freud's general view of deviant behavior of a variety of sorts manifested by women resulted from the "masculinity complex." The masculinity complex, as described by Freud, resulted from an unsatisfactory resolution of the women's discovery of her lack of a penis. Rather than making a "healthy adjustment," she overidentified with maleness and involved herself in a variety of phallic activities, presumably including criminal acting-out.

These biological notions persist even in the writings of the theoretician whose primary explanations of female criminality address cultural and social roles. One of the most important and oft-quoted theoreticians is Pollak,[4] whose exploration of female criminality utilized an interactional model. He occupied a rather intermediate position between those writers whose focus was primarily biological and those writers whose focus centered on social roles. Pollak believed that a major facet of criminality in women began with their natural deceitfulness. To buttress his conclusion that women were inherently deceitful, he presented both physiological and sociological rationales. He alleged that the female anatomy allowed women to practice deceit more readily than males. He contended that the physiological fact that a man could not conceal an erection contrasted with a woman's ease in concealing lack of sexual arousal or interest. He stated, "It cannot be denied that this basic physiological difference may well have great influence on the degree of confidence which the two sexes have in the possible success of concealment and thus on their character pattern in this respect."[4] He also supported this inference of natural female deceit on the basis of social norms. He contended that not only sexual mores, which forced concealment of menstruation, but also more general cultural beliefs, which required women to conceal aggressive impulses, specifically trained women in the practice of deceitfulness.

In his examination of the patterns of variation in female criminality, Pollak fundamentally maintained that female crime had been consistently underestimated, a notion that was unique at the time he stated it. He attributed this underestimation to the operation of four major variables. The first involved the crimes to which women were "inclined." He viewed female crime as being manifested largely in crimes of prostitution, shoplifting, and forgery. These were charges that were traditionally underreported and rarely result in convictions. Thus, the true extent of women's involvement in crime was concealed. The second factor leading toward underestimation involved social roles. The author believed that many of the social roles attributed to women allowed them to become accomplices, and therefore, their involvement in a given crime was harder to detect. Third, he argued that such social roles as nurse, mother, or housekeeper augmented the natural deceitfulness of women, reducing the public nature of their crimes. He maintained that in her role as nurse or housekeeper, a woman could murder with considerably less likelihood of detection (e.g., surreptitiously increasing or decreasing dosages of medication.) Last, Pollak maintained that female crime was underestimated because of chivalry. He maintained that even should a woman be arrested, there was greater leniency in both conviction and sentencing. He attributed this leniency to the conventional prejudices of the culture regarding women. This alleged observation of greater leniency in the courts is a theme that occurs in much of the subsequent literature.

In discussing the causes of female criminality and the changes in its incidence, Pollak focused on the possible impact of social emancipation. However, he also looked to biological factors, particularly surrounding the issue of menstruation. While he was circumspect about the relevance of such biological factors, he felt that it was a viable source of the explanation of female crime.

More recent theories of female criminality have focused on the importance of social roles or socioeconomic factors. Adler clearly stated the primacy of social roles in both conformist and deviant behavior: "How else can we understand the female (or for that matter, the male) offender, except in the context of her social role? The mother becomes the child beater, the shopper the shoplifter, and the sex object the prostitute."[5] Adler maintained that as the social and economic disparity between females and males decreases, female criminality increases. A corollary of this position is that as the social roles become more similar, so do the types of crime in which women are found to be involved. Thus, it would seem that the same forces that impel equality in the culture and the labor force also compel equality in the underworld. The association of changing rates in female crime with feminism was clearly stated by Adler, who reflected, "Women have lost more than their chains. For better or worse, they have lost many of the restraints which kept them within the law."[5] We also see a similar discussion in the work of Simon,[6] who has focused largely on the influence of socioeconomic variables. Simon noted that any changing rates in female crime may not be attributed to differences in propensity but to differences in opportunity. She noted that women's increased participation in the labor force increases the scope and extent of opportunity. She postulated that as this opportunity increased, it would be reflected in the incidence and type of female crime.

Some Statistical Considerations

From the above discussion, it can be seen that much of the theoretical exploration of female crime assumes, at least for the purposes of discussion, an increasing rate in the criminal involvement of women. Recent newspaper and television coverage of female crime has widely disseminated the belief that women are currently committing more crimes of all kinds than in the past. Regrettably, the statistical documentation of such a conclusion, along with other statistical inferences, is open to question.

National crime statistics, primarily collected by the Federal Bureau of Investigation, are beset by a variety of difficulties that hamper conclusive interpretations. FBI statistics do not take into consideration changes in the population, nor do they consider the possible influence of other factors that may affect arrest rates, such as increased police efficiency or better record keeping. Other explorations of changing female crime rates have utilized conviction rates that also hamper interpretation because conviction rates do not reflect the actual incidence or the specific nature of crimes. In evaluating statistical inference in this area, the reader must keep in mind that there are errors in the basic data on crime in the United States and must take with a grain of salt the statistical inferences drawn by the various writers on female crime.

In general, women's involvement in crime still accounts for only a relatively small percentage of reported crimes. In 1974, the Uniform Crime Reports indicated that only 16.1% of all those arrested for crimes were females; this percentage represents some increase over preceding years. A careful study by Ward, Jackson, and Ward[7] drew conclusions about the changing rates in the trends of female crime. Their conclusions were based on statistical data spanning an eight-year period from 1960 to 1967. They drew several conclusions:

1. Arrests of women for all serious crimes have increased faster than the population.
2. The percent that women represent among persons arrested in the United States for violent crimes has been declining for homicide and assault— from 16.1% in 1960 to 14.8% in 1967 and from 15.3% to 12.9% respectively. The proportion women account for among robbery arrestees has increased from 4.6% to 5.2%.
3. The percentage of women arrested for violent crimes out of the total number of women arrested has remained fairly stable over the last eight years.[7]

Thus, the findings of Ward, Jackson, and Ward would suggest that while there has been some increase in the arrest rate of women for serious crimes, their involvement in crimes of violence has changed little.

Simon[6] also disputed the popular impression that women are becoming increasingly involved in violent crime. Simon utilized as her raw data statistics taken from the FBI Uniform Crime Reports. Her analysis of these data reflects several trends. In her opinion, the increase in the proportion of female arrests for serious crimes resulted largely from the fact that women seemed to be committing more property offenses than they had in the past, particularly larceny. In 1953, according to Simon[6] roughly 1 out of 7 arrests for larceny involved a woman. In 1972, the proportion had risen to 1 out of 3 arrests. She noted that female arrest rates for homicide, the most violent of crimes, had been the most stable among the arrest rates for all offenses. Additionally, she commented that further examination of the female arrest rate revealed that the greatest statistical increases were involved in embezzlement, fraud, forgery, and counterfeiting. Simon, while noting some increase in women's involvement in crime in general, reflected that this increase was due to increases in property offenses as opposed to crimes of personal violence. As previously noted, she explained this increased involvement as being a result of increased opportunity flowing from increased participation in the labor force.

In summary, statistical inferences that can be safely drawn seem to reveal that women still account for a relatively small percentage of the criminal arrests but that they are increasingly involved in crimes. Their increased participation does not appear to reflect an increasing propensity for violence. The percentage of women arrested for violent crimes has been noted by several authors as having remained relatively unchanged over time.

WOMEN AND VIOLENCE

While there is no statistical evidence to support the popular notion that violent crime among women is increasing, women are involved in crimes of violence. We now turn to an exploration of the possible etiology and dynamics of such involvement.

Violent behavior is multidetermined and results from a complex interaction of psychological, social, cultural, environmental, and biological determinants. While much of the following discussion focuses on one or another of these factors, the reader is cautioned to bear in mind that a violent crime is the end product of a host of factors.

The operational definition of *violence* has been widely discussed and varies from researcher to researcher. *Violence* can be defined as destructive aggression involving the infliction of physical damage on persons or property. Some writers extend the concept of violence to include the infliction of psychological damage and the infringement of human rights. This broadened meaning of *violence* has been seen as resulting from the social equivalence of violence. Boelkans and Heiser defined violence as "any variety of behavior which threatens damage, attempts to damage, or, in fact, does damage another individual or his property."[8] They commented that violence is deliberately vindictive and deals only with observable behavior, reason, motive, or purpose. An operational definition offered by the American Psychiatric Association is laid out in the report of the Task Force on the Clinical Aspects of the Violent Individual.[9] These clinicians defined the violent patient as a patient who acts or has acted in such a way as to produce physical harm or destruction. This definition emphasizes the patient's behavior rather than his or her thoughts, fantasies, or verbalization. Daniels, Gilula, and Ochberg[10] defined *violence* as destructive aggression that inflicts physical damage on person or property. They included property because the human often equates property with the self. They added that such violence and infliction of damage often appear to be intense, uncontrolled, excessive, furious, sudden, or seemingly purposeless. Furthermore, violence may be collective or individual, intentional or unintentional, and apparently just or unjust.

While violence and dangerousness thus appear to be intimately linked, depending on one's definition of *violence* this link may or may not actually exist. If the violent person is defined narrowly, as simply committing acts that produce physical harm or destruction, then such a person is, indeed, dangerous. If, however, one uses a broader definition, including threats, thoughts, and fantasies, the violent person may or may not exhibit dangerous behavior. It is *dangerous behavior* by women with which we are primarily concerned in this paper. Such behavior results in such criminal acts as murder, felonious assault, and armed robbery.

Before considering the various etiological explanations for female violence, it is useful to review the characteristics of women involved in such aggressive behavior. It is regrettable that little sound research has been conducted in this area. The most carefully done and succinctly presented examination of crimes of violence committed by women is the study conducted by Ward, Jackson, and Ward.[7] This study was based on the demographic characteristics, the personal histories, and the institutional experience of a large sample of women incarcerated at the California Institute for Women. The population cited included all the inmates of that institution housed there between 1962 and 1964 and a comparable sample collected in 1968. Women committed to prison for homicide were more likely to be white, and they

tended to come from homes that were relatively stable, with little reported previous criminality and little separation of the parents by divorce. They tended to have drinking problems but not to be involved
in narcotics abuse. Few had an extensive prior criminal record, and a
large percentage were diagnosed as having some type of psychological
disability. Women committed for assault, on the other hand, were much
more likely to come from minority groups and from families disrupted
by previous criminal acting-out and the separation or divorce of the
parents. Like the women committed for homicides, the women committed to prison for assault also had serious drinking problems, but
unlike the homicides, they were involved in narcotics. This group had
a history of previous criminal involvement, and to a lesser extent than
the homicide group, they were diagnosed as having psychological disabilities. Women committed on charges of robbery also had histories
of alcohol abuse. These women had a 50–50 chance of having come
from homes disrupted by death or divorce or by criminal acting-out
by other family members. Of the three groups, the women committed
for robbery had the smallest percentage of diagnosed psychological
disorder.

Ward *et al.* then went on to look at some characteristics of the
violent act itself. The woman involved in homicide or assault tended
to be the sole perpetrator. However, women convicted of robbery were
more frequently involved as accessories or partners to men. The victims of the homicides and assaults tended to be persons known to the
assailant, either her children, her spouse, or a friend. The women involved in robberies, on the other hand, tended to victimize strangers.
It should be noted that the American Psychiatric Association (APA)
Task Force on Clinical Aspects of the Violent Individual[9] viewed
women's involvement in violent crime as a passive one. The Ward
data suggest that this view applies only to robbery. Totman,[11] Resnick,[12,13] and others have also commented, as noted by Ward *et al.*,[7]
on the connection between violent crime, the family, and interfamilial
violence. It should be noted, however, that this relationship of violence within a close social network is not the exclusive province of
women, and, indeed, most homicides involve a relative or friend as
the victim.

Totman[11] also addressed the study of the characteristics, both
psychological and social, of women convicted of homicide. The author
analyzed the responses of 129 murderesses who were interviewed during their prison stays. The author found that her data supported the
notion that such women are largely unsuccessful and unsatisfied with
their previous educational and vocational ventures. The author found
that these women's lives, for the most part, had focused on wifely or

maternal activities. Her respondents frequently rejected the idea that satisfactions, outlets, pleasures, or relief were possible through employment or education. They were found to be poorly educated and poorly trained. The author commented that these women did not share personal concerns, nor were they able to get support or help from any significant relationships or community resources. Ultimately, in a time of crisis, these women defined and reinterpreted their negative situation so that it called for actions that they had previously not considered, including murder. The author saw these women as having exhausted all possible courses of action for solving their personal dilemmas and as having seen no recourse but murder, either in actuality or in fantasy.

In turning to etiological discussions of female violent behavior, themes of an organic or physiological nature or notions focusing on social roles or on psychodynamic explanations predominate. Organic or physiological explanations for violent behavior have been put forward by researchers exploring brain dysfunction and genetic variants. It is clear that the destruction or stimulation of certain brain areas, either experimentally or as the result of a disease process, may cause behavior to become disordered, particularly in the direction of the expression of aggression. The control of aggressiveness is an extremely complex matter and incompletely understood. Many research studies provide evidence implicating brain mechanisms in the initiation, modulation, inhibition, and control of aggressive behavior. In the area of brain dysfunction, most of the specific literature addresses the clinical experimental evidence correlating epilepsy, epileptoid behavior, and violence. Mark and Ervin [14] described a discrete clinical entity called the *dyscontrol syndrome.* This syndrome is characterized by four indexes: (1) senseless brutality; (2) pathological intoxication (a clinical phenomenon in which a relatively small amount of alcohol releases uncontrolled behavior); (3) sexual assault; and (4) multiple serious automobile accidents. This particular syndrome has been associated with focal brain disease of the temporal area. In their study of women prisoners, Climent et al. [15] reported a disproportionately high incidence of medical disorders among violent women. They noted an especially high prevalence of head injuries, headaches, and seizure disorders. Although a body of literature touching on the relationship of organic brain disease to violent behavior does exist, much of this material is useful for neither prediction nor prevention.

Another aspect of the physiologically based research literature on violence addresses the issues of chromosome variance. The role of Klinefelter's syndrome, a genetic anomaly consisting of an XXY chromosome pattern, is discussed by the APA Task Force on Clinical As-

pects of the Violent Individual.[9] This syndrome is thought to be related to aggressiveness and violence in certain institutional populations.
A statistically less frequent anomaly, that of the XXY pattern, or su-
permale syndrome, has led some researchers [16] to consider the possibility that the extra male chromosome may cause high "supermascu-
line" behavior, increased aggressiveness, and violence in women. In
general, there is insufficient evidence to make possible the valid prediction of aggressive or violent behavior on the basis of genetic information.

Regarding psychodynamic explanations of violence, the focus of
most of the literature has been on the control of aggression. In addressing the problem of the handling of aggressive impulses, many
clinicians have commented on either the overcontrol or the undercon-
trol of aggression as it relates to violent acting-out.[17] Lion *et al.*[18] described a diffuse awareness of anger that, in many cases, may be defensive and may prevent the violent person from realizing the true
single target of her or his anger. In situations of crisis or stress, such
defenses may break down and result in a violent act. Other authors
have described jealous murderers, depressed murderers, and masochistic murderers. Others have suggested that the central dynamic displayed by violent persons is helplessness.[19] They see these patients as
defending themselves against passivity, helplessness, and possible
underlying homosexual needs by adopting a hypermasculine stance,
whereby they become aggressive. Other authors comment on the involvement of jealousy in violence.

Solomon[20] has discussed the phenomenon of aggression in violence from a psychoanalytic perspective. He developed the concept of
primary reactive aggression. *Primary aggression* means hostility and attack that are reactive and proportional to the frustrating event. *Secondary defensive aggression* means hostile and violent behavior that is entirely disproportionate or even unrelated to the current provocation.
Senseless killing, this author suggested, can be a manifestation of secondary aggression in its most extreme form. Such aggression occurs
in conjunction with emotional conflict and maladaptive, unrealistic
behavior. However, it is not specific to any form of psychiatric disorder and may be manifest in the immature, the psychotic, the neurotic,
or the psychopathic individual. Solomon saw secondary defensive
aggression as developing from several sources involving the process
of identification. He noted that such aggression may develop if there
is a total failure to establish a successful identification or if, in the
process of maturation, the person identifies with the aggressor. This
form of identification occurs developmentally when the child allies
himself or herself with the cruel or hostile parent or parent substitute

and becomes the tormentor rather than the tormented. Also, the child may identify with an unconscious component of the parent that is hostile and indirectly expressed. Such a process of identification leads to aggressive problems, as the person may develop a bad self-concept and may see himself or herself as an evil person.

However, while the above gives some overview of the psychodynamic explanations for violent behavior, one must be careful to discriminate a psychodynamic motivation or explanation for violent crime from an attribution of violence to the process of mental illness. A dynamic understanding of behavior is not equivalent to a finding of profound psychological pathology. While there is no such equivalence, the involvement of mental illness in female violence, as noted in the introduction of this paper, has been of great interest both in the past and more recently.

Mental Illness and Violent Crime

As we discuss the role of mental illness and violence, we must be careful to define what we mean by *mental illness.* Since precise definitions have varied from researcher to researcher, it is difficult to make accurate cross-research comparisons. Definitions used by researchers have covered behavior disturbances diagnosed as character disorders; in some cases, mild neurotic conditions; and in almost all cases, psychotic disturbances. We believe that *mental illness,* particularly when one is examining its relationship to violence, should be relatively narrowly defined, and we define it as "A substantial disorder of thought or mood which significantly impairs judgment, behavior, capacity to recognize reality and the ability to cope with the ordinary demands of life."[21] Such a definition excludes alcohol-related diagnoses and those related to substance abuse. While previous authors, particularly Ward *et al.*[7] have noted that the involvement of drugs or alcohol is a common contributing factor to violence, we do not address that issue here. Rather, we would like to examine what little is known about the interface of violence and mental illness, particularly in women.

In the previously quoted study on murderesses, Totman[11] explored the role of psychiatric disability in murder. She noted that there is a distinction to be made between women who murder their children and women who murder their spouses and that in self-report data, child murderers feel that they should have been placed in a mental hospital or should have received psychiatric or psychological counseling rather than a prison sentence. Mate killers, in contrast, consider themselves mentally healthy. Diagnoses of these same mate killers revealed a higher frequency of psychotic illness, schizoid or borderline schizophrenic disturbance, whereas in the case of child murderers, diagnoses were more frequently of personality and character disorders. Studying psychiatric disorders in criminal recidivism, Kloninger and Guze[22] commented on the high percentage of character disorders in their group. Climent *et al.*,[15] also looking at psychiatric variables related to violent behavior, noted a disproportionately high prevalence of emotional disorders of all kinds in their population of women prisoners. They also commented on the strong evidence they found of psychodynamically significant events in the lives of violent individuals, such as the loss of parents at an early age.

Ward *et al.*[7] also commented on the high percentage of female felons diagnosed as suffering from some variety of psychological disability, and indeed, they commented that the percentage so diagnosed appeared to increase over time. They found that women incarcerated for homicide or assault were described as disturbed significantly more often than other female felons. They noted, in 1968, that 81% of the women committed for homicide had been diagnosed either as giving evidence of psychosis or as displaying behavior that was disturbed, though not psychotic. Similar statistics for women charged with assault and robbery were 78% and 45%, respectively. This rather high incidence of psychiatric disturbance of one variety or another in female offenders has been mentioned by several other authors, including Cowie, Cowie, and Slater[23] and Kloninger and Guze.[22] Despite this concordance of studies, it should be noted that there is great disparity in the definition of *mental illness* used by each researcher and in the indexes used to operationalize that definition. Much more research is needed before a complete understanding of the relationship of violence to mental illness can be understood. Nevertheless, that a relationship exists is clear, and indeed, it is in those instances related to mental illness that the basic dynamics of violence may most clearly be seen. Therefore, let us turn to some clinical examples.

EXAMPLES OF FEMALE CRIMES RELATED TO MENTAL ILLNESS

We have previously noted that most violent crime committed by women is personal in nature, directed at an intimate victim. In this section, we describe through clinical examples three common violent female crimes associated with mental illness. Following the clinical examples, we discuss what seems to be common in the personal, family, and social histories of women committing violent crimes associated with their mental illness. The most common homicide committed by women is spouse murder.

Ms. J, a 35-year-old white woman, was seen by clinicians at the Center for Forensic Psychiatry, an agency of the Department of Mental Health in Michigan charged with evaluating and treating mentally ill offenders who have been charged with the murder of their husbands. Ms. J was the oldest of four children, born in Arkansas. She remembered her parents as thoroughly unpleasant. Her father was a confirmed alcoholic who has been married twice. Ms. J's victim was her second husband. She described him as someone who was "good to everyone but his family." She alluded to his possessiveness and violent temper. Sexuality was a conflictual issue in their marriage, and she had ambivalent feelings about her sexual relationship with her husband. On the evening of the offense, the patient noted a 20-minute gap in her memory. She was able to recall that she and her husband had gone out to dinner and that they had shared a peaceful meal. On their return home, they went to bed together. Her next memory was being awakened from a fitful sleep by her husband's calling another woman's name while performing gross sexual movements. She alleged that this was the last thing she remembered. The next memory was of herself in the living room with her husband; he had his hands over his stomach, and he was calling for assistance. She remembered a policeman's saying to her, "Get out of the chair, lady," and her response being to continue to sit and stare at the police. A psychiatric diagnosis of an acute psychotic episode in a patient with a hysterical personality disorder was made. Ms. J presented a clear demonstration of the dynamics preceding a dissociative reaction and the clinical course from a hysterical personality to a brief hysterical psychosis. Her clinical picture clearly showed the importance of anxiety and rage, the emergence of a dissociative episode and the importance of these in facilitating a period of violent assaultive behavior.

Another type of violent crime is either infanticide or neonaticide. *Neonaticide* is defined as the killing of a neonate on the date of its birth; filicide is operationally defined as the murder of a son or daughter older than 24 hours.[12] In the literature, all child murders by parents are usually lumped together under the term *infanticide*.

Ms. S also had a traumatic early childhood and family history. She was an unwanted child, raised by a mother who abused her verbally and beat her physically. Her mother attempted to introduce her to prostitution at the age of 13. Her childhood was marked by feelings of uselessness, unworthiness, and little self-esteem. She was taunted by peers for her dumbness and her hearing defects. She was married at an early age to a man who provided her with material goods and little emotional support. From the age of 10, she had complained of auditory hallucinations, but she was offered no treatment. She became seriously depressed after a second unwanted pregnancy, and the extent of her depression frightened her husband, who finally sought psychiatric treatment for her. On the day of the murders, she called her psychiatrist, who was unavailable. She then strangled her two daughters at the insistence of internal voices. She was hospitalized and responded to psychotropic medication. The diagnosis was chronic schizophrenic illness.

A third clinical example will serve to illustrate another crime of violence directly related to mental illness:

> Ms. Z, a 40-year-old divorced woman, began her criminal career after an extensive hospitalization for a traumatic back injury. She was the unwanted product of an unhappy marriage. Her adjustment, though marginal, was adequate until the time of her accident. During that hospitalization, she developed an all-encompassing delusional system that centered on what she saw as the unexpressed love of her physician for her. That first psychotic episode was resolved after a period of supportive psychotherapy and medication, but it was followed by a series of multiple hospitalizations for other delusional episodes that centered on her view of herself as being on a special mission. She was designated as a leader to help all other women in their fight for equality. To this end, she had participated in three armed robberies to obtain funds for her unknown women colleagues, who she believed were calling to her for aid.

Abstracting from the histories and interviews of many mentally ill women offenders involved in violent crime, the clinician sees many similarities. A composite picture of the mentally ill woman offender often reveals a disturbed early childhood and scanty or absent relationships with parents and relationships marked by physical and emotional abuse or inconsistency. In adolescence, this patient might be unhappy and have few friends. She would have difficulty with the expression of any degree of aggression or assertiveness. Her personal history would show her to be concerned with academic achievement; she might have a marginal employment record and a possible history of alcohol or substance abuse. She might have been treated for mental illness in the past and might either be in treatment or requesting it prior to committing her violent crime. Her marriage would be marked by trauma, and her husband may bear certain marked similarities to the abusive parents. The crime of this patient is clearly a product of her mental illness and offers one form of resolution for her difficult intrapsychic and interpersonal struggle. What is especially important for professionals is to realize that our composite patient would have been giving indications of her internal turmoil to friends, family, and professionals either verbally or nonverbally prior to the final resolution of her conflict by committing a violent crime.

What seems to be clear (and common) as we look at the various categories of crimes committed by mentally ill women is that these women can be so ill for such a long period of time and not be recognized by the helping professions. Many of these women have verbalized their intent to commit crimes to physicians, social workers, and other professionals. Is it, as Pollak suggested, that as a society, we are so chivalrous that we refuse to recognize the incidence of crime in

women, or is it that the crimes proposed are so heinous that we wish
to deny them?

Summary and Some Further Research Questions

When one views the literature addressing itself to female violence,
one is immediately struck by the regrettable lack of data. Ward et al.[7]
aptly noted, "Our knowledge of the character and cause of female
criminality is at the same state of development that characterized our
knowledge of male criminality some 30 or more years ago." Indeed,
there are few conclusions that can soundly be drawn about the involvement of women in crimes, particularly violent ones, because there
is a notable lack of research in the area of women and violence and
because much existing research suffers from clear investigator bias
and/or methodological difficulties. Current statistical studies suggest
that, in general, women account for only a small percentage of criminal arrests. A trend toward increasing involvement can be seen in
property crimes, but not in crimes of violence. Women's violence tends
to be directed at persons close to them, often within the family. There
is little else that can be concluded, particularly in the area of the etiology and the psychodynamics of violence in women.

Much of the literature addressing female violence is hypothetical
in nature, and it is only since the early 1960s that any systematic research studies have been done on the causes and character of the violence of women. While all writers have acknowledged the complexity
of this social phenomenon, few have mounted research designed to
examine the interaction of biological, social, and psychological factors
in female crime, and a great deal of very basic research remains to be
done before this matter can be meaningfully cleared up. First, it is
clear that more sound statistical studies need to be conducted on the
incidence of crime and the changes in women's crime rate over time.
While demographic explorations in this area have been popular, only
such rather simple factors as marital status or employment have been
examined. Demographic materials would certainly be of use in examining the hypothesis that female criminality is the result of socioeconomic factors. Demographic methodology would also assist in assessing, both in an interactional model and independently, the role of
undereducation in the etiology of female crime.

In addition to these more statistical areas of inquiry, considerably
more research is needed on the psychodynamics of aggression. Much
of the theoretical and some of the research literature on violence in
women relates this violence to the difficulty that women have in handling aggressive impulses. It is theorized that this difficulty results not

only from intrapsychic circumstances but from cultural stereotypes as well. Research on the roles of women within families and in other social contexts might serve to clarify the phenomenon of female violence and the use of violence to resolve interpersonal conflict. Also, some cross-cultural studies on the development and handling of aggressive impulses by women might shed some light on this interaction. Little is known about the psychosocial circumstances that transform simple aggression or hostility into a violent act of major proportions. Along these lines, an exploration of female motivations for crime might assist in a clearer understanding of how various factors combine to produce violent behavior.

Last, some attention needs to be addressed to differential treatment models. In recent years, considerable attention has been given to the problem of male violence. The use of psychosurgery, chemotherapy, psychotherapy, and a variety of behavioral paradigms specifically designed for the male violent offender has been explored. However, for the violent woman, whose offense is frequently committed within the small circle of family and friends, little has been done along the lines of specific treatment. While this may be understandable owing to the relatively small percentage of homicides, assaults, and robberies committed by women, nevertheless it is clear that this population possesses special problems that warrant specific treatment designs.

In time, one hopes, a complete understanding of the violent woman will emerge. This understanding should give us all better insight into the nature of violence in its social and psychological manifestations. It should allow the mental health professions to provide more meaningful treatment for the individual, as well as recommendations for a society increasingly concerned with the prevention of violent behavior.

REFERENCES

1. Lombroso C: *The female offender.* New York, Philosophical Library Edition, 1958.
2. Klein D: The etiology of female crime: A review of the literature, *Issues in Criminology,* 8(2):3–29, 1973.
3. Freud S: *New introductory lectures.* New York, Norton, 1933.
4. Pollak O: *The criminology of women.* Philadelphia, University of Pennsylvania Press, 1950.
5. Adler F: *Sisters in crime.* New York, McGraw-Hill, 1975.
6. Simon RJ: *Women and crime.* Lexington, Mass., Heath, 1975.
7. Jackson DA, Jackson M, Ward R: *A staff report to the national commission on the causes and prevention of violence,* Vol. 13. Edited by Mulvihill DJ, Tumin MM, Curtis LA. Washington, D.C., Superintendent of Documents, U.S. Government Printing Office, pp. 843–909, 1969.

8. Boelkans R, Heiser J: Biological bases of aggression. In *Violence and the struggle for existence.* Edited by Daniels DW, Gilula MF, Ochberg FM. Boston, Little, Brown, pp. 15–22, 1970.
9. American Psychiatric Association Task Force on Clinical Aspects of the Violent Individual: *Clinical aspects of the violent individual,* Report 8. Washington, D.C., 1974.
10. Daniels DW, Gilula MF, Ochberg FM: *Violence and the struggle for existence.* Boston, Little, Brown, 1970.
11. Totman J: *The murderess: A psychosocial study of the process.* Ann Arbor, Mich., University Microfilms, 1971.
12. Resnick PJ. Child murder by parents: A psychiatric review of filicide, *American Journal of Psychiatry 126*:325–334, Sept. 1969.
13. Resnick PJ: Murder of the newborn: A psychiatric review of neonaticide, *American Journal of Psychiatry 126*:1414–1420, April 1970.
14. Mark VH, Ervin FR: *Violence and the brain.* New York, Harper & Row, 1970.
15. Climent CE, Rollins A, Ervin F, Plutchik R: Epidemiological studies of women prisoners. I: Medical and psychiatric variables related to violent behavior, *American Journal of Psychiatry 130*:985–90, Sept. 1973.
16. Kessler S, Muse RH. The XYX karyotype of criminality: A review, *Journal of Psychiatric Research 7*:153–170, 1970.
17. Megargee EI: Undercontrolled and overcontrolled personality types in extreme antisocial aggression, *Psychological Monographs 80* (Whole No. 611):1–29, 1966.
18. Lion JR, Bach-y-Ritta G, Ervin FR: Violent patients in the emergency room, *American Journal of Psychiatry 125*:1706–1711, 1969.
19. Lion JR: *Evaluation and management of the violent patient.* Springfield, Ill., Charles C Thomas, 1972.
20. Solomon GF: Psychodynamic aspects of aggression, hostility and violence. In *Violence and the struggle for existence.* Edited by Daniels DW, Gilula MF, Ochberg FM. Boston, Little, Brown, pp. 53–78, 1970.
21. Michigan Mental Health Code 1974.
22. Cloninger CR, Guze SB: Psychiatric disorders and criminal recidivism: A follow-up study of female criminals, *Archives of General Psychiatry 29*:266–269, August 1973.
23. Cowie JV, Cowie, Slater E: *Delinquency in girls.* London, William Heinemann, 1968.

Chapter 4

Wife Abuse: Culture as Destiny

Elaine (Hilberman) Carmen

This chapter describes the psychological and behavioral consequences of wife beating, as derived from clinical work with a group of battered women.[1] The general medical clinic setting in which victims were identified differs from that of other samples[2] in that the abused women were not selected out by virtue either of admission to a shelter or of awareness that the abuse they suffered warranted attention. This, then, is a sample of "silent" victims.

A summary of historical, cultural, and family information is presented, with a focus on the psychological impact of marital violence on the women and children in these families. Although this report is about individual women, family violence and wife abuse must be viewed as an alarming and pervasive societal problem. We live in a violent society that legitimizes and permits wife beating, and society, in turn, suffers the consequences.

The Social Context

Until recently, violence within the family has received little attention, although there has been great public concern and fear about violence in general. While the concept of family is cherished as the source of serenity and nurturance, the family is also the most frequent single locus for all kinds of violence, including homicide.[3,36,37,38] Violence is said to occur in 50% of American families, so that the marriage license is also a "hitting license."[3,4,5]

Family violence, in contrast to violence outside the family, is likely to be perceived as normal, legitimate, and instrumental.[3,4,6] This is most clearly seen in the corporal punishment of children; it is believed

ELAINE (HILBERMAN) CARMEN, M.D. ● Associate Professor, Department of Psychiatry, University of North Carolina School of Medicine, Chapel Hill, North Carolina.

that children need and deserve to be hit for moral reasons (e.g., "Spare the rod and spoil the child.") As Gelles noted, individuals do not label the use of physical force on children as "violence" because of the "powerful pro-use-of-physical-force-on-children norms." He further suggested that if violence is defined as an act with the intent of physical injury of the victim, then the physical punishment of children is violent.[4]

Violence between spouses is also socially condoned and is not limited to any particular social class or ethnic group. Although the highest *reported* incidence of spouse abuse is found among the poor, this finding is felt to reflect a reporting bias in that poor people are more likely to come to the attention of public agencies, while middle- and upper-class women have their privacy protected.[6,7] Harris and associates, in their 1979 survey of wife abuse in Kentucky, concluded that "the collective portrait of the abusive and violence-prone family is hardly distinguishable from the profile of the average family on the street."[8] Income levels were not good predictors of family violence in this survey, in which school dropouts with less than an eighth-grade education appeared to be less violence-prone than those who had some college education.

Family violence has several important societal ramifications beyond the suffering of individuals[9]:

1. Family violence culminates in serious injury or death. Of all murders, 20%–50% take place within the family.[6,7,10,11,12] As Dobash and Dobash pointed out, family violence is not randomly distributed among family members but is disproportionately directed at women. Female homicide victims are more often killed by their spouses, while most male victims are killed by someone outside the family. About 40% of all female homicides are committed by husbands, while only 10% of male victims are killed by wives. Among those who murder spouses, wives are seven times more likely than husbands to have murdered in self-defense.[13,36]

Police are called to intervene in domestic disputes more often than in all other criminal incidents combined, and one-fifth of all police fatalities occur while intervening in family fights.[7,9] In a Kansas City police study, 40% of the city's homicides were between spouses; in more than 85% of these homicides, police were called at least once prior to the fatal episode, and in half of these cases, police were called five times in the two-year period preceding the murder.[14]

2. Gelles and Straus observed that the family is the primary training ground for violent behavior: "A person is more likely to observe, commit, and to be the victim of violence within the family than in any other setting."[3] The beating of women in the home is usually

accompanied by the physical and/or sexual abuse of children in the home.[1,2,15,37,38] An English study of 100 battered women revealed that 37% of the women abused their children, while 54% claimed that their husbands committed violence against the children.[2] Children who are abused grow up to abuse their offspring, and children who see parents interact violently will very likely have physically abusive relationship themselves. Thus, violence breeds violence.[3,4,8,16]

3. Surveys by social scientists of populations of homicidal adolescents[17,18] and convicted murderers[19] suggest that in all categories, the offenders were themselves victimized by their families, usually as children. Thus, intrafamily violence is not only an individual problem but a problem for the general public, who will ultimately be victimized by the offspring of violent families.

The sexist organization of the family contributes heavily to the acceptability of wife beating.[7,20,21] Men who lack superiority or competence in their personal resources are allowed to use violence, without fear of legal reprisal, as a way of maintaining a superior power position in the family. Their wives understand that neither separation nor the law will necessarily protect them from further violence.[9,22] The man is protected, and the abused woman comes to believe that marital violence is the norm and that she deserves the abuse. This self-blame is reinforced by the attitudes of "helping" agencies, which ignore and demean the victim or accuse her of provoking the assault.[7,16,23]

Finally, women are trapped by cultural norms that dictate that men are responsible for the economic support of families, while women must bear the full responsibility for child rearing. Women learn the mythology that their rightful place is in the home and that single-parent families are damaging to children. Violent marriages are maintained by pervasive patterns of sex discrimination. Women who leave violent homes are denied child-care facilities; equal educational, vocational, and economic opportunities; and legitimate self-supporting and autonomous roles outside the home.[20,21,38]

THE CLINICAL SETTING

Half of all women referred by the medical staff of a small rural health clinic for psychiatric evaluation were found to be victims of marital violence; that is, 60 women suffered serious and/or repeated physical injury as the result of deliberate assaults by their husbands or cohabitees.[1,23] The history of marital violence was known to the referring clinician in only 4 of the 60 cases, although most of these women and their children had received ongoing medical care at the clinic. This finding has profound implications for case identification by clinicians and is discussed later in this chapter.

This report was not the result of a preconceived plan to study battered women. Rather, the authors gradually became aware of striking similarities among referred clients and found that physical abuse played a central causative role in paralyzing anxiety and symptom formation. While information about the women was acquired by dialogues with them, material about their husbands was almost always acquired indirectly. Attempts to engage the husbands in either medical or psychiatric treatment were met with adamant refusals. Involvement with the husbands was further limited by the women's need to maintain silence about their clinic visits and their concern that conjoint treatment in the absence of provisions for safety might result in an escalation of violence.[4]

CHARACTERISTICS OF SAMPLE. The 40 black and 20 white women ranged in age from 19 to 82, with the majority evenly distributed in the 20–40 age group. At the time of referral, 46 of the women were living with their husbands. During the course of treatment, 27 women left their husbands; of this group, 14 separated or divorced, and 13 returned to their marriages. Economic, educational, and social deprivation was the norm for these mill and tenant-farm families, which were characterized by high unemployment rates, poverty-level incomes, and severe stress associated with basic survival needs.

Lifelong violence was the pattern for many of these women, who gave remarkably similar histories. Violence between their parents (usually the father assaulting the mother), paternal alcoholism, and physical and/or sexual abuse as children were described by half of the women. The men, also, were said to have had early exposure to emotional deprivation, alcoholism, lack of protection, and violence, both as witnesses and as abused children. Suicides and homicides among family members and neighborhood acquaintances were common occurrences and were usually committed with guns.

Most of the women had left home at an early age to escape from violent, pathologically jealous, and seductive fathers, who kept their wives and daughters imprisoned at home. The usual age of marriage was 16, and many of the women had been pregnant or had had children prior to marriage. Pregnancy was viewed as the only way out of the home. Once married, they found themselves with alcoholic, battering husbands who also kept their wives and daughters at home, thus replicating exactly their lives prior to marriage. Alcoholism was said to be a significant problem for all but four husbands in this sample, this rate being somewhat higher than that reported elsewhere.[2,4] Because drinking is not always accompanied by violent behavior, and wife abusers who drink also beat their wives when they are sober, it has been suggested that individuals become intoxicated in order to carry out violent acts and thus to avoid personal responsibility for their deviant behaviors.[4]

The Marriage

The violent relationship is one of extraordinary intensity. When not aggressive, the men were described as childlike, remorseful, and yearning for nurturance; this picture of fragility was confirmed by the occasional reports of the husband's suicidal or psychotic behavior when there was any threat to dissolve the relationship. The women, understandably, felt quite sorry for them because they often shared similar histories of deprivation and abuse. Since the men could never understand or acknowledge a termination without murderous rage, these marriages became life sentences for their wives.[16] When the husbands threatened homicide, they were taken at their word because threats and wishes became a reality with explosive suddenness. For example, one woman made active plans to leave her marriage despite her husband's threats of violence; she abruptly retreated when her closest friend, also an abused woman, was murdered by a violent spouse.

Walker has described a cycle of violence in these marriages, with three components that may be predictable for a given marital dyad: a tension-building phase, followed by a brief phase in which the violence erupts, and finally, the postviolence phase. During this third phase, there is relief from tension, and the batterer is often attentive, loving, and quite remorseful. During this postviolence reconciliation, the husband's affectionate behavior and promises to be "good" validate his wife's belief that he can and will change, and consequently, this phase serves as a powerful reinforcement for the victim to remain in the relationship.[24,25] Generally, battered women are seen by clinicians toward the end of the first phase or in the postviolence period. Awareness of this cycle is important for clinicians, who may easily misinterpret the victim's behavior as masochistic or "asking for it." For example, toward the end of the tension-building phase, women may act to precipitate the violence when the anticipatory anxiety becomes intolerable. By contrast, in the reconciliation phase, the victim may seem unconcerned about the violence and protective of her husband.[23]

In this study, many women had left their marriages for brief periods, but they inevitably returned.[26] Their return was related to economic dependence on their husbands and threats of further violence, from which they had no protection. Some sought recourse through the criminal justice system, but these attempts were frustrated by the lack of response of magistrates, law enforcement officers, and the courts, as well as by the husband's retaliative violence. Families of origin were not supportive of efforts to leave, especially when violence was the norm there as well: "My mother told me to go back home for the sake of the children"; "I was told to take the good with the bad so I shut up." Shame was prominent and made it difficult to ask for help: "I didn't want anyone to know. I put up a front to convince them I had a perfect husband and marriage." Low self-esteem was coupled with the belief that the abuse was justified, even when they were assaulted while asleep: "It's all my fault . . . he is supposed to be the boss in the marriage"; "I asked for it. I shouldn't have talked back to him."

PATHOLOGICAL JEALOUSY. Extreme jealousy occurred in 57 marriages, and the husbands made active and successful efforts to keep their wives ignorant and isolated. Leaving the house for any reason resulted in accusations of infidelity, which culminated in assault. Clinic visits were often made in secrecy, and some women were regularly beaten when they returned from the clinic. Other channels of communication were also prevented. Friendships with women were discouraged either by embarrassing the wife in front of her friends or by accusations that her friends were lesbians or "trash," and their entry to the home was denied. Many husbands refused to allow their wives to work, or when the women did work, efforts were made to ensure that both partners would work at the same place so that the women's activities and friends could be monitored. Thus, for these rural women, isolation was complete and potential support unavailable. The women were quite aware of this, one commenting: "He'd do anything he could to get me down to where I would not go out in the world."

MARITAL VIOLENCE. The husband's alcohol intoxication, low tolerance for frustration, poor impulse control, and pathological jealousy constituted a lethal mix. He was usually drinking at the time of the assault, but this was not always the case. Some women were assaulted daily, while others were beaten intermittently, and the women lived in constant anticipatory terror.

Violence erupted in any situation in which the husband did not immediately get his way. A common pattern was for the husband to come home late after having been out with another woman and to goad his wife into an argument that ended in violence. The assaults usually occurred at night and on weekends, and the children were witnesses and participants. Frequently, the oldest child had not been fathered by the husband, so that violence toward the wife was extended to include the "bastard kid." Older children were also involved when they attempted to defend or protect the mother. The assault weapons included hands, feet, fists, rocks, bottles, phones, iron bars, knives, and guns. Scratching, slapping, punching with fists, throwing down, and kicking were prevalent, and faces and breasts were the most frequently mentioned sites of assault. A broad spectrum of injuries was sustained that included multiple bruises and lacerations, black eyes, fractured ribs, subdural hematomas, detached retinas, and gunshot wounds. Strangling and choking until consciousness was impaired were also reported. Sexual assaults were common, and the women described being beaten and raped in front of the children. Guns were available in most homes and were constant threats; some of the men kept guns in bed to intimidate their wives. One woman slept with her shoes on for a fast getaway, and another was hospitalized with a heart attack that occurred when her spouse was threatening her with a gun.

Changes in the pattern of violence during pregnancy were noted by most women. There was increasing abuse for some, with the pregnant abdomen replacing face and breasts as the target for battering, and abortions and premature births were the result. It has been hypothesized that this kind of battering represents a prenatal form of infanticide or child abuse.[4,27] Other women reported less abuse with pregnancy, one woman deliberately staying pregnant to avoid violence.

The most frequently employed coping strategy for the woman during the assault was to get away temporarily, although there were few places to go. The few women who resorted to counterviolence did so as an act of desperation associated with the failure of other options. The combined effect of their fear and rage and the use of weapons to compensate for their lesser size and strength sometimes resulted in potentially lethal actions. They fought back with kitchen knives, broom handles, frying pans, hot grease and lye, hammers, screwdrivers, and, rarely, guns. In contrast to the husbands' violent behavior, the use of violence by the women was related to a direct threat of life and usually came as a surprise, since they themselves were unaware of the extent of their rage.

THE CHILDREN

Physical and/or sexual abuse of children was identified in 20 families and was suspected in others. There were two styles of child abuse: the husband beat the wife, who beat the children, and/or the husband beat both his wife and the children. In either case, the children in violent homes are quite vulnerable.[2,4,15,25,37] Whether the children were themselves battered or were onlookers to parental violence, they were deeply affected by the climate of violence in which they lived. They were witnesses to drunken rages, savage assaults, strangling, shooting, stabbing, and rape. Emotional neglect and abuse were the norms, as was the chaos of frequent separations, so that the children were never certain who would leave and when.

Chart surveys revealed patterns of terror of physical examinations, anxieties about dying, unkept appointments, families lost to follow-up, and medical problems involving suspected abuse and neglect. For example, one violent family was identified when a youngster panicked during a neck examination, believing that the physician was trying to strangle him. Evidence of somatic, psychological, and behavioral dysfunction was documented for a third of the 209 children and was suspected for many more. Psychosomatic illness and symptoms were prominent, somewhat more frequently in females, and included headaches, abdominal complaints, asthma, peptic ulcer, rheumatoid arthritis, stuttering, and enuresis. Depression, suicidal behavior, and overt psychosis occurred in a smaller number of the children and adolescents.

The following portrait of the children emerged. Preschool and young school-age children had somatic symptoms, school phobias, enuresis, and insomnia. The insomnia was often accompanied by intense fear, screaming, and resistance to going to bed at night. This behavior was time-related, much of the wife beating occurring when the children were in bed. Older children began to show differential behavior patterns, which divided along sex lines. Aggressive disruptive behavior, most usually fighting with siblings and schoolmates, and temper tantrums when frustrated were the most frequently reported cluster for the boys, this style being notably absent in the girls. In contrast, the girls continued to have an increasing array of somatic symptoms and were likely to become withdrawn, passive, clinging, and anxious, this pattern also occurring with a smaller number of the boys. Most of the children had impaired concentration spans and difficulty with schoolwork. Teenage girls further suffered from the perpetual surveillance and accusations of sexual activity by their fathers, who were seductive if not overtly incestuous. Finally, there were reports of married daughters who were battered and of grown sons who were alcoholic and violent, thus completing the cycle.

BATTERED WOMEN: PSYCHOLOGICAL CONSEQUENCES

The reasons for psychiatric referral generally clustered around marital problems, somatic concerns, or mixed anxiety and depressive symptoms. The marital problems were generally defined in terms of the husband's alcoholism, financial irresponsibility, and promiscuity, with the battering never mentioned. Those with physical symptoms were referred because of chronic tranquilizer or analgesic use, unremitting symptomatology, treatment noncompliance, and frequent clinic visits.

Somatic complaints, conversion symptoms, and psychophysiological reactions were abundant as evidenced by frequent clinic visits for headaches, choking sensations, hyperventilation, asthma, chest pain, gastrointestinal symptoms, pelvic pain, back pain, and allergic phenomena. The symptoms were often connected to previous sites of battering. One husband regularly scratched and gouged his wife's back to the point of bleeding and scarring; whenever there was increased tension at home, her back "broke out" with giant urticaria. For other women, the treatment of preexisting chronic diseases was complicated by their affective states such as uncontrolled diabetes. An epileptic required multiple hospitalizations for seizures; noncompliance in the use of anticonvulsants was her only escape from a savagely brutal husband who refused to allow her to leave the house unless she needed medical attention.

Psychiatric histories provided evidence of prior psychological dysfunction for more than half of the women. Depressive illness was the single most frequent diagnostic category, with manic-depressive psychosis, schizophrenia, alcoholism, and personality disorders all represented in lesser numbers in this sample. Of these women, 13 had been hospitalized in mental institutions, some repeatedly, with violent and psychotic behavior often the precipitant for hospitalization. Others had utilized crisis lines, outpatient mental-health facilities, and emergency rooms for treatment. Almost all the women had made frequent visits to local physicians for the treatment of somatic symptoms, anxiety, insomnia, or suicidal behavior, usually by drug overdoses. Most had been treated, either intermittently or chronically, with sedative-hypnotics, tranquilizers, and/or antidepressants.

THE CLINICIAN'S RESPONSE. Despite multiple contacts with many clinicians over the years, the psychiatrists and the nonpsychiatrist physicians were not directly told of the violence, nor did they ask.[1,28,39] As with rape, there is a complex cultural mythology about wife beating that protects the assailant and accuses the victim. Health professionals share the societal bias and respond to the abused woman's complaint with blame or disbelief. Since women themselves are aware of and even share these attitudes, they are likely to remain silent about their victimization. Thus, there is a covert collusion between clinicians and victims, in which symptomatic treatment is offered as an alternative to the direct identification of the problem and the more appropriate interventions.[23]

Blame. Clinicians have been notably uncharitable in their attitudes toward battered women. This attitude is reflected in the literature on masochism, which lends legitimacy and reinforcement to prevailing social attitudes. One study concluded, "We see the husband's aggressive behavior as filling masochistic needs of the wife and necessary for the wife's (and the couple's) equilibrium."[29] Another report offered the following advice: "The masochist must be forced to bear responsibility for his plight. A woman who had been choked several times phoned me late one night to say that her husband was again choking her. I replied 'what right do you have to place your neck between his hands?' "[30] These instances are reminiscent of the myth that the rape victim not only provoked the assault but "really liked it." Just as the rape victim stands trial in the court, the abused woman is scrutinized by the mental health professional. Her motivation and her contribution to marital conflict are explored, while the violent expression of the conflict is ignored.[7,21,23]

The "masochistic" label not only locates the problem within the victim but further implies that abused women are unwilling and unable to change and are therefore hopeless. As Waites argued, "Female motivation, like motivation generally, must be studied in the context of external constraints such as actual choices available and the consequences of particular choices."[31] Thus, theories of female masochism are inadequate as explanations of actual behavior because "in situations in which choice is externally restricted, the question of internal motivation approaches irrelevance."[31]

Disbelief. The apparent inattention of psychiatrists to marital violence was confirmed in a review of psychiatric-hospital discharge summaries for the 13 abused women who had been hospitalized.[32] The summaries contained frequent references to violence and murder in their families of origin, and the descriptions of the women suggested that concerns about violence had a primary causative role in their psychotic decompensation. The marital violence was not addressed during these hospitalizations; psychotropic medication constituted the primary—and, in some cases, the only—form of treatment. The following statements from the discharge summaries convey the disbelief and denial of the professionals:

> She also related that her husband hit her in the eye and ran on at great length explaining other maltreatment . . . she first noted the mistreatment at home sometime in June when she began to feel certain that someone was trying to kill her.

Physical examination revealed bruises on her right arm, leg, and side, presumably inflicted during a scuffle with her son as he attempted to get her hospitalized.

Her chief complaint was that she began to feel strange after her husband gave her a cup of coffee, and she was concerned that he might have been trying to harm her . . . she reported that her husband beats her and doesn't want her around, but this was not substantiated by the children who said they had not seen any abuse since they had been small.

She had a paranoid flavor to her feelings about her boyfriend, also a heavy drinker.

She became progressively more anxious and agitated, pacing the floor, staying up all night, and being unable to eat. She complained on admission of bad thoughts, wanting to curse, to kill herself and wanting to kill her husband.

This last woman, in her ninth hospitalization at age 65, was discharged early to care for her ailing husband, who demanded her release. Six months later, in secrecy, she sent a desperate letter to a clinic provider, requesting help for her "nerves" and her "bad thoughts" and apologizing for not keeping clinic appointments because "I want to come and see you but he won't let me come."

The battered woman, although usually a silent victim, is more likely to provide direct verbal and behavioral evidence of her victimization when she loses control. At such times, however, she is judged unbelievable by mental health professionals.

THE RESPONSE OF VICTIMS: DENIAL OF RAGE. The variety of presenting complaints and diagnoses notwithstanding, there was a uniform psychological response to the violence, which was identical for the entire sample. The women were a study in paralyzing terror, which was reminiscent of the rape trauma syndrome[33] except that the stress was unending and the threat of the next assault ever-present. Indeed, many women sought help just prior to the next assault, for example, at a time when the husband had been on "good behavior" for a while, with evidence of increasing tension at home and perhaps a return to drinking.

Agitation and anxiety bordering on panic were almost always present: "I feel like screaming and hollering but I hold it in"; "I feel like a pressure cooker ready to explode." They described being tense and nervous, by which they meant "going to pieces" at any unexpected noise, voice, or happening. Events even remotely connected with violence, whether sirens, thunder, people arguing, or a door slamming, elicited intense fear. The woman who had been shot by her husband panicked at any loud noise. There was chronic apprehension of imminent doom, of something terrible always about to happen. Any symbolic or actual sign of potential danger resulted in increased activity, agitation, pacing, screaming, and crying. They remained vigilant, unable to relax or to sleep. Sleep, when it came, brought no relief. Nightmares were universal, with undisguised themes of violence and danger: "My husband was chasing me up the stairs . . . I was trying to escape but I kept falling backwards"; "There was a man breaking in the house . . . trying to kill me"; "Snakes were after me . . . in my bed."

In contrast to dreams in which they attempted to protect themselves or to fight back or to escape, their waking lives were characterized by overwhelming passivity and an inability to act on their own behalf. They felt drained, fatigued, and numb, and without energy to do more than minimal household chores and child care. There was a pervasive sense of hopelessness and despair about themselves and their lives. They saw themselves as incompetent, unworthy, and unlovable women and were ridden with guilt and shame. They felt that they deserved the abuse, had no vision that there was any other way to live, and were powerless to make changes.

Like rape victims, these battered women rarely experienced their anger directly, although their stories elicited anguish and outrage in the listener. It is likely, however, that the constellation of passivity, guilt, intense fear of the unexpected, and violent nightmares reflected not only fear of another assault but also a constant struggle with the self to contain and control aggressive impulses. The violent encounter with another person's loss of control of aggression precipitates great anxiety about one's own controls. We know from rape victims that *one* such encounter is sufficient to bury aggression.[34] In the life experiences of battered women, there is not much perceived or real difference between affect, fantasy, and action. It is not surprising, then, that fear of loss of control was a universal concern. These fears were often expressed in vague abstract terms but were unmistakably linked to aggression.

This was clearly seen in the minority of women who were more overtly enraged. Although some women presented when the violence had escalated to the point where their lives were endangered, others came because they were losing control of aggressive impulses toward their spouses or their children; for example, one woman was seen after she tried to strangle her infant daughter, and another, after she bought a gun. Some women became frankly homicidal; one woman served a prison term for the shooting death of her husband, and another went to trial for assaulting her husband's lover. Some women fantasized detailed plans for murdering their husbands as a way of coping with their anger. One woman, who had been explosive in the past, began throwing the shotgun at her husband instead of firing it. Still others locked up guns and knives to prevent easy access to weapons without knowing why they did so. Some displayed outward aggression by becoming adept at verbal retaliation, while others fought back physically.

These cases were the exceptions, however, and passivity and paralysis of action more accurately described the majority. Their aggression was most consistently directed against themselves: suicidal behavior, depression, grotesque self-imagery, alcoholism in a few, and self-mutilation in one woman, whose face and body were covered with self-induced scratches and scars. Passivity and denial of anger, then, do not imply that the battered woman is adjusted to or likes her situation. It is the last desperate defense against homicidal rage.

TREATMENT ISSUES

Clinicians must be aware of the prevalence of family violence and the variety of ways in which victims may present themselves so that victim identification is facilitated.[23,39,40] Once established, marital violence tends to escalate, and the possibility of a lethal outcome must be considered throughout the diagnostic and treatment process. This consideration is especially important in the usual clinical situation, in which only the abused wife is in treatment and the violence at home is continuing. Most violent husbands do not willingly enter treatment because they do not perceive their behavior as a problem requiring intervention. Removal of the women and children from the home to a safe environment is often essential to adequate long-term treatment and rehabilitative efforts, and it is important for the clinician to be aware of community resources that provide protection and safety.[23,35]

Women are trapped in violent homes for a variety of complex intrapsychic and situational reasons. They are often economically dependent on their husbands; they have few job skills and difficulty finding work outside the home; and if they come from violent families of origin, these families give them little emotional support for separation. They are paralyzed by fear, are threatened by further violence to themselves and to their children if they leave, and have learned from experience that law enforcement will not protect them. Thus, clinicians must work to identify those internal and external barriers to self-protection, so that abused women can take action to terminate the violence or, more likely, the relationship.

The battered woman has often experienced a lifetime of abuse and neglect by significant others and by previous contacts with medical, social, and criminal justice agencies. She comes to believe that she deserves such treatment and expects no empathy from clinicians. Her feelings of helpless rage, which she may well have acted out against her children or herself, only intensify her belief that she is unworthy or bad. To tell the clinician of the violence against her or of her own frightening impulses is to risk yet another person confirming her own judgment of guilt. The core issues for psychotherapeutic work, then, are the woman's markedly impaired self-esteem, emotional isolation, and mistrust.

There is a complex mythology about wife beating that must be identified and challenged early in the work with battered women:

1. The violence is perceived as a norm; this is most likely when the victim comes from a violent family of origin.
2. The violence is rationalized; he is not responsible because he is sick, mentally ill, alcoholic, unemployed, or under stress.
3. The violence is justified; she deserves it because she is bad, provocative, or challenging.
4. The violence is controllable; if only she is good, quiet, and compliant, he will not abuse her.

The victim utilizes this group of beliefs to "explain" the brutality. This "explanation" reinforces her tenuous denial and protects her husband and her marriage, at the expense of her self-esteem and autonomy—and possibly her life. It allows her to remain totally enslaved while believing that she is in control.

A second group of myths serves to prevent the dissolution of the marriage even when she perceives the violence as inappropriate: she loves him; she can't survive without him; she stays "for the sake of the children"; he will change. There is usually ample information to confront these beliefs with a multitude of broken promises and betrayals, blatant evidence of disturbed or abused children, and the reality that she is surviving in spite of a husband who provides neither emotional nor financial support for his family.

An elaboration of the mythology begins the process of challenging her denial, altering her self-concept, and raising her consciousness about sex roles. Certainly, much of the mythology is based on rigid stereotypical cultural norms for a woman's behavior as passive, male-dependent, and masochistic, and for a woman's place being in the home. This is also a time when it is helpful for a clinician to provide information about the widespread incidence of wife beating, so that it is seen not only as a personal dilemma but as a broad social problem that affects the lives of many women. One of the positive outcomes of treatment has been the beginnings of women identifying with women, and a wish to provide assistance, information, and support to other abused women.

As she begins to feel less deviant and more trusting, the battered woman may tentatively begin the work of looking at the extent of her rage and the relationship between her anger, her fear of loss of control, and her passivity. This work is accompanied by great anxiety, both for the clinician and for the patient, because the violence and provocation by the husband are continuing, and incitement to homicide by either party is obviously not the desired outcome. With a more direct focus on the affective impact of the violence, the woman may share information, for the first time, about other aggressive acts against her, so that the clinician must be prepared to deal with an earlier rape, an incestuous relationship, or abuse as a child. One may also hear about aggression directed toward her children and her confusion about mothering. Basic work on the differences between limit setting, discipline, and battering is necessary, and this may require the involvement of child-protective services and/or direct work with the children.

Understandably, beginning a therapeutic relationship may be a crisis point for some women, who may require hospitalization or intensive outpatient work to support their controls. This is also a time that one sees dissolution of the passivity in favor of a more active position, with embryonic plans for employment, vocational training, education, and termination of the marital relationship. Because of the real possibility of escalating violence as a result of the changes in her behavior, it is stressed that the woman should not be pushed to move beyond what she feels are safe boundaries in terms of her acknowledgment of anger or actions to confront her husband. The clinician must assume that her assessment of her own controls, the extent of the danger to herself and children, and her husband's potential for violence are accurate.

CONCLUSION

Wife beating is not a new phenomenon, but one that has been largely ignored by mental health professionals. Extensive research and service efforts focus on child abuse and alcoholism, but in neither instance has there been a recognition of the savage aggression that is directed toward the mothers and wives in these same family units. Prevailing social norms and public policies reinforce the wife's role as her husband's property, so that violence that occurs in the privacy of one's home is not considered a public issue. The relationship between the violent home and another generation of violent individuals is not addressed, while medical, social, and criminal justice institutions unwittingly conspire to preserve the integrity of home and family, whatever the costs.

Until attitudes change, battered women will continue to remain silent about the crimes committed against them, so that clinicians must assume the responsibility for identifying the violent abuse. The following constellation of symptoms and circumstances is closely correlated with wife abuse [1]:

1. Violence and/or child abuse in families of origin.
2. Suspected physical or sexual abuse of children in the family.
3. Multiple somatic, emotional, behavioral, and sleep problems in the children.
4. Aggressive and destructive behavior in teenage sons.
5. Alcoholism and pathological jealousy in the husband.
6. Multiple somatic complaints, frequent medical visits, and chronic use of tranquilizers and analgesics by the wife.
7. Severe agitation, anxiety, insomnia, and dreams with violent themes reported by the wife.
8. Chronic depressive symptoms and a history of repeated suicidal behavior.

While not all of these items apply to every battered woman, this checklist has been extremely useful in identifying "silent" victims of marital violence. Of 60 battered women, 56 were identified only because they were asked about the battering.

REFERENCES

1. Hilberman E, Munson K: Sixty battered women, *Victimology: An International Journal* 2(3/4):460–471, 1977–1978.
2. Gayford JJ: Wife battering: A preliminary survey of 100 cases, *British Medical Journal* 1:194–197, 1975.
3. Gelles RJ, Straus MA: Family experience and public support of the death penalty, *American Journal of Orthopsychiatry* 45(4):596–613, 1975.
4. Gelles RJ: *The violent home: A study of physical aggression between husbands and wives.* Beverly Hills, Calif.: Sage, 1974.
5. Straus M: Wife-beating: How common, and why? *Victimology: An International Journal* 2(3/4):443–458, 1977–1978.
6. Steinmetz SK, Straus MA (eds.): *Violence in the family.* New York, Harper & Row, 1974.
7. Martin D: *Battered wives.* San Francisco: Glide, 1976.
8. Schulman MA: *A survey of spousal violence against women in Kentucky.* Conducted for Kentucky Commission on Women by Louis Harris and Associates, 1979.
9. Gates M: *The battered woman: Criminal and civil remedies.* Presented at annual meeting of the American Psychiatric Association, Toronto, 1977.

10. Boudouris J: Homicide and the family, *Journal of Marriage and the Family* 33(4):667–682, 1971.
11. Goode W: Force and violence in the family, *Journal of Marriage and the Family* 33(4):637–648, 1971.
12. Truninger E: Marital violence: the legal solutions, *The Hastings Law Review* 23:259–276, 1971.
13. Dobash RE, Dobash RP: Wives: The "appropriate" victims of marital violence, *Victimology: An International Journal* 2(3/4):426–442, 1977–1978.
14. Kansas City Police Department: Conflict management: Analysis/resolution, 1973.
15. Scott PD: Battered wives, *British Journal of Psychiatry* 125:433–441, 1974.
16. Pizzey E: *Scream quietly or the neighbors will hear.* Middlesex, England, Penguin, 1974.
17. Easson WM, Steinhilber RN: Murderous aggression by children and adolescents, *Archives of General Psychiatry* 4:47–55, 1961.
18. Duncan JW, Duncan GM: Murder in the family: A study of some homicidal adolescents, *American Journal of Psychiatry* 127:1498–1502, 1971.
19. Duncan GM, Frazier SH, Liten EM, *et al:* Etiological factors in first-degree murder, *Journal of the American Medical Association* 168:1755–1758, 1958.
20. Straus M: Sexual inequality, cultural norms, and wife beating, *Victimology* 1(1):54–76, 1976.
21. Straus M: A social structural perspective on the prevention and treatment of wife-beating. In *Battered women.* Edited by Roy M. New York, Van Nostrand-Reinhold, 1977.
22. Field MH, Field HF: Marital violence and the criminal process: Neither justice nor peace, *Social Service Review* 47:221–240, 1973.
23. Hilberman E: Overview: The "wife-beater's wife" reconsidered, *American Journal of Psychiatry* 137(11)1336–1347, 1980.
24. Walker LE: Battered women and learned helplessness, *Victimology: An International Journal* 2(3/4):525–534, 1977–1978.
25. Walker LE: *The battered woman.* New York, Harper & Row, 1979.
26. Gelles RJ: Abused wives: Why do they stay? *Journal of Marriage and the Family* 38:659–668, 1976.
27. Gelles RJ: Violence and pregnancy: A note on the extent of the problem and needed services, *The Family Coordinator* 24:81–86, 1975.
28. Dewsbury AR: Family violence seen in general practice, *Royal Society of Health Journal* 95(6):290–294, 1975.
29. Snell JE, Rosenwald RJ, Robey A: The wife-beater's wife, *Archives of General Psychiatry* 11:107–112, 1964.
30. Kaunitz PE: Sadomasochistic marriages, *Medical Aspects of Human Sexuality* 11(2):66–80, 1977.
31. Waites EA: Female masochism and the enforced restriction of choice, *Victimology: An International Journal* 2(3/4):535–544, 1977–1978.
32. Hilberman E, Munson K: unpublished data.
33. Burgess AW, Holmstrom LL: Rape trauma syndrome, *American Journal of Psychiatry* 131(9):981–986, 1974.
34. Hilberman E: The impact of rape. In *The woman patient,* Vol. 1. Edited by Notman MT, Nadelson CC. New York, Plenum Press, 1978.
35. United States Commission on Civil Rights: *Battered women: Issues of public policy.* Proceedings of a consultation published by the Commission, 1978.
36. Dobash, RE, Dobash RP: *Violence against wives.* New York: Free Press, 1979.
37. Herman, JL: *Father–Daughter incest.* Cambridge: Harvard Press, 1981.

38. Carmen EH, Russo, NF, Miller JB: Inequality and women's mental health: an overview. *American Journal of Psychiatry* 138(10):1319–1330, 1981.
39. Stark E, Flitcraft A, Frazier W: Medicine and patriarchal violence: the social construction of a "private" event. *Int. J. Health Serv.* 9:461–493; 1979.
40. Herman J, Hirschman L: Families at risk for father–daughter incest. *American Journal of Psychiatry* 138(7):967–970, 1981.

Chapter 5

Incest

Veronica Tisza

Definition of Incest

The dictionary definition of *incest* is sexual intercourse between persons too closely related to marry legally. In its restricted application, this definition would include relations between parents and their children. However, this restricted concept of incest melds into the wider concept of intrafamilial sexual abuse when one considers the frequency with which children, primarily little girls, are sexually exploited by adult members of their extended families, especially those living under the same roof. The aggressor may be a stepfather, a grandfather, an uncle, an older cousin, or any other close relative to whom the child is bound by love and trust, and by whom the child desires to be loved.

There is a significant qualitative difference between the emotional impact of intrafamilial sexual abuse and the emotional impact of incestuous relationships within the nuclear family. In cases of intrafamilial sexual abuse, the children suffer from the betrayal of trust invested in the adult, from feelings of helplessness, and from the consequences of the age-inappropriate sexual stimulation. However, if they can turn to the parents for understanding, compassion, and protection, their basic emotional relationships and the understanding of their natural role within the family may remain unharmed. It is different when the incestuous exploitation of children occurs within the nuclear family. This difference is due to the quality of the early reciprocal relationship that develops between parents and their children. While tending to their young children's needs, parents develop strong attachments, bonds arising from deep biological sources. Ba-

VERONICA TISZA, M.D. • Lecturer, Department of Psychiatry, Harvard Medical School; Consultant, Department of Child Psychiatry, Massachusetts General Hospital, Boston, Massachusetts.
65

bies, in turn, also respond early with strong and exclusive attachments, and this early "bonding" between parents and their children is a relationship of extraordinary intensity. Any breach of the trust implicit in these relationships has tremendous emotional impact because of the depth and the intensity of the feelings involved. Furthermore, the emotional betrayal of children through incestuous exploitation within the nuclear family is a significant symptom of the deterioration of family life. It occurs when there is an extension of genital eroticism from its careful restriction to the marital couple, across the generational boundaries, resulting in the erotic involvement of parents with their children. This involvement represents a socially and psychologically regressive phenomenon and has serious implications for the child's psychosexual development.

The erotic involvement of a parent with a child, or a family member with a child in the household, may not be limited to sexual intercourse. It may include a whole range of inappropriate and sexualized physical contacts, like the fondling of breasts and genitals, mutual masturbation and fellatio. These are violations of erotic restraints within the family and an exploitation of the trust and respect that children feel toward their elders.

Cuddling, touching, and loving appreciation of the child's charm increase the youngster's self-esteem and reassure him or her about being good, pleasing, and valuable. If the adult has sexualized fantasies, and the intensity of the physical stimulation of the child transgresses the usual boundaries, the intensity of the encounter may create such heightened excitement in the child that the physical contact, instead of reassuring the child of parental love, may become a frightening and overwhelming experience. At the same time, it is important to keep in mind that the socially sanctioned physical manifestations of endearing contact between parents and children are different in different cultures and in different cultural subgroups.

FACTORS LEADING TO A BETTER RECOGNITION OF INTRAFAMILIAL SEXUAL EXPLOITATION OF CHILDREN

Until quite recently, the problem of incest and the sexual abuse of children commanded little attention. Cases of incest came to professional attention when they were reported to the courts, usually by a mother or sometimes by the social agency to whom a hurt and desperate daughter turned for help. Incest was seen by professionals and the public alike as a rare and repulsive sexual deviation restricted mainly to the disadvantaged and disorganized section of the population. Blind faith in the effectiveness of the incest taboo interfered for a long time with the recognition of reality. Recent social and cultural changes, however, have created an atmosphere that permits the recognition of the frequency and the nature of incestuous relationships and an examination of the social and psychological structure of the incestuous family.

The upsurge of professional interest in the sexual mistreatment of children followed the recognition of the frequency of child abuse within our culture. The appreciation of the widespread nature of the physical abuse of children was a shocking experience for professionals and the public alike. Once the veil of ignorance was lifted, experts learned to recognize cases of abuse and were forced to reevaluate many haunting experiences from the past. They diagnosed, retrospectively, many puzzling and tragic accidents as cases of physical abuse inflicted by desperate parents on helpless children. Child advocacy was strengthened, and increasing sophistication made it clear that child abuse was not restricted to lower-class or disorganized families, but that it occurred in all social classes and was a symptom of serious family difficulties.

In addition to the recognition of child abuse, another factor in the recognition of incest has come from the women's movement, which has led the way toward the recognition of the sexual exploitation of women in society in general, and within their families in particular. The new freedom to discuss sexuality opened the eyes of professionals and the public to the realities of people's lives and helped to dispel old and stubbornly held convictions. The present-day interest in the study of the psychological forces operating within families has made it possible to approach the sexual abuse of children with increasing sensitivity and understanding.

The dissemination and sharing of knowledge and experience also brought relief to women who had been sexually exploited when they were young. The understanding that they were not unique has helped them to feel less lonely, as well as less guilty about their painful secret. Communications from incest victims have become increasingly frequent in clinical encounters, and families have become less defensive about discussing intrafamilial sexual problems in which the child is the victim.

The increased awareness of the problems of incest and the intrafamilial sexual abuse of children tempts one to believe that the incidence of such abuses is increasing. Nothing in the history of childhood, however, permits us to believe that children are worse off now than they have been throughout the history of Western civilization. Thus, it is likely that the incest taboo has been broken throughout history, with unsuspected frequency.

Origins of the Incest Taboo

Prohibition of incest is a common feature of all known societies. As Parsons pointed out, it would be difficult to attribute something as general as the incest taboo to one specific cause. It is more probable that a combination of multiple sociological and psychological considerations, which are basic to human societies, are also involved in the evolution of the taboo.[2]

Historical and anthropological studies reveal that in some instances, incestuous unions have been permitted under highly exceptional circumstances. The immortal gods of Greek mythology were united in incestuous unions. The royal families of ancient Egypt, Iran, and pre-Columbian Peru symbolized their divine descent and exalted status, as well as serving their economic and political goals, by practicing marriage between siblings. Incestuous unions are permitted in some contemporary tribal societies, but only under highly exceptional, religious and ritualistic circumstances.[1]

Among the theories proposed to explain the evolution of the incest taboo, Lévi-Strauss's anthropological-sociological theory[3] and Freud's psychological theory occupy[4,5] prominent positions. Van Lawick-Goodall's[6] observations of primate behavior raise interesting questions; Westermarck's[7] theory points out factors that may enhance the effectiveness of the incest prohibition; and the biological theory of the evolutionists is an important and interesting contribution to the solution of the problem.[8]

Lévi-Strauss based his theory on the well-documented observation that in primitive societies, relationships are regulated by the exchange of reciprocal gifts. The exchange of gifts occurs at ceremonies celebrating important events in the lives of individual families and the tribe. The exchange of gifts brings no economic advantages to either party, but the skillful use of the exchange seals friendships and alliances and fortifies the individuals and tribes against risks threatening their security and prosperity. The objects of exchange are food, manufactured objects, and women. Nuclear families give up their daughters as objects of exchange to ensure safety and prosperity through alliances. Daughters sexually used by their fathers and their families are tarnished and lose their value as gifts of exchange. Such losses lead to the impoverishment of individual families and diminish the ceremonial gift-giving ability of the tribe. Such transgressions could not be tolerated because they reduced the strength, the influence, and thereby the security of the whole community. To quote Lévi-Strauss, "the prohibition of incest is a rule of reciprocity."

The exchange of reciprocal gifts is not limited to primitive societies; it pervades, in more-or-less symbolic forms, all aspects of contemporary life. Invitations are extended and gifts are exchanged at specific occasions and according to well-regulated customs. Women, especially daughters, have maintained their position as the most valuable gifts of exchange in the service of forming alliances and ensuring the continued flow of services. Thus, the reciprocal exchange of gifts is an archaic custom, but as Lévi-Strauss pointed out, its "reason for existing is so fundamental that its transformation has been neither possible nor necessary."

Psychiatric interest in incest began with Freud's psychological studies of hysteria. Freud became interested in incest when he repeatedly heard memories of incestuous childhood experiences from his patients. He did not believe that incest could be such a frequent occurrence, and thus, he began to recognize that unconscious incestuous fantasies were a normal part of psychosexual maturation. This recognition led to his theory of infantile sexuality and the development of the concept of the Oedipus complex. This theory, in turn, led to his interest in the origins of the incest taboo. He related it to violent sexual rivalries within the nuclear family. The clinical experience of psychoanalysts supported the thesis that patients in treatment recalled and related fantasies dating back to the first years of their lives. The universality of unconscious incestuous fantasies, however, should not blind the clinician to the possibility that some of the memories of incest may, in fact, relate to actual historical events in the patient's life. There is an increasing conviction that at least some of Freud's patients recalled the memories of actual sexual abuse in early childhood, committed either by the father or by some other trusted and feared male member of the household.

An ethological view of incest offers challenging observations. Since the word *taboo* has religious and moral overtones, we use here the term *incest avoidance* in discussing primates. There is a definite pattern of inhibition of mother–son mating among rhesus macaques.[9] An examination of the social relations of mother–son pairs showed that the mothers maintained a protective attitude toward their sons well into adulthood and remained dominant over them. The social rank of the mother in relation to that of the son seemed to be a very important variable in the degree of dominance maintained. Van Lawick-Goodall[6] described definite mother–son incest avoidance in chimpanzees, and according to her observations, the young female chimpanzee was also reluctant to mate with her male siblings. Whether there is some biological predisposition underlying the social and environmental stimuli in the development of incest avoidance among chimpanzees is a hypothesis that cannot be answered at the present time.[10]

Westermarck[7] based his theory of the development of the incest taboo on the observation that prolonged social familiarity decreases sexual desires among family members. He hypothesized a natural aversion that arises from the continual association of persons living closely together from early childhood. Westermarck's thesis was supported by the observations of social anthropologists. It seems, however, that he failed to evaluate sufficiently the effect of social disapproval on the development of sexual expression within the family.

The biological theory of the development of the incest taboo in human families is based on the observation that inbreeding often produces damaged and nonviable offspring. The congenital damage is caused by the pairing of two mutant recessive genes; the probability of such an occurrence is much higher in genetically related than in unrelated persons. There is considerable research concerning this problem, including the Adams and Neel study,[11] in which 18 incest babies, 6 of which were the products of father–daughter incest and 12 of brother–sister incest, were compared with the matched controls of 18 children of unwed mothers under the care of the same agency. By 6 months of age, 7 of the incest babies appeared normal; however, 3 were dead, 3 had severe congenital defects and 5 showed significantly retarded development. Of the matched controls (all were living), there was no case of recognizable congenital abnormality, and though some showed somewhat slower development, there was no evidence of significant retardation.

In the largest reported study, Seemanova[12] collected 161 incest offspring of 141 mothers. The average age of the mothers at the time of the birth of these children was 14–15 years. Of the 141 mothers, 116 had normal intelligence, 20 were judged to be of "subnormal" intelligence, 2 were deaf-mutes, and 3 were schizophrenic. Of the 138 related fathers, 8 were mentally retarded. Of the 161 children, 88 were the products of father–daughter incest, 72 of brother–sister incest, and 1 child of a mother–son incest. As controls, Seemanova used a group of 95 children of the same mothers by unrelated fathers. By the time of the birth of the second group of children, the mothers were older. The average maternal age was 20 years. Of the incest children, 21 died, 10 of them from evident congenital malformations. Of the control group, 5 children died, only 1 from a recognized congenital defect.

These studies indicate that children born from incestuous relationships suffer from a higher-than-average mortality rate, an increased incidence of congenital malformations, and a higher-than-average risk of mental retardation. Incest children, however, are not only potentially biologically disadvantaged. They are also handicapped in their development by being the unwanted children of adolescent girls living in a chaotic environment, who are unable to extend the care and nurturance necessary for the optimal development of their children.

The recognition of the increased incidence of congenital abnormalities among children born from incestuous unions may have played a supportive role in the enforcement of the incest taboo. Even without the recognition of the causal relationship between sexual relations and pregnancy among primitive tribes, the birth of a deformed and non-viable baby may well have been regarded as punishment for the commitment of specific sins. Incest avoidance protects the survival of the species because it increases the genetic pool. In spite of its significance, it cannot be regarded as the only and basic explanation of incest avoidance. The incest taboo is a basic rule of all known human societies, and it serves not only biological but important social and psychological purposes.[13] Once established within the nuclear family, its pattern changes from culture to culture presumably depending on the kinship system of each society.[14]

Weinberg[15] elaborated the sociological view. He stated that there is a set of socializing influences within the structure of the contemporary family that serves as a protection against incestuous behavior. Social obligations, affectionate ties, and common socialized living conditions within the family all contribute to the dulling of sexual desires for family members. They help to establish social intimacy, sexual privacy, and distance between the generations. The hierarchical arrangement of family life places the parents in the role of providers and protectors; it permits the children to reach out to their peer groups for companionship and provides them with freedom within well-regulated channels. Whatever their discipline and theoretical background, anthropologists, sociologists, and professionals in the psychological disciplines all agree that the breakdown of the incest taboo is a symptom of severe family dysfunction.

The following discussion focuses on cases in which the incestuous sexual abuse of the child was an undeniable reality, including father–daughter incest, mother–son incest, incestuous relationships between siblings, and homosexual incest.

DIFFERENT TYPES OF INCEST

FATHER–DAUGHTER INCEST. This most frequently occurring infraction of the incest taboo has been studied from many perspectives. One of the first studies was Weinberg's psychosociological project in the early 1950s. This project investigated 203 father–adolescent-daughter incest cases that had come to the attention of the courts. The investigator interviewed not only the fathers, but other members of the families. He tried to understand the individual and the family dynamics of the incestuous family groups. Within this population most of the fathers belonged to the lower socio-economic strata and had a low educational level and a high percentage of unemployment at the time of the incest.

From this group, Weinberg described two main types of incest initiators:

1. The "endogamic" incest fathers were men confined emotionally within their families, unable to deflect their sexual desires to persons outside the family. These men were the products of inbred, socially isolated families, and they perpetuated this lifestyle throughout their adult existence. Incest appeared to them to be less frightening than the possibility of adultery. These fathers felt guilty about their actions. The rehabilitation of their problem-ridden but functioning families was found to be a rather hopeful task.

2. The so-called exogamic incest initiators were impulse-ridden, frequently sadistic men, often reared in families where incest was tolerated and promiscuity accepted. These fathers failed to internalize the sexual constraints of family living; they lacked the capacity for affection and felt little guilt. Such men abused their wives and children and forced themselves on their daughters. The rehabilitation of their families, as complete and functional units, could not be viewed as a promising task.

More recent studies come from many different settings. There are reports by psychiatric teams and mental health professionals working at medical centers, community clinics, and acting as consultants to protective service agencies and parent groups.[16] From a survey of the recent literature, one observes a spectrum of cases of sexual misuse, that is, the exposure of the child to sexual stimulation inappropriate to the child's natural role in the family and the society.[17] At one end of the spectrum are cases where the adults are by no means malicious assailants, and the intent of their behavior does not appear to have been malevolent. At times, there is not even a conscious awareness that the child is being used to satisfy the parent's dependent-erotic needs. Fathers and daughters, for example, may be involved in exciting physical games like "horseplay" and wrestling; lonely mothers may engage in undue physical contact with their young sons. These activities are inappropriate and potentially damaging to the child because in these type of activities, it becomes difficult to separate actions from underlying fantasies. These games may generate more excitement and stimulation than a child is able to manage without feeling overwhelmed. It is also difficult to ascertain at what point such experiences engender an individual child's reaction of anxiety and guilt with the

possibility of psychological and psychosomatic symptom formation.
On the other end of the spectrum of sexual misuse is the frank sexual abuse of the child. Because of spreading enlightenment about incest, professionals are beginning to deal with cases coming from a wide social and psychological spectrum. Most of the fathers involved appear to belong to the category of so-called endogamous incest aggressors, and the cases demonstrate that the main characteristics of the incestuous family are social isolation, emotional deprivation, and inadequate parenting.

CASE ILLUSTRATIONS

The angry and depressed wife of an alcoholic man withdrew from her husband and refused sexual relations with him. The father turned to their 14-year-old daughter with his sexual and dependency needs. After some months, the mother "heard" the signals of her daughter. When the truth was admitted, she pressed charges against her husband. As a result of the daughter's testimony, the father received a five-year prison sentence. The mother obtained a divorce, and on the advice of the court, she and her daughter entered psychiatric treatment. In treatment, the mother recalled some of the warnings voiced earlier by the daughter, and she wondered how she could have failed to understand the signals. The anger and guilt reverberating between mother and daughter was never completely resolved.

A 15-year-old girl, the oldest of three daughters, was brought to a psychiatric clinic with complaints of social isolation, lack of communication, insomnia, and multiple aches and pains. At home, she took care of her chronically depressed mother, who suffered from a host of psychosomatic symptoms. During the psychiatric evaluation, the girl's sustained incestuous relationship with her weak, deprived, and angry father was disclosed. The incest situation had appeared to solve the family's problems temporarily; however, the daughter had become increasingly conflicted and incapable of satisfying the roles assigned to her, that is, as the father's wife and as the caretaker of the entire unhappy and isolated family. In fear of exacerbating her mother's illness and causing her death, the girl turned her guilt and anger inward and became increasingly depressed and withdrawn. The mother found this withdrawal intolerable and had thus initiated a referral to the psychiatric clinic. The daughter correctly understood the referral as permission to reveal the family secret. Protective services and individual and family psychotherapy helped this family to reorganize and work together for a successful rehabilitative outcome.

The oldest daughter of an upper-class professional family was exposed to her father's intermittent sexual advances throughout her adolescence. The relationship culminated in actual sexual intercourse when she was 17 years old. Some weeks later, the daughter, who harbored much resentment toward the successful socialite mother, revealed her secret and requested that the mother get a divorce. The father denied her accusations, and her mother accused her of attempting to break up her parents' marriage. The relationships within the family remained extremely tense. When the daughter entered college, she sought psychiatric treatment to relieve her pain and outrage.

A young mother brought her severely congenitally abnormal child to the clinic. The mother was one of nine children, the second oldest daughter, and was away on a farm with her family. Her father, a severe, moralistic, and withdrawn man initiated sexual relations with her when she was in her mid-teens. When she became pregnant, it became clear that the meek and exhausted mother had known all along what was happening, and she accepted her daughter's pregnancy and the handicapped baby without question or protest. On a visit to the city with her child, the young mother managed to get in touch with her older sister, who had run away from home a few years earlier. She found out that the sister had run away because she could not tolerate the sustained sexual relations with the father.

The Incestuous Family in Father–Daughter Incest. The initial studies examining father–daughter incest focused on the individual personality patterns of the incest participants. Increasingly, however, a family-oriented approach has evolved. This has helped to bring about a better understanding of the intrapsychic conflicts, as well as the interpersonal determinants of the psychological behavior patterns within the family. Weinberg defined incest as a sign of family disorganization.[15] Kaufman *et al.,*[18] working in a child psychiatry setting, studied a group of incest cases, all of which had had long-term psychiatric treatment, and recognized the multigenerational family dynamics leading to the incest.

Incest has been seen as a homeostatic device for families suffering from intense fear of separation and abandonment. The fear of loss in such families overrides all other concerns, and when the family group senses that there is a distance developing between the parents, incest becomes a way of keeping the family together. At least initially, and then for a shorter or longer period of time, every member of the family group cooperates because the equilibrium of the group depends on the maintenance of the ingrown family structure.[19]

For an understanding of this family constellation, it is necessary to describe briefly the psychological characteristics and emotional needs of the members of the incestuous family.

The fathers, as noted above, were characterized as rather isolated and passive men whose emotional needs remained confined within the nuclear family. They were described not as psychotic, but as markedly anxiety-prone and often addicted to alcohol. They turned for the satisfaction of their great dependency needs to women, and when they felt deprived or disappointed, women also became the recipients of their frustrated anger. These men had difficulties with their masculine identity and not infrequently were sexually inadequate. Their identity problems and possible homosexual fears interfered with their relationships with men, thus adding to the intensity of their successive dependence on mother, wife, and eventually daughter. They turned to their daughters when they felt deprived by their wives, and they seemed to perceive unconsciously that their wives' ambivalence gave them permission for the incestuous relationship.

The mothers were described as women whose early needs for nurturance and dependency had never been met. During their growing years, they learned to distrust their fathers, who had some nurturing abilities but were unreliable. They overidentified with their mothers, who gave them all the warmth they were capable of giving. Because of their early deprivations, however, the emotional supplies of these mothers were limited, and their capacity to relate to their daughters was also limited and deeply ambivalent. Eventually, the daughters chose husbands who were quite similar to their fathers. These men, in turn, confirmed their lack of trust in men. When these women become mothers, they may also perpetuate the same pattern within their families. So it proceeds through successive generations, a line of women who play out their destiny more or less according to a pattern resulting from early deprivation and low self-esteem.

As mentioned above, there is usually one "chosen" daughter whom the mother identifies with her own mother, and this daughter starts early to carry the burden of her mother's needs. She assumes, early in life, some of the caretaking responsibilities within the family, and the family lives tightly bound together, preserving the rigid intrafamilial system that assures for everyone at least a modicum of well-being. When, for some reason, the mother's depression deepens and she withdraws in hurt and disappointment from her husband, she leaves the way open for her daughter to become involved in the multigenerational identification pattern. The mother's ambivalence, her identification with her daughter, and her displaced anger toward the daughter are acted out as she unconsciously paves the way toward the incestuous union. This constellation prevents her from becoming conscious of the reality of the incest. The incestuous relationship and the shared secret assure the stability of the nuclear family, and for a variable period of time, no one in this emotionally deprived group can afford the loss of nurturance and the possible abandonment that would result from the revelation of the secret.

The daughter's overidentification with her mother and her unconscious rivalry and anger toward her mother prepare her for the incestuous relationship. The precipitating event in disturbing the family's equilibrium appears to be the mother's relinquishment of her caretaking function. Her withdrawal drives father and daughter toward each other for care and dependency gratification and simultaneously provides an outlet for them to act out their anger toward her. In these emotionally deprived families, touch and even genital sex are perceived as care and nurturance; and while the needy young daughter is "giving" and also "receiving," she has the satisfaction of ensuring the stability of the family.

The incestuous relationship, however, usually offers the needy family only temporary relief from fear. The daughters are the members of the family group who pay the heaviest price for the incest and the attending confusion of roles. They suffer from guilt because of the strong though ambivalent bond with their mother. They feel anger and revulsion toward the incestuous fathers, but more often than not, there is compassion mixed into their feelings. They perceive their father's neediness and see him as the more available parent.

Eventually, the daughter may feel overwhelmed by the responsibilities she is carrying. Her feelings of emotional deprivation may not find relief in the incest itself; on the contrary, anger and guilt may add to her emotional burden. Additionally, since her adolescent strivings and needs may increasngly find satisfaction in the company of her peers, she may find the strength to revolt against the role assigned to her within the nuclear family.

There are, presumably, countless incestuous relationships that are a part of a family's lifestyle and never come to the attention of outsiders. The revelation of the family secret, when it occurs, is usually made by the daughters, either alone or in cooperation their with mother. What motivates mothers suddenly to hear and to understand the family drama defies generalization. In our experience thus far, only the frequently explosive and punishing anger turned toward their husbands gives some indication of the change that has occurred in the wives' emotional economy. This anger may lead to criminal prosecution of the father, making the daughters feel extremely guilty about breaking up the family. The daughters also feel guilty because of a vague understanding that their fathers were not the only culprits. At times, when these mothers are finally ready to hear the truth, they may turn their anger toward the girls, accusing them of lying or of having seduced their fathers in order to break up the family. Some daughters, feeling deprived of help from their mothers, may then talk to trusted older friends, who help them to get assistance for themselves and for the rehabilitation of the family. Some deeply hurt daughters of incestuous families may run away from home or attempt suicide to call attention to their predicament and the plight of their family.

Besides families that carry the burden of long-standing incestuous relationships, there are families of similar psychological structure, but better impulse control, in which incest is not expressed in clearly genital terms but finds a symbolic expression in many aspects of the families' life. In these families, the daughter occupies a special position in relation to her father and may become his confidant and partial caretaker. Although the physical contact may not exceed hand holding and "horseplay," there is usually an undue amount of exhibitionism, a lack of respect for the daughter's physical privacy, and an intrusive interest in the daughter's physical functioning. The true nature of the relationship is further expressed by the father's strivings to interfere with the daughter's peer relationships, especially her relationships with boys, where the father expresses suspicious jealousy and angry prohibitions of her every attempt to participate in an age-appropriate social life. There are also cases in which, under unusual circumstances, the father's rigidly maintained impulse control breaks down and incest is consummated. Such an occurrence leaves both partners extremely frightened and guilty, and with the firm resolve that it will never happen again. These cases never come to the mother's attention, but psychotherapists learn about them much later, when the daughters developed sufficient trust to talk about their traumatic secret.

Effects of an Incest Relationship on the Child. Clinical experience with the different types of incestuous relationships is relatively limited, and there are no large-scale studies available that examine the effects of incestuous involvements on the incest participants and their families. Therefore, the following discussion is restricted to an examination of the effects of sexual exploitation in the most commonly reported and best-studied type of incestuous relationship, that between a father and his daughter.

In an incest relationship, the daughter is always the victim. Even if she submits to the father's demands, her immaturity excludes realistic judgment. Especially in the case of younger girls, their participation is never optional because of the confusing mixture of love, trust, respect, and fear that children feel toward the parent. The daughter may want to be close to the father and may even be seductive, but she does not want actual sexual relations. She usually feels safe in giving expression to her need for love and closeness because of her trust in the generational boundaries and the protective role of the parent. In an incestuous relationship, the daughter is caught in the web of aberrant and destructive family relationships. She also has to handle the effect of sexual stimulation, which is inappropriate in view of her age and developmental phase.

It is difficult to discuss the effect of incest on the child's person-

ality development from a clinical vantage point because data from longitudinal studies are just beginning to accumulate. There are a number of retrospective clinical reports in the literature describing the
psychological effects and the emotional sequelae of incest in the girl
victims. These reports are important and interesting contributions, but
their evaluation becomes difficult because of two major methodological handicaps: (1) most retrospective studies work with a small and
rather specific population, and (2) the outcomes are usually not defined
by a comparable set of criteria. Some studies claim that childhood incestuous experiences have had seemingly no harmful effects on the
woman's "normal adult adjustment." The majority of the reports,
however, consider the incestuous experience a harmful factor in the
girl's subsequent psychological development. In his study of 204 mid-
adolescent daughters of lower-class families who were incest participants, Weinberg found that some became promiscuous; some needed
psychiatric treatment, presumably as a result of the incestuous experience; and some whose social freedom had previously been severely
curtailed by the father's jealousy within the dysfunctional family
emerged as young women very shy of men.

A more recent psychiatric study points out that the degree of the
psychological trauma caused by seduction and incest depends on (1)
the youngster's developmental phase; (2) the nature of her relationships and the strength of her personality at the time of the event; (3)
the nature, the duration, and the extent of the sexual experience; and
(4) the victim's relationship to the seducer.[20] In accordance with this
thinking, evaluations of the effect of the incest experience on the victim await longitudinal studies of such children and studies of their
family process.

There is rich clinical material accumulated by practicing psychiatrists about the psychological difficulties of adult women who suffered
incestuous experiences in childhood and adolescence. Not infrequently, they enter psychiatric treatment because of depression, and
the history of incest comes to light only during the treatment process.
Many have problems centering on their difficulties in developing
trusting relationships; and many complain of sexual problems, including frigidity. It is a recurrent observation that mothers who suffered
incestuous experiences during their early years have the tendency to
expose their daughters, especially the one to whom they feel the closest, to similar experiences during the girl's growing years. This clinical
finding supports the multigenerational pattern of incestuous relationships previously described.

Reports from this distressed population, however, are not confined to psychiatric clinics. In recent years, there have been many books

and articles in which women have accused their incestuous families for the sexual abuse they suffered and for their subsequent psychological and social ills.

BROTHER–SISTER INCEST. Clinicians are aware that mutual exploration and sexual play among prepubertal brothers and sisters occurs frequently, not only in overcrowded and poorly supervised homes but among the children in all socioeconomic groups. Sexual desires between brothers and sisters are not always repressed when they enter adolescence. Brother–sister incest involving postpubertal partners is probably a more common type of infraction of the incest taboo than is generally recognized. One cannot even estimate the frequency of brother–sister sexual unions because they are rarely reported to outside agencies. The whole family has a vested interest in maintaining this family secret, and as there is no triangle, there is no angry third person looking for revenge. Adoption agencies tend to suspect incest when a young mother steadfastly refuses to divulge the name of the child's father. In the Adams and Neel's study sample, the authors found that there were twice as many babies born from brother–sister unions as to daughters impregnated by their fathers.[11] Sibling incest cases come to clinicians' attention only accidentally and in unusual situations, for example, while becoming acquainted with a patient who comes to a medical clinic for reasons that, at least in the patient's mind, have nothing to do with the incest relationship.

CASE ILLUSTRATION

> A mother brought her 18-year-old daughter to a medical clinic. The girl was complaining of a host of medical problems and appeared emotionally immature and slightly retarded. The internist felt that many of the somatic complaints had no organic basis and referred the girl for psychiatric evaluation. The girl talked without much prompting about having had a history of several years of sexual relations with her older brother and, after he had married and left home, having had sexual relations with her younger brother. The mother, a dull and distraught woman, had been aware of both relationships, but as she was worried about the daughter's potential promiscuity, she preferred to have her daughter's sexual involvement confined to the home. There was no history of pregnancy. On psychological testing, the girl's retardation appeared to be a hysterical defense against "knowing."

HOMOSEXUAL INCEST. Mutual genital exploration and masturbation is a rather common practice among boys, including brothers. Very little is known, however, about brother–brother incest, including homosexual practices, and the few reports in the literature do not lend themselves to generalizations.

Somewhat more is known about incestuous relationships between fathers and sons. The literature on the subject is limited, but such cases increasingly come to the attention of practicing psychiatrists. In most instances, grown-up sons talk about the experiences of their childhood and adolescence. They describe the fathers as the incest initiators, and some, though not all, picture him as a perverted, sadistic abuser.

The length of the homosexual relationship depends both on the father's insistence and on the son's cooperation. Among the sons who enter psychiatric treatment in early adulthood homosexual fear seems to be a frequent complaint.

MOTHER–SON INCEST. Mother–son incest is considered the least frequently occurring infraction of the incest taboo. It is a betrayal of a powerful emotional bond, the relationship between the mother and her young and growing child. The mother's continued caring and protective function helps the child to harness his aggressive and sexual drives and gives the child the strength to develop increasing autonomy and independence. The mother's attitudes influence her child's human relationships throughout his lifetime. A sexual relationship between mother and son represents regressive distortion when primitive erotic aspects of the early mother–child interaction become expressed in adult, sexual, genital terms.

Nevertheless, rural health and social agencies convey the impression that there are many cases of mother–son incest among people who live in deep social isolation, especially when there is no adult male in the home. There is no collection of cases published on mother–son incest, and the few single case reports available do not lend themselves to generalization. Mother–son incest indicates severe psychopathology in the participants if it occurs in a community that presents opportunities for social interactions. However, among people who are deprived of neighbors and friends, it may represent not a symptom of mental illness but a regressive phenomenon due to the isolation.

Although actual mother–son incest is presumably a rare occurrence, the veiled sexual exploitation of sons by lonely mothers occurs frequently in the form of inappropriate and prolonged infantilization of the child. In clinical practice, one encounters lonely mothers who keep their only sons very close. The mother may devote exaggerated and age-inappropriate care to the boy's physical care and bodily functions, and they may share the same bed well into school age. This type of exploitation of the child borders on sexual abuse, because even in the absence of active sexual relations, the sons grow up in an atmosphere of physical overstimulation and social deprivation; they are overly dependent on their mothers and frequently without available male identification figures. Some rebel in adolescence and demonstrate their strong ambivalent feelings and poor impulse control in outbursts of aggression toward their possessive mothers. Others may become social and emotional cripples who live their lives in a love–hate relationship with the mothers whose neediness interfered with their sons' strivings toward independence and emotional and social maturation.

IMPLICATIONS OF INCEST IN MODERN SOCIETY

The reporting of physical abuse is mandatory in all states. Almost half of the states, however, do not specifically mention sexual abuse in their mandatory reporting laws, despite the growing evidence that the sexual abuse of children is a much greater problem than was previously suspected and that incest occurs in a wide spectrum of families. Poor social conditions, unemployment, crowded living conditions (with resulting demoralization), disorganization, and lack of privacy interfere with the protection of children. This population, however, is also more exposed to public scrutiny through the use of public clinics and social agency supervision and intervention, factors that may facilitate the identification of incest. Middle- and upper-class families, through the use of private resources, are in a better social position to guard family secrets, and intimate aspects of family life remain buried until a family member reveals the truth. The revelation of incest, however, may have grave consequences. The father may be put in jail; the parents may become permanently separated or divorced; and the members of the family may become scattered.

Clearly, there is a need for an interdisciplinary support system working with the entire family. Liaison with judges is helpful—in fact, necessary—when the authority and the protection of the courts is needed for the rehabilitation of incest victims and their families. Medical and mental health specialists, attorneys, and protective-service agency workers are needed to serve as consultants on most cases. Recently, private and public medical and social service agencies have been making efforts to cushion the impact of legal proceedings with the ultimate goal of the possible rehabilitation of the family. The therapy of the children is directed toward relieving feelings of guilt over the part they have played in the incest relationship and the possible dissolution of the family. The therapy of the parents is aimed at helping them to recognize and remedy marital difficulties. The purpose of work with the entire family is to effect change in their aberrant emotional relationships and dysfunctional lifestyle.

REFERENCES

1. Murdock GP: The social regulation of sexual behavior. In *Psychosexual development in health and disease*. Edited by Hock PH, Zubin Y. New York, Grune & Stratton, pp. 259–260, 1949.
2. Parsons T: The incest taboo in relation to social structure. In *The Family, Its Structures and Functions* (2nd ed.). Edited by Coser RL. New York, St. Martin's Press, pp. 13–20, 1974.
3. Lévi-Strauss C: *Reciprocity, the essense of social life sociological theory.* Edited by Coser C, Psenberg, New York, Macmillan, pp. 84–94, 1957.
4. Freud S: *The origins of psychoanalysis*, Letter #29 (8-10-1895) and Letter #30 (15-10-1895). New York, Basic Books, 1954.
5. Freud S: *Standard edition.* Volume 13. *Totem and taboo.* London, Hogarth Press, pp. 1–162, 1955.
6. van Lawick-Goodall J: *In the shadow of man.* New York, Delta, pp. 182–183, 1971.
7. Westermarck EA: *Three essays on sex and marriage.* London, MacMillan, 1934.
8. Lindzey G: Some remarks concerning incest, the incest taboo, and psychoanalytic theory, *American Psychologist* 22:1051–1059, 1967.
9. Sade DS: *Inhibition of son-mother matings among free-ranging rhesus monkeys.* Paper presented at the Annual Meeting of the American Academy of Psychoanalysis, May 7, 1967.
10. McConnell TW: Incest avoidance: A primatological approach, *Papers in Anthropology* 15:55–65, 1974.
11. Adams M, Neel YV: Children of Incest, *Pediatrics* 40:55–61, 1971.
12. Seemanova E: A Study of Children of Incestuous Matings, *Human Heredity* 21:108, 1971.
13. Meiselman KC: *Incest: A psychological study of causes and effects with treatment recommendations.* San Francisco, Jossey-Bass, 1978.
14. Murdock GP: *Social structure.* New York, MacMillan, 1949.
15. Weinberg KS: *Incest behaviors.* Secaucus, N.J., Citadel, 1955.
16. Summit R, Kryso J: Sexual abuse of children: A clinical spectrum, *American Journal of Orthopsychiatry* 48(2):237–251, 1978.
17. Brand RS, Tisza VB: The sexually misused child, *American Journal of Orthopsychiatry* 47(1):80–90, 1977.
18. Kaufman I, Peck AL, Taguiri CK: The family constellation and overt incestuous relations between father and daughter, *American Journal of Orthopsychiatry* 24:266, 1954.
19. Lustig N, Dresser JW, Spellman SW, Murray TB: Incest: A family group survival pattern, *Archives of General Psychiatry* 14:31, 1966.
20. Lewis M, Sarrell PM; Some psychological aspects of seduction, incest, and rape in childhood, *Journal of the American Academy of Child Psychiatry* 8:(1):606–619, 1969.

Chapter 6

The Adolescent Girl in a Group Home

Mirjam Mathe and Nancy Rudes

> *In point of fact, adolescence is life between a saddening farewell—i.e., to the self and the objects of the past—and a gradual, anxious-hopeful passing over many barriers through the gates which permit entrance to the, as yet unknown, country of adulthood.*
> Edith Jacobson, *The Self and the Object World. Part III. Puberty and the Period of Adolescence*, 1964

Relatively little has been written about the development of the adolescent girl who has been separated from her natural family and environment. [1,2,3,4]. In this chapter, we consider some observations of adolescent girls who have been placed in an environment away from their families in group homes. Our data are based on five years of observation in one such group home, as well as on our long-term clinical experience in working with adolescents, children, and families.

The Group Home

Group homes were developed as a result of a child-care crisis that occurred in the 1970s. A burgeoning adolescent population that showed increased acting-out and aggressive behavior demanded a new approach. Many established institutions were unable to provide enough individualized management and treatment or had no space available. A number of programs were established by New York City to serve adolescent girls. The program described here was mandated by New York City to care for 12 female adolescents (ages 13–18) in an unlocked home in the community. Special schooling was secured as needed in

Mirjam Mathe, M.D. • Department of Psychiatry, Albert Einstein College of Medicine, Bronx, New York.   Nancy Rudes, M.S.W. • Private practice, New York.

the community's schools; individual psychotherapy was provided for all; and work with the families of the girls was part of the total program. An attempt was made to sustain a general family atmosphere in the group home.

Girls were referred to these group homes by the family court and/or by the child welfare department. They generally became known to the family court when their parents or other institutions brought charges against them or when they were arrested for various crimes, for example, shoplifting. They often became known to the child welfare department when complaints of neglect or abuse were reported by schools or other social agencies. The girls were separated from their parents because of either the parents' inability to cope with the girls' behavior in the community or in the school, or the need to protect the girls from neglect or abuse when their parent(s) were violent, alcoholic, drug-addicted, or severely emotionally disturbed and unable to provide consistent and adequate care.

The most constant past experience of this group of adolescent girls was continuing aggression from and rejection by "parenting" figures. In many homes, no father was present, and numerous males entered and left the household. Most of the mothers had had similar experiences as children. During these girls' development, their mothers often withdrew in response to the independent behavior of their daughters, or they inconsistently reinforced their daughters' aggressive behavior.

For example, one girl was referred by family court because she refused to attend school and stayed out past the time she was due home or all night. At the same time, she was responsible for three younger siblings who were left unattended if she did not return home. Another girl took black-market pills and other drugs that she found at home. Both her mother and her mother's boyfriend were drug abusers.The home was found by the child-welfare social worker to be without any furnishings so that the girl slept on the floor. No food was in the home. Another girl was referred because her mother was a prostitute and brought her customers into the home; some of these men had approached the girl.

Since some of the most damaging experiences in these girls' lives were the shifts in their attachments from one person to another over long periods of time in their early childhood, strong attempts were made to keep the girls in the program regardless of the difficulty that a particular case might present for the staff. The staff was composed of experienced child-care workers, a resident director, a social worker, a part-time child psychiatrist, and an overall director of several group homes.

In the past, the girls' behavior would have provoked their removal to other facilities—often locked institutions—as a means of control. Such behavior included physical violence directed toward each other and not infrequently toward staff members, destruction of property in the home, running away for two or three days, smoking marijuana in the home, bringing in alcohol, and frequently bringing their boyfriends into their rooms through rear windows.

The philosophy of the treatment approach was to keep them at the home, to provide therapy, and to attempt to tolerate their behavior, rather than trying to control it by separation or threats of separation. Their behavior provided a focus for discussion in a group therapy program designed to be supportive and explorative. The development of strong relationships between the workers and the girls was encouraged. These relationships, along with regular staff training, supportive supervision, and close communication among the staff members, resulted in stable staffing patterns. Our goal was for each girl to establish a special, trusting relationship with a staff member of her choice. In this context, damaging past experiences could be explored and approached therapeutically. Another important advantage of the program was that each girl had the opportunity to remain in the same school for several years. This relative permanency facilitated the stabilization of peer relationships and provided other adult models and another consistent environment.

Girls who were referred were screened; those were selected who would most benefit and grow through this kind of treatment. All girls under 18 were considered except those who were mentally retarded or actively psychotic and who were referred elsewhere, since this setting was not judged optimal to meet their needs. Most of the girls who were referred to us were diagnosed by family-court or child-welfare psychiatrists as having (1) unsocialized, aggressive reactions; (2) inadequate personalities; (3) antisocial personalities; or (4) group delinquent reactions.

They had certain characteristics in common, including difficulty in their relationships with others and fear of abandonment or rejection. They had problems in peer relationships and were unable to confide in a "best friend" or in anybody outside of themselves. Their relationships with boyfriends were fleeting and seemed meaningless. They had poor self-images, and their sexual contacts were relatively devoid of feeling, although they attempted to get close to others through sexual encounters.

Another feature repeatedly observed was depression. Acting out, such as running away and assaultive behavior, and the constant need to change relationships and environment appeared to be an effort to ward off the painful experience of underlying depression. In cases where this particular defense mechanism was not successful, the depression emerged and was intense and debilitating.[5] High levels of anxiety were also seen, and in some cases, this anxiety bordered on states of panic, especially at such times as there were changes in attachments (e.g., during staff vacations or during the development of peer relationships or an increasing closeness in heterosexual relationships).

We also observed a great deal of ambivalence toward parental figures. For example, the girls would idealize certain staff members, primarily those with whom they had long-standing relationships. Often, they exhibited clinging and demanding behavior; that is, they might not let the staff person ("the cherished object") out of their sight. Then, within a short period of time, the worker would become the object of vicious, hateful, and angry attacks. This kind of behavior often lasted for a long period of time and became more pronounced as the treatment continued. It appeared to be the result of "splitting," whereby an integrated image of the worker's characteristics, including the "good" as well as the "bad," could not be maintained simultaneously. Only when the girls were able to become more aware of themselves and this aspect of their emotional response in the context of the psychotherapeutic process did this behavior subside.

In therapy these girls were able to talk about their early memories of being angry at their mothers and at the same time feeling sorry for them. They talked about how they "had to love" their mothers and also wanting them, as well as the dread of losing them. Sometimes, early memories of their fathers were also discussed, including their fears and anxieties when their fathers stopped coming home. They also explored their feelings about their placement and the program. They expressed feelings of hatred toward the staff, which in time they were often able to connect with similar feelings toward their mothers. They could express these negative feelings when they trusted that they would not be abandoned by the staff so that this expression of feelings was less dangerous. Once they reached this point, they became better able to deal with the staff in a more stable way and also to be alone on their own and not feel rejected by the termporary absence of a staff member.

Another, almost universal, characteristic was their very low frustration tolerance and their need for immediate gratification. Their poor impulse control was manifested most often by running away and suicidal gestures, such as superficial wrist cutting. Frequently, when a girl's needs could not be met at the moment they were expressed, she would become angry and behave impulsively. Phobic reactions were also frequently observed. All of these features changed in the course of treatment.

These girls also demonstrated many strengths. Many of them desired change, and this desire enabled them to make an initial adjustment to the structure of the setting relatively quickly. In addition, despite their behavior problems, they valued education, most of them were concerned with their appearance and they were able to physically take care of themselves well.

A DEVELOPMENTAL FRAMEWORK

When we examined the major common features in the behaviors and histories of these girls, we were impressed by their problem relationships with adults and peers and the limiting effect that these had on their functioning. We focus here on their aggression in the context of their relationships.

In searching for a useful theoretical explanation, we have found Mahler's developmental framework most helpful in elucidating the problems of these girls.[6,7] She described a process of separation–individuation occurring between the ages of 5 months and 3 years. During this time, there are several tasks to be accomplished in periods that she termed "subphases":

1. Differentiation, or hatching (5–8 months).
2. Practicing (8–10 months).
3. Rapprochement (16–25 months).
4. Movement toward object constancy (25 months–3 years).

During the first subphase, hatching, the infant begins to pull away from the mother* and to develop body differentiation ("first tentative steps toward breaking away in a bodily sense, from the hitherto completely passive lap-babyhood"[7]). The next subphase, practicing, occurs as the infant begins to move away from the mother, initially by crawling and later in the all-important upright position: "The child concentrates on practicing and mastering his own skills and autonomous capacities."[7] The child begins to become less concerned with his or her mother's whereabouts but returns to her side for "refueling."

In rapprochement, the third subphase, instead of appearing to be oblivious of the mother's presence, the child is consistently concerned with the mother's whereabouts. Rather than moving away, more approach behavior is observed. This subphase appears to be characterized by an ambivalence between fear of engulfment and a need for the

---

*The word *mother* is used here to mean the primary mothering person.

love of the "object" (mother). Mahler further divided rapprochement into three parts. During early rapprochement, the child gains awareness of his or her separateness in the world and no longer feels as omnipotent as he or she did earlier. In middle rapprochement, anxiety about separation is at its height. An internal struggle ensues between the desire for autonomy and the desire for closeness. In the last period of rapprochement, the distance at which the child functions best is established.

The fourth subphase, during which "consolidation of individuality and the beginnings of emotional object constancy" occurs, is unique in that it is open-ended. *Object constancy* refers to the ability to retain a relationship with a person (called an *object,* technically) regardless of fluctuations in internal perceptions of needs, to retain a firm sense of self, and to view others as whole persons rather than only as need gratifiers. Theoretically, object constancy implies that there is a fusion of the "good" and the "bad" parts of the "object" into one whole representation as well as "establishment of a mental representation of the self as distinctly separate from representation of the object."

When there are disturbances in rapprochement, there is a failure of fusion of the "good" and "bad" parts and "splitting" occurs. In one of her clinical reports, Mahler[7] noted that "the relationship [between mother and daughter] was at that early stage beset by many precursors of serious developmental conflicts giving rise to marked ambivalences and the splitting of 'good' and 'bad' objects and probably also of self-representation."

A more detailed description of the various theoretical perspectives regarding the etiology of the splitting process is beyond the scope of this chapter.[8,9] However, as the child develops, by a process of internalization, consistent representations or images of the object and of the self also develop. The child experiences both need gratification and need frustration, which must be integrated. When a synthesis of these two aspects fails to occur, and the integration of good and bad self and object representations or images is coupled with an inability to cope with ambivalence about people, severe psychological handicaps occur.

Thus, from our perspective, as well as from interviews with mothers and other caretakers, many of the youngsters in the group home program were at a developmental disadvantage from early in their lives because they generally had not established reliable attachments, nor had they worked through the process of separation–individuation because their mothers were emotionally unavailable or unable to allow the process to occur during their early years. During the practicing phase, these often needy and immature mothers would perceive their child's moving away as a personal rejection and would meet the child's exhilaration with resentment. During the child's attempts at "refueling," the mother would not be responsive and the child would feel rejected. It seems, then, that this interactional failure had resulted in failure to establish a close relationship with a loved mother.

During the rapprochement subphase, Mahler emphasized the importance of the optimal emotional availability of the mother and her acceptance of the child's ambivalence. However, the mothers of the girls in this group had remained unavailable and had pushed their children away or had remained distant when encouragement for independent or individuating behavior would have been helpful. Instead, these mothers had rewarded regressive and clinging behavior, but even these responses were inconsistent and unpredictable, depending on the mood of the mother.

The period between the end of early childhood and the beginning of puberty is theorized to be a state of relative inactivity of the sexual drive in our society.[10] It is during this time that there is supposed to be a major displacement of drive energy into socially approved channels. During this period, the child learns socialization in school, is expected to develop relationships with peers, concentrates on learning, etc. The girls in this group changed schools and friends very frequently, and their ties with their mothers were ambivalent and conflicted. The onset of adolescence was extremely disruptive, and there were no resources for stability or nurturance.

The following cases illustrate the impact of disruptive early relationships that hamper the normal process of separation–individuation. The resultant lack of object constancy affects subsequent adolescent development.

Clinical Example A

Mary was 14 years old when she was admitted to the group home. She was the unwanted, out-of-wedlock child of a mother who was 16 when she was born and who lived alone. Mary was conceived as the result of a fleeting sexual liaison, and although she never knew her father, she continually searched for him. Occasionally, Mary discussed her wish to find her father, and she even claimed to have seen him.

Mary's first year of life was filled with deprivation. She was left alone for long periods of time and often not fed. At times, she was left with a variety of neighbors, while her mother drank, engaged in prostitution, and experimented with drugs. Within less than 11 months, a second child, a boy, was born to the mother. He had been fathered by a different man, who immediately removed the boy to his own family. There was no further contact with father or son.

Mary's mother moved almost monthly during the first three years of Mary's life. There were no other family members because her mother was the "black sheep" of the family and was ostracized by them. When Mary was 8 years old, another brother was born, and Mary was immediately forced to assume responsibility for him. Although she was enrolled in public school, she rarely attended. Eventually, her mother's sister intervened, and the boy was returned to his natural father while Mary remained with her aunt. During the next two years, Mary was constantly reminded of her mother's faults. When Mary was 14, she was sexually accosted by her uncle and was accused of being a seductress by her aunt, who took her to court for placement.

When Mary arrived at the group home, she wore hiking boots, a black leather jacket, and overalls. Her face was locked in a permanent scowl and she did not make eye contact. Initially, she resisted involvement in the program. In fact, she stayed out of the home as much as she could and broke many rules, but always with a sense of remorse. She had no peer relationships, and she related to the staff superficially, in an angry and threatening manner. She assaulted a teacher at school and in the first year was transferred to four different schools.

From the beginning, however, she kept her appointments with her social worker and sought extra meetings. The most striking feature in the treatment was the intensity of Mary's ambivalent feelings toward her mother. She would often leave the home after sessions to look for her mother. She felt that her mother needed her and wanted her help. Then, she would return in a rage after seeing her mother, who was unresponsive and rejecting. She would calm down after talking with a trusted staff member.

She often spoke about being "in pieces" and "all over the place." She communicated both her sense of desperation and her desire to help herself. She demanded immediate gratification, and if her needs were not met, she responded explosively. At the beginning of the second year, she accepted special schooling and was able to remain in this setting for four years, until she graduated. Although she continued to have explosive outbursts, they were now spaced between long periods of quiescence. Her relationships with others in the house began to improve, and she slowly committed herself to becoming a group member. She began to believe that this was not a temporary situation, as her past homes had been. Her relationship with her peers, however, were distant, her choice of boyfriends was poor, and her relationships were fleeting. She would discuss men in a derogatory way, seeing them only as a threat to women, impregnating them and then abandoning them.

Her mother's sudden death (as the result of an overdose of drugs) in the third year of her stay, when Mary was 16 years old, caused a severe setback. Her schoolwork suffered, as did some of the very tenuous relationships she had recently formed. She was in a continuous rage. She cried, remained in her room, felt guilty and remorseful for not taking care of her mother, and blamed the home for not doing so. She promptly became pregnant, and this proved to be a turning point.

She was able to express her desire not to follow in her mother's footsteps by having a child without a father. She decided to have an abortion.[11] During the next few months, her therapy was intensified. She began to develop rigid defense mechanisms and obsessive-compulsive traits to control her intense anxiety and impulses. It became evident that she was beginning to internalize controls, but that she had to do it in a very rigid and harsh way, because she could not risk the breakthrough of her impulses.

At the time of the first anniversary of her mother's death, Mary began to act out again. This behavior was interpreted as her effort to deal with the sadness and the sense of rejection that was revived at this time. In the following year, however, she began to deal more openly with these issues in therapy, and by the second anniversary, her acting out was minimal.

At about this time, she formed a relationship with a boy, and she continued to see him for two years. Although the relationship was not always consistent, it was continuous. Mary related to him as her mother had treated her: demanding, clinging, punitive, equally hateful and loving. Since he was a reformed drug addict, she was able to fulfill her wish to rescue her mother through this relationship. During this time, Mary also graduated from high school, entered a business training program, graduated and obtained a good job.

Clinical Example B

Ann was the first of five children, each of whom was fathered by a different man. She and her siblings were placed in foster care when she was 13 years old because her mother was unable to care for the children. The youngest one was 11 months old at the time and suffered from retardation, malnutrition, and neglect.

Her mother, Ms. B, had been an alcoholic from the age of 14, and was herself an out-of-wedlock child. Her own mother had died when she was a child, and she had lived with a neighboring family, where she was treated cruelly. She completed the sixth grade and lived a lonely, isolated life.

Ms. B was unable to recall anything about the development of her children. When home visits were arranged, the social worker often found her drunk. Prior to the placement of the children, the neighbors bought food, since Ms. B used her money to buy alcohol. While there was no evidence of physical abuse, the children regarded her as emotionally unavailable. Ann, as the oldest, assumed the responsibility for her mother and siblings.

When Ann was placed in two foster homes, she was unable to relate in these situations, and she was eventually placed in the group home. During the placements, Ann was described as depressed and withholding most of the time, although she had verbally explosive, angry episodes.

Ann's first year in the group home was filled with turmoil. She attempted to separate from her mother by refusing to allow her to visit. While in the past she had been very protective and loving toward her mother, she now became enraged and hateful toward her mother. She had problems making contact with the staff, in contrast to the other girls, who tended to become intensely involved. When Ann did choose a particular worker to whom to relate, she found a woman who was not intrusive, who did not foster physical closeness, and who allowed Ann to relate from a distance. Yet, the worker maintained an undercurrent of warmth that permitted Ann to develop the relationship she needed at a very slow pace, which was possible for her.

In her interactions with others, she repeatedly protected the underdog; this behavior appeared to be related to her interaction with her mother. Ann had few friends. Those friendships that she did have were superficial; they were usually with girls who got into trouble, and she would feel the need to protect them.

It took two years for Ann to establish close ties with one girl, who was passive and dependent. The friendship broke up when this girl became independent and withdrew from Ann. Ann was angry and disappointed and began to drink.

Her relationship with male peers followed a pattern that was similar to her relationships with female friends. After approximately four years, Ann began to date. She eventually developed a positive attachment to a boy at school.

DISCUSSION. In addition to Mahler's framework, Blos's theoretical perspective on adolescence is helpful.[12,13,14] He has emphasized the developmental opportunity to rework early issues in adolescence. The adolescent achieves autonomy and a level of maturity by separation from early objects. The process of detaching from infantile objects requires periodic regression. Since these girls appeared to have been unable to achieve a level of object constancy, this regression, or the defense against it, was severe and unabated. There was little to fall back on internally, and they could not count on the support of a stable, caring environment or stable, caring parents.

Since adolescents identify with persons in their environment whose roles are similar to those of parents, if their experience is not a repetition of their early experiences of rejection, abandonment, and deprivation, it is possible for change to occur through attachment to new objects. The group home, and the treatment provided in it, permitted regression within the limits and structure of the milieu so that regression could occur with enough support to prevent acting out that was destructive. The adolescent could, through positive identification with the staff and through psychotherapy, gain awareness, grow, and develop. Psychotherapy helped these girls to look at their behavior and to recognize some of the factors and forces that affected them. They learned to understand their feelings and even to reorganize some of their adaptive and defensive coping mechanisms.

Other modalities successfully serving adolescent girls in group homes range from those based on a behavioristic model to treatment from a sociological perspective.[15,16,17] The approach described here was found to be effective for many. It facilitated growth and enabled the girls to demonstrate more age-appropriate and gratifying behavior. Their motivation for school work showed marked improvement, as evidenced in their attendance and their scholastic achievement. Meaningful and lasting friendships developed, and dating and future planning took on new importance. They also developed a sense of responsibility in the group home, where they were protective of each other, fulfilled their chores, kept curfew, etc.

The group home, with its stable staff and population, provided a positive experience. Staff members, who could become loved persons, remained steady in their roles as adults. They were emotionally available, despite the girls' regressive behavior, and they encouraged positive steps in the direction of maturation, as parental figures. In addition, these competent and autonomous women served as role models.

Although demographic and statistical data were not obtained about this population, the clinical evidence is that most of these girls maintained regular contact with the home for three or four years after leaving. (When girls entered the home, there was an understanding, as specified by the funding source, that they would be required to leave by age 18 or age 21, depending on their status as students. This requirement was considered in treatment planning, and attempts were made to work within that time frame.) There were many gratifying successes, although there certainly were some failures. Some girls ended up psychiatrically hospitalized, incarcerated, or repeating their mothers' past histories. Others, however, reported that they maintained employment, often acquired more skills, and, contrary to the parental history, married and remained married to stable, employed men.

References

1. Taylor J: *A group home for adolescent girls: Practice and research.* New York, Child Welfare League of America, 1974.
2. Kasowski E: *A follow-up appraisal of process and change in a group home treatment program for disturbed adolescent girls.* Dissertation Abstracts International, Vol. 36, City University of New York, 1974.
3. Carey TR: *An adolescent therapeutic community and its effect on subsequent academic performance.* Dissertation Abstracts International, Vol. 35 (9a), University of New Mexico, 1975.
4. Redl F, Wineman D: *Children who hate.* New York, Free Press; London, Collier Macmillan, 1951.
5. Freud A: *The ego and the mechanisms of defense.* London, Hogarth Press; New York, Basic Books, 1936.
6. Mahler MS: *On human symbiosis and the vicissitudes of individuation.* Volume 1. *Infantile psychosis.*
7. Mahler MS, et al: *The psychological birth of the human infant: Symbiosis and individuation.* New York, Basic Books, 1975.
8. Kernberg O: *Borderline conditions and pathological narcissism.* New York, Jason Aronson, 1975.
9. Masterson JF: *The treatment of the borderline adolescent: A developmental approach.* New York, Wiley, 1972.
10. Freud S. (1905): *Standard edition.* Volume 7. *Three essays on the theory of sexuality.* London, Hogarth Press, pp. 135–243, 1953
11. Gilligan A: In a different voice: Women's conceptions of self and morality, *Harvard Educational Review* 47(4)481–517, 1977.
12. Blos P: *On adolescence: A psychoanalytic interpretation.* New York, Free Press of Glencoe, 1962

13. Blos P: *The young adolescent: Clinical studies.* New York, Free Press, 1970.
14. Blos P: *The adolescent passage: Developmental issues.* New York, International Universities Press, 1979.
15. Phillips EL, *et al.*: Behavior shaping for delinquents, *Psychology Today* 7(1):74–79, 1973.
16. Cross A: *The black experience: Its importance in treatment of black clients.* New York: Child Welfare Services, March 1974.
17. Kadushin A: *Child welfare services.* New York, Macmillan, 1974.

Chapter 7

Juvenile Delinquency in Girls

Susan M. Fisher and Irving Hurwitz

> This essay is dedicated to Dr. Elizabeth Makkay, a distin-
> guished psychiatrist, psychoanalyst, and teacher, who did
> pioneer work in research, programming, and conceptuali-
> zations in the area of delinquency and adolescent devel-
> opment. It has been our great privilege to work with her.

Introduction

Since the scope of characteristics and problems encompassed under
the term *juvenile delinquency* is vast, for the purposes of this chapter
we define a *pathological delinquent* as

> an individual suffering from an impulse-ridden character disorder with
> origins of pathology in pre-school years . . . we find that children with
> delinquent character formation have suffered the trauma of a serious dis-
> turbance in object relationships.* We have found that many of the parents
> are disturbed, and are also acting-out, impulse-ridden people with a ten-
> dency toward sado-masochistic† patterns of relating (in which they are
> both victim and oppressor in alternation). There is, then, neither a nor-
> mally adequate parental model for identification and reality orientation,
> nor the security and support necessary for the development of the ego
> mechanisms to cope with both the inner and the external threats that con-
> front the child.[1]

In addition, recent evidence reveals significantly greater physical abuse
of girls who later become delinquent.

---

*Object relations are the extent and quality of the interaction with other human beings.
†*Sadomasochistic* is term applying to relations characterized by giving and receiving pain
admixed with pleasure.

Susan M. Fisher, M.D. ● Lecturer, Department of Psychiatry, University of Chicago
School of Medicine, Chicago, Illinois.   Irving Hurwitz, Ph. D. ● Professor of Edu-
cation, Boston College, Chestnut Hill; Consultant, Division of Child Psychiatry, New
England Medical Center, Boston, Massachusetts.

"Normal" versus Pathological Delinquency

It is important to differentiate "normal delinquency," part of the rebelliousness of adolescence, from problem delinquent behavior.* Some phase of what has been called *delinquent activity* is to be expected in the healthy development of adolescence. It is part of tempting fate, of moving into the larger community, of moving from being controlled to controlling, of testing the boundaries of one's own self as part of identity formation, and of testing society's controls. The expression of aggression is an important part of the process of normal ego development. The question is: How far can an adolescent go and be safely "delinquent" or rebellious in order to express aggression and to be in touch with it so that it can be sublimated later? Such normal delinquency resolves the difference between acting up and acting out— to separate the "me" from the "not me" and to locate the limits of the self.

For girls, the normal delinquent phase—the testing and the excitement of the forbidden act—gradually diminishes with heterosexual contact. In boys, the normal delinquent phase has more to do with group acceptance through the breaking of rules.

Some stealing, vandalism, and sexual exploration are often seen in boys of around 7 or 8. They have been observed less often in girls. One explanation suggested is the lack of a "gang tradition" among girls, as well as the fact that aggression in women (when it does erupt) has been more self-directed and often has a more primitive and less socialized character. Female aggressive activities have simply not "lived" in the world, channeled by social conventions, and have not been tempered over time.

It is possible to distinguish normal delinquent behavior from malignant delinquency. Essentially, there is a lack of compulsion about normal delinquency; there is a quality of playacting, a lightheartedness. There is also a component of "cultural conformism"[2] in it, in that children who really know what they want are playing the part of delinquent. We are not including those forms of delinquency in which economic need, peer pressure, or neurological or other physiological factors have etiological significance; we are restricting our comments to the conditions delineated in the definition given here.

We shall report, informally, a variety of research findings and observations of delinquent girls. There is relatively little published information about female delinquency. The major published findings are

*The traditional definition of *normal delinquency* has stressed its being socially sanctioned antisocial behavior. In this context, we are referring to normal delinquency as an expectable component of adolescent rebellion.

from male populations; these studies report a number of dynamic features and intrapsychic conflicts and note the symptom of depression. They imply such etiological factors as inadequate identification processes, a distorted and malformed ego or supergo structure, and conflict over sexual identity.[1] More recent approaches to delinquency have centered on the importance of neurological contributions,[3,4] ineffective social learning,[5,6,7,8,9] and genetic factors.[10,11] We shall report material that is drawn essentially from clinical data derived from work with acting-out boys and girls in delinquency control programs at the Tufts–New England Medical Center, Boston, Massachusetts. These findings reflect shifting orientations over time from the narrow emphasis on single factors, to a more comprehensive, ecological point of view of delinquency that encompasses and integrates the biological, sociological, and psychodynamic issues. These changes have profoundly influenced both our clinical and our theoretical perspectives.

In our observations, the girls who became delinquent appeared to have experienced significantly more physical punishment by their fathers than a comparable group of boys who became delinquent. The difference was evident in the early school years but was even more pronounced in adolescence. Numerically, four times as many boys as girls are judged delinquent, but there has recently been a greater incidence of delinquency in girls. Our explanations for this increase are only speculative. In general, there are currently more internal and external sources of conflict for girls in our culture than in previous generations. More new options and alternatives are presented, particularly to lower socioeconomic groups. The "frustration-leading-to-aggression"[12] hypothesis speaks to these changes; that is, the buildup of energy when an activity and/or a desire is frustrated in its expression leads to sudden explosive outbursts in the form of aggressive behavior.

There is also a fluctuating pattern of expressed aggression in delinquent girls. These girls fight openly during the early school years, and then, in early adolescence, there is a period when aggression directed against people is suppressed. They seem to renounce manifest aggression between age 12 and age 15 and begin to try out passive, receptive modes, which resemble their passive responses to their fathers' brutality. These girls are caught between extremes. Later, they are again reported to begin to display open aggression. They give up their passivity and become more active, attacking in gangs and stealing cars. This pattern, which had been more typical of boys, has been observed more frequently in girls in recent years.

Delinquent behavior in girls is different from delinquent behavior in boys. While boys get tough and hard-nosed and know when they are in trouble, girls, even in the aggressive phase of later adolescence, do not see themselves as so purely engaged in the expression of anger. Our clinical observations of delinquent girls reveal that they talk tenderly of younger siblings and seem to be able to tolerate many more cross-currents of feeling. While peer-group pressure plays some part in influencing delinquent behavior in girls, for boys the father, as a model for identification, and the peer group, also as a masculine model, seem more significant.

The pattern of sexual behavior is different from the pattern of aggressive behavior. It is linear and there is not a period of change of behavior. If there is orginally any sexual acting-out behavior, it continues for a fluctuating period of time. The time span reflects the length of time it takes the "anchor worker" (see below) to solidify his or her relationship with the girl.

Girls seem to be more vulnerable to addiction to marijuana and alcohol (economic factors usually preclude the use of hard drugs), and there is more flight than fight in them. There appears to be an underlying depression that motivates delinquent behavior, and it is much more intense in girls than in boys. The depression correlates with the decrease in overt aggression in early adolescence and with an increase in somatization.

From our data, it appears that female delinquents often later become the mothers of delinquents. Without therapeutic intervention, they stop being delinquent when they marry and have children, but frequently, they provoke their husbands and bring them into court for petty crime and assault. Some delinquent girls who have received therapy bring their 5- or 6-year-old children in for treatment, saying, "He's the way I was; we have to do something for him."

The Tufts–New England Medical Center has developed a preventive program using juvenile delinquency "anchor workers." These are therapists who "anchor" the lives of these children and are available 24 hours a day to each child in the program. The worker acts as a combination therapist and ombudsperson. He or she becomes a one-person therapeutic environment. The worker does this by active outreach and energetic engagement—on the street, in school, on the electronic beeper. The worker sees the child everywhere, at home, at school, and at the center, and shares experiences, night and day, in the larger metropolitan area. The girl who is vacillating between the extremes of aggression and passivity achieves a middle ground via her identification with the worker. This results in an altruistic concern for other girls in the group and a change from competition and aggression toward concerns about caring and nurturance derived from this identification.

As told by a group of delinquent girls to an experienced street worker, the subjective sense of what a delinquent girl feels is as follows: For generations, the destiny of a girl of working-class parents was sealed. She'd marry a man who, like her father, inclined toward physical abuse. Now she is beginning to sense that as a female, she has other options, though they are beyond the range of her immediate experience and run counter to the internalized values of her family and community, which may cause her to deny many of the new pathways open to her. She feels pushed to progress but she also feels that she will encounter innumerable obstacles from peers and family. Their values direct her to maintain close ties within the family, with a strong sense of "inside versus outside," a narrow definition of achievement, and a general anti-exploratory attitude. The titer of her aggression rises, and since her internal controls are less than adequate, she may begin to act out, using fighting and stealing cars as an outlet. This car stealing is highly symbolic of the underlying wish to escape from the confining community. Many of these girls have never been outside their local area. They live with rising expectations and without fulfillment. When a career development program of training sessions and trips outside their neighborhood was introduced by their anchor worker, there was a precipitous drop in fighting and car stealing. Delinquency workers speculate that these girls feel free and in control in a car. This description arises from our own observations. Further data about these same girls are in the transcript at the end of this chapter.

The anchor worker establishes contact and a relationship through active outreach and ready availability in school, on the street, wherever the girls are "hanging out." Initial contacts with these highly unstable yet needy girls require tactful, gradual, and sensitive interactions. Clinical contact follows a distinctive pattern. When they are first engaged, they are depressed and passive. A period of acting out follows, which appears to mask an underlying depression. In response to the support of the worker, over time, the girls return to school and begin to progress in human relationships. They attain a greater sense of self-worth, yet they feel comfortable only in choosing friends who have had similar experiences. One evidence of their ongoing instability, however, is that they are frequently in court in the company of their anchor workers. Over time, an embryonic trust evolves, though expressions of feelings still seem very frightening to these girls, as is any sense of being out of control. They need to be continually reassured that they "aren't crazy." Their anxiety about "craziness" is so great that some girls have even made suicidal gestures out of their fear of being passively overwhelmed by their inner feelings.

As suggested earlier, physical violence at the hands of the father is common to these girls. The experience of brutality by their fathers leads these girls to become extremely angry at their mothers. In fact, their mothers are the key figures in their lives. They convey little sense that their mothers care for them, and their social behavior seems directed towards punishing their mothers. Being in trouble and having to go to court with their mothers, who frequently appear to be depressed and withdrawn, are ways of involving their mothers in their lives and forcing a demonstration of concern.

MIDDLE-CLASS VERSUS LOWER-CLASS FEMALE DELINQUENCY

Based on our own clinical and professional experience over fifteen years, including unpublished research studies,[13] we have reached the following conclusions. Despite some areas of overlap in etiology and behavior, there are major differences in delinquent behavior between middle-class and lower-class girls. The issues with middle-class delinquents are much more ones of intrafamilial stress than with the lower-class girls, for whom social and cultural factors play a significant part. Although the father is important in middle-class delinquent families, it is conflict with the mother that predominates in setting the stage for antisocial behavior.

Clinical observation suggests that a large number of middle-class girls become overtly delinquent when, as they reach adolescence, their mothers resume their careers. From the vantage point of the development of these daughters, this return to work is often premature. The girls continue to have intensely strong dependency needs. They seem to suppress and avoid open competition with their mothers. This avoidance can result in a decline in effective school performance that appears to be a learning deficit. With emancipation (their own and their mother's), they are furious at their mothers for "being what they are." A young shoplifter said, "I'll get what I want my way." With these girls, there is a history of unstable relations within the family, a desire to escape, and a feeling of rejection. The mother is experienced not as a role model for the girl but as the opposite: "She is the way I do not want to be." The fathers are often absent and are passive even when physically present.

In the delinquency of middle-class origin, we have identified girls who struggle with basic narcissistic* issues that originate in the fact that they do not feel that they have experienced adequately the early infant phase of total care, of unconditional acceptance at the relevant

---

*The term *narcissistic* is based on the Greek legend of the boy to whom nothing was more pleasing than his own image; the term relates to the attachment to the self.

time developmentally; and they define experience as it has been defined for them—in terms of partial gratifications. They feel bombarded by *quid pro quo* feelings, that is, "Do this in order to get that response." Interactions about giving and receiving are entirely conditional. One receives only what is deemed to be commensurate with what one gives. When the delinquency erupts, it is far out of proportion to the seeming intrafamilial injuries—but so, it seems to the delinquents, is what they must yield up in order to get the indulgence they seek.

Middle-class female delinquency may be in the service of self-differentiation (i.e., the establishment of a separate identity), since indulgence and nurturance have had strings attached and have created excessively tight bonds between mother and daughter. The delinquent acts are acts of deep rebellion and therefore make prognosis poorer for middle-class girls than for lower-class girls. Because middle-class delinquents frequently have more elaborate and complex inner psychological defensive structures, they can find and accept substitute gratifications that lower anxiety levels. This characteristic creates a far more flexible structure, which can be used to avoid coming to terms with core conflicts about self-esteem. This avoidance may diminish the self-confrontation necessary to resolve their struggle either in treatment or by self-generated efforts. Lower-class girls are more directly in touch with (i.e. have greater conscious access to) anaclitic or early-life depressive issues as the source of their delinquent inclinations, and they can resolve their conflicts through obtaining sufficient nurturant gratification through close ties to a giving, accepting, and trusting adult.

Some advantaged girls experience guilt and reverse their sense of entitlement; that is, they feel they deserve unlimited punishment and more discipline. They feel that their demands are inordinate, in spite of counterbalancing feelings that they do, in fact, deserve to have the gratification they seek. They are angry about being given too much and feel that they have not been asked for much themselves. They see the indulgence they have experienced as a buying off or even as deprivation of self-sufficiency. These girls have been inappropriately overindulged by their parents. They are stuck in mid-adolescence and can neither study nor work, and they have meager social relations. They may turn to alcohol and drugs out of a sense of being directionless and a deep feeling of being misled—of having been promised a great deal and being inadequately prepared for frustration. Diagnostically, they occupy a position close to what have been defined as "borderline" disorders in adolescence.[14] To recapitulate at this point, it appears that middle-class female delinquent behaviors have significant antecedents in the configuration of the early parent–child relationship, particularly in the management of dependency needs; mothers make rigorous demands without compensatory emotional gratifications, and fathers are out of the picture, actually or effectively.

These girls are depressed, but their depression is very different in quality from the deep anaclitic depression of many lower-class girls. Often, the lower-class girls have been given enormous practical and emotional responsibilities prematurely. Frequently, they have had to assume a precocious caring responsibility toward their own mothers and have rarely experienced adequate mothering themselves. Their needs are very deep. Stealing, promiscuity, and pregnancy often represent attempts to re-create a rapprochement with the mother through identification with the mother's perceived negative characteristics. There is often a replication in the delinquency of the mother–daughter style of pairing, so that these girls are more frequently delinquent with a partner or a group. The depression in lower-class girls is not due to realistic deprivation. Were that the case, the incidence of depression in lower-class children would be much greater than it is.

An enormous amount of abuse and exploitation is experienced by such female delinquents. They easily become the victims of pimps who are a new version of their cruel fathers, and the longing for strong fathering is very great in these girls.

A significant compounding factor observed in both middle- and lower-class delinquents is the presence of learning problems. Reading is particularly vulnerable, and school testing reveals deficiencies of two to three years in this area. These girls are often pushed to achieve when they could not. The disproportionately high incidence of learning disabilities in prisons has been demonstrated repeatedly. The senior author (SMF) was struck over and over by the calming effect on violence in a children's detention center when one-to-one tutoring was introduced.

One question to be raised is whether "normal delinquency"—the trying out of delinquent behavior—is more common now that there is no frontier, no adventure, so that these testing games become the only area in which to show one's mettle. For those for whom learning is inhibited, the frontier of knowledge is not available.

An interesting contrast was observed in the following setting: "Normal delinquents" who were placed in an Outward Bound-type program were challenged to find their way out of a forest. A worker took two groups of her more extremely acting-out, violent teenagers on a mountain-climbing trip. Both groups loved the experience. However, the "normal delinquents" were gratified by the opportunity to demonstrate their independence and self-sufficiency. In the new, challenging situation, the seriously delinquent girls regressed and needed to be gratified on an infantile level by the protective care that the anchor worker offered them. This caretaking accounted for their pleasure in the experience.

A normal delinquent, when caught, worries about the feelings of his or her parents and has a neurotic response. A pathological delinquent, when apprehended, worries most about *being caught,* and the delinquent behavior itself is ego-syntonic: it feels acceptable to his or her self-image.[2]

At the present time in our culture, delinquent behavior is far more a problem for girls than for boys. The culture has created structures that safeguard boys in their access to aggression: the clubhouse, the peer groups, the gang, the notion of "Boys will be boys," or "Oh, he'll grow out of it." For girls, there is nothing institutionalized to put the brakes on, and when aggressive impulses are overwhelming, there are far fewer sublimated, social options to provide deceleration or escape from the impulsive thrust.

There is also the simple present-day social fact that aggression is syntonic with male identity, while issues of aggression in connection with feminine identity produce far more conflict these days among women than do issues of sexuality.

One question worth speculating on is this: Our culture does, as noted above, give more channels for aggressive behavior, and the acceptance thereof, to boys than to girls. How is this fact tied to sexual acting-out in teenage girl delinquents? It could be an alternative open to girls. It also could be a backup option if aggressive behavior fails to bring relief. What happens is a primitive collapse between sexuality and aggression, and sexual behavior becomes an aggressive instrumentality or its equivalent.

A key point to emphasize in the pathological delinquency of many girls is their underlying depth of despair, depression, and emptiness and the *direct* relationship of these feelings to their getting into trouble, by denying depression or being self-destructive.

A moving tape recording of the conversation of several lower-class girls who had been in an intractable gang of car thieves and runaways follows. Joan is their worker.[5]

This transcript reveals many of the themes discussed in this presentation: the inner emptiness of the girls, the mixed feelings toward their mothers, the longing for close and meaningful contacts with grown-up figures, the underlying depression, the need for continuous care, and the capacity for growth when their needs for human relationships are met and channeled.*

---

*All names and identifying data in this transcript have been altered to ensure privacy.

Joan: (anchor worker)   There are reasons why kids get into trouble today and one of those reasons isn't just because they're bad.

Mary: Sally, what was it like hanging on streets and not doing anything?

Sally: It was boring.

Mary: Why was it boring?

Sally: There was just nothing to do but sit around on the street corner and cause a lot of trouble.
          [*Boredom and lack of stimulation accentuates the depression.*]

Mary: Well, what about the schools—didn't they have any programs?

Sally: None of the public schools I went to had any programs at all. The school I'm in now and the one I went to last year did.

Mary: What if they did? Would you have gone?

Sally: Yeah, I would have. I went to some of them that they had in the school.

Mary: You said they had programs in some of the schools. Were they after school or during school time?

Sally: Most of them were during school; you know, we went a lot of places and stuff. They had some things after school.

Mary: What kinds of things did you do?

Sally: Well, we went on a lot of trips out. They took us apple picking and stuff. It was something to do, anyways. After school, we went to Sturbridge Village, museums, and stuff. We went a lot of places.

Mary: And how did you feel about the teachers?

Sally: I liked them a lot. They're really good. They really help you a lot, and you can talk to them and stuff.

Mary: Did you feel like they wanted to help?

Sally: Yeah, they were always trying to help. You could sit down and talk all the time and joke around. They always take you places and everything. This was only like in the school I'm in now. *In the public schools they didn't have none of this stuff. The teachers were just there and teaching. They wouldn't take time to talk to you or nothing. They just didn't care what was goin on.* They just give you work; school I went to last year was CAP. It was really good. We would talk whenever we wanted to. And the school I'm going to this year isn't that bad either. They used to go on trips and stuff. But they ran out of money so they can't do it anymore—*the John Smith School. They can't go on trips like they used to. It gets you*

depressed and stuff. They used to give the kids jobs after school during the summer, cleaning the school and stuff. And they can't do that anymore. They have no money left. *I think they should try and get money for things like that. They're trying to get it but they can't.* They're trying to help the kids and everything, but they can't get the money. They're running out of money. It would be good if they could keep on giving the kids jobs during the summer and stuff. At least it would give us some money to go places.
[*This demonstrates need for adult interest and involvement in a caring way.*]

Mary: What was it like before you got into these schools?

Sally: Well, I was in the public school. I was in the seventh grade and they threw me out the third day of school and that's when I first met Joan. They threw me out 'cause it was the first time I ever went to a different school like that where you had to change classes and stuff. I wasn't doing enough work. I was doing some work, but I wasn't doing enough. So they threw me out the third day of school. They suspended me for three days. And that's when I got Joan. I've known her since the seventh grade.

Mary: What about you, Julie? How do you feel about school?

Julie: When I first started going to public schools, I didn't really care about the school. I mean, it's important to care about school; I know that. But I don't know, I just didn't like school, I guess. So anyways, I started not going to school a lot. And really missed out on a lot of school which I'm sorry about it now. I missed out on a lot of school. I was really far behind and I started staying back and then I realized what I was doing. And then I figured, "Oh, what the heck. I have too much to catch up on. Forget about it." I just said, "Forget about the whole thing."

Mary: Well, what made you start thinking about it?

Julie: I don't know. Because I stayed back so many times.

Mary: I mean, what made you start thinking you should go and stuff?

Julie: Well, I stayed back a lot. I already said that—O.K.
[*tape erased.*]

Mary: What was the difference between the public school and the one you're going to now?

Julie: Well the difference is the public school—if you need help in math or reading or whatever—if you need help in that, they won't help you with it. If you don't know it that once, that's

it. That's just too bad for you. At the John Smith School,
they're good in that stuff. They'll teach you it and teach you
it until you know it. And then they'll give you private tutoring after school or whenever it's a good time for you. I
really like the John Smith School. I wish there was more
schools like it.

[*Demonstrates the helplessness and longing for assistance in developing coping mechanisms.*]

Mary: What kinds of programs and stuff do they have there? What
did you do?

Julie: Well, on Thursdays, they have trips and stuff or going to
the show, going bowling, and stuff. And they have jobs
after school. I really like my job. I have extra money. And
they have movies and stuff.

Mary: Let's talk about courts.

Sally: All right, Mary, what did you get arrested for?

Mary: For several things. Like B-and-Es [breaking and entering],
disorderly, shoplifting, and stolen cars.

Sally: How did your mother feel when you got arrested?

Mary: I imagine she must have felt really bad, but I didn't really
care.

[*Shows strong sense of alienation and isolation from mother's
interest and willingness to help.*]

Sally: Why?

Mary: I didn't really care about anyone else, because I had a good
time doing it.

[*Demonstrates ego-syntonic quality of acting-out behavior.*]

Sally: What did you think would happen when you went to
court?

Mary: I didn't think nothing would happen to me, 'cause it was
my first offense. And I really didn't care what would happen, 'cause I knew they wouldn't put me away or nothing.
I knew I'd get away with it.

Sally: What did you think about the cops then?

Mary: The cops? Well, the first time I thought they were all right.
The first couple of times. But then after I was getting arrested a lot, I thought the cops were jerks, because they used
to encourage us to do things. For instance, there was this
cop who always came down the corner and say to us kids,
"If I catch one of you kids in a hot box, or pulling a
B-and-E, you know, I'm gonna catch you, and you can't get
away from me." So we thought we were smart. Big bad kids
hanging on the corner. We'd jump in a car and go around

the block, we'd lose him, and we thought it was funny; so
we used to do it all the time. I thought they were really
jerks, you know. *They should have been helping, talking and
trying to help instead of encouraging the kids. They should have
been explaining to the kids that it's wrong.*
[*Direct expression of need for limits.*]

Sally: Was there anyone there to help you in court?

Mary: At first, there wasn't. There was like this idiot lawyer. He
was the type that would say. . . . The judge would say,
send her away for life. He would say OK. But he was all
right for the time being 'cause I wasn't in that much trouble
then. Then I started getting into deeper trouble; then I had
to get another lawyer. He was really good. His name was
Joe Jones. He was 100% for the kids, and there was Joan
there. I really took advantage of it; rather, *we* took advantage of it because we didn't have that help before and we
were scared to trust people then. We figured why should
we start now. Now they're both good friends of mine. Sally,
how do you feel?

Julie: What did you get arrested for, Sally?

Sally: Just about the same things she [Mary] did, really. B-and-Es,
stolen cars, disorderlies, shoplifting. Just the same things, I
guess.

Julie: How did your mother feel when you got arrested?

Sally: Well, she was mad, and then she felt bad, too. But then it
was just fun to us. No one could stop us. There was nothing
else to do. We had no place to go.

Julie: How did you feel when you got arrested?

Sally: I thought it was one big game. I didn't care about nothing,
then.

Julie: What did you think would happen in court?

Sally: I didn't really think anything was ever going to happen. I
was never in court before or nothing. I didn't really care
anyways, but I didn't know. When I did go to court, we
had to go back and everything. They kept continuing the
case again. And they dismissed it and everything, and then,
after a while, after we got arrested a couple of times, it was
like a hangout, the court; it was. There was a whole bunch
of our friends. And even if we weren't supposed to be in
court, we could go anyways, you know, just to talk. Stay
home from school 'cause school was bad, and we'd just go
up there and start talking and fooling around in a courtroom. We'd be in a courtroom or sitting out there with all

our friends who are supposed to be there, talking and having fun and stuff.

Julie: What did you think about the cops?

Sally: The cops, oh, boy. I got beatings from almost all of them. They're really jerks and stuff. They aggravate you into getting into cars and stuff, stealing more cars. They always say, "If I catch you again, I'll do this, or that's it for you, or I'll beat your brains in and stuff." They're always saying all kinds of stuff to us. Then a couple of them really started to help, really wanted to help. We ignored them all.

Julie: Was there anyone in court to help you?

Sally: If there was, I didn't care. Not really. At the end of it, there was a lot of people there, like Joan and our lawyer Joe was there. Some of the people that worked with him would be up there, and they would be talking to us. At first, we took advantage of everything. We really didn't care who was there to help us or not. We didn't want to listen to no one. We wanted to do what we were doing. No one was going to tell us not to. They told us a lot. We didn't care anyways.

Julie: Did you ever get sent away?

Sally: Yeah, I got sent away a lot of times. I was at Lancaster, Roslindale, a halfway house at Charlestown "Y."

Julie: What did you think about them places?

Sally: Lancaster wasn't that bad, except you were all closed in. They were pretty clean. The halfway house, that was clean 'cause you had to clean it yourself. Then you come to Roslindale. Now that's a mess. You sleep with the cockroaches. It's really dirty out there. Oh, I hated that place. It's really filthy rotten and everything. It's just sleeping out in the gutter with the bums on Broadway. It's like being in a dump. There's paint falling off the walls and stuff. It's really awful.

Julie: How were the people up there? Social workers, whatever, how were they?

Sally: I don't know. I ignored them, too. I didn't do nothing. When I first went in there, they were saying, "All right, did you take a bath today?" I just looked at them. I said, "No, I went into the shower and I walked back out," and I said, "Yeah, I did." The shower was filled with mud and dirt. It looked like they swept the floors and dumped it in there a couple of years ago. They didn't sweep them while I was there. The place was really. . . . I didn't eat or nothing when I was up there. The food and everything just looked awful.

It was really dirty. It was really rotten. I never seen no place so dirty in my whole life besides the dump on "A" Street.

Julie: How did your mother feel when you got sent away?

Sally: *Well, most of the time she was the one that said she didn't want me home or around the house. She was telling them to go ahead and take me.* She didn't want me home. She was the one that told them to send me up Lancaster twice. She just didn't know what to do. She just had given up all the time. She told me that I should go away someplace to try to smarten me up, and it didn't do me no good. They threw me out of the halfway house I was in.

[*Again the strong sense of maternal rejection appears here.*]

Julie: Do you think your mother's pride was hurt by you doing those things?

Sally: It probably was, if she was always sending me up places and stuff.

Julie: How do you feel about those things now? Do you feel bad about them, do you feel good about them?

Sally: It didn't bother me as much as. . . . Like, it does bother me if someone sits there and starts talking about it; then it bothers me a lot, 'cause I'd like to just forget, you know. I hope they get more things for kids to do, so that when they get older, they won't have to look back at the things they did when they were small.

Julie: We'd really like to thank Joan.

Sally: For all the things she done for us. God bless her, there should be more like her.

Julie: I don't know, I just didn't like school that much. And all the kids were ahead of me in school and everything. I just didn't feel like going, maybe because I felt funny going to school 'cause I was in such a low grade. People say I should have tried harder. Maybe then, it wouldn't have been so bad, you know.

[*Learning problems and low self-esteem are communicated here.*]

Sally: But how could you try harder, if no one was willing to help you?

Mary: If they helped you, you would have been ahead.

Julie: But no one cared, so . . . . If nobody else cares about how you do in school, then you don't care really. It's wrong to feel that way, but that's how I felt. I wish I wouldn't have felt that way, 'cause now I have a lot of catching up to do. I went to school as less as I could. I didn't like school. Even

| | thinking about doing schoolwork really got me mad. I really hated it. |

Mary: Do you think they could have helped you catch up a little more?

Julie: Yeah, they could have. But why should they help me? That's what they figured.

Sally: I know. They were there to get their week's pay. That's about all they were there for.

Julie: Why should they waste their time on one student? That's what they figured. I never went to school. I never cared. Why should I care about anything? Why should anybody care about how I do in school? I really did care. I don't know where to begin with my schoolwork. I didn't know where to start, and no one would help me with it. I asked people who were giving me work. How could I do the work they were giving me when I was so far behind that I needed to go back in my school years? I was in third grade, and how old was I? I stayed back three times, and I really felt bad about the whole thing. I didn't like the teachers. Some of them were just like us. Some of them used to come to school driving stolen cars, and they used to say it's a big joke. It's kind of bad when you think about it that the teachers felt that way. Why should they care? They were getting paid. If you are going to be a teacher, you should get into it. You shouldn't do it just for the pay. Things were boring where we live. What else was there to do but go out and steal cars, which is the wrong way to think—now that I think about it now. But then you didn't think that way. If we weren't doing that, we were standing on corners or something and starting trouble.

[*Sense of despair and helplessness around academic experience and its relation to delinquency.*]

Sally: I think if they had more recreation centers or something open, then we wouldn't had had to do all that stuff. We would have had more stuff to do. . . .

Julie: It was boring. There was nothing to do. It was boring and everything else. Everybody figured there was nothing else to do.

Sally: We would have to go out on the corners and we would start wise-mouthing and the cops would bust us for disorderly and stuff. And then we would go to court and the judge would let us get away with it. They were too easy on us and all the whacks on the heads we got didn't help us at all. Our parents used to make us stay in and stuff, but that didn't help either. . . . We didn't get enough discipline that we should have got.

Julie: And plus there was nothing to do around. Maybe if they had more things to do. . . . What else can you do? A lot of people can think of a lot of things to do. Those things were boring, that people thought of. Oh, why don't you go play jump rope. Fourteen years old and they wanted us out playing jump rope.

Sally: Jacks or something. Ice skating, down there with all the holes in the ice. Or sledding, there was no place to go sledding or even if there was, no snow, or there was a place to go sledding and it was all rocks. . . . Over any stupid little thing. Just because we were bored or something, it was something to do and they thought it was a big joke. Half the time they wouldn't even break it up. They would just sit there and watch us. They'd just go by, and like it was an everyday thing. Of course, then it was.

Julie: And then we met this lady, Joan. And then we started getting to know her and everything else.

Sally: Things were so bad we didn't really trust anyone. We just wanted to stay by ourselves and have everyone leave us alone while we were running around tearing up the place. [Clear example of mistrust and anger in relationships.]

Julie: We met this lady named Joan. We didn't know her that good, and then we started getting to know her, and then she started doing things with us. And then we started thinking about what we were doing, like she was talking to us about what we were doing.

Mary: And then we felt like someone cared, so we were willing to stop, slow down, on half the stuff, but we didn't completely stop. We just felt a little better, I guess—'cause someone was there helping us.

Sally: Then she started bringing us out on the weekends on camping trips and stuff with her and everything.

Julie: And she would talk to us and stuff like that. And then I was out of school for a while. For about a couple of years. And then Joan got me into this school which was really nice. It's a really nice school. I like it a lot. The name is the John Smith School. I thought the school would be like all the other schools, but this school is like—I didn't think there was any other people around, and then I started meeting these teachers in the John Smith School. They really helped me a

lot. They spent time with me helping me do school work
and everything. And now I don't miss school anymore. I
always go and everything else. I didn't like it. And they're
tutoring me and everything. I feel like I'm wanted to go to
school. I want to go to school. I get up on my own and
everything. I really like this school.
[*Here the impact of a trusting and supporting relationship has
had major significance in developing self-image response to environment.*]

Sally: And I think they should have more people like that to help
           kids, and more schools and things.

Julie: I didn't think there was any schools around like that be-
           cause the teachers are really nice. It's just I really like that
           school. My three girlfriends go and I think it helped them.
           This girl I know that came from all these homes goes there,
           and they didn't think the school would help her out. But it
           really helped her. And she likes it, too. It's a really good
           school. I can't explain it—how I feel about it. I'm really glad
           that I'm finally starting to go to school and starting to
           smarten up and everything. Before, I could care less about
           school. I never thought I'd ever get to like school. Now I'm
           going everyday. I'm trying now, more than I ever did be-
           fore. I care now and I never cared before.

A number of key themes are reflected in this excerpt. They point to
some of the issues with which these girls were struggling, including
the sense of alienation and rejection they experienced in relation to
their mothers and their difficulties with boredom, which appeared to
be a real threat to their meager controls. Boredom confronts such girls
with the intensity of their needs and their reliance on external stimuli
to draw awareness from inner processes, which generate an enormous
burden of anxiety. Also, they are frequently bored because they are
unable to use or further develop their own skills. In addition, the need
for control and limits to be imposed from outside sources is clearly
evident from the transcript, along with the lack of insight regarding
the possibility that they might *themselves* develop control mechanisms
that would be effective.

The importance of the academic deficiencies of these girls, as both
primary and secondary factors in depressive expressions of low self-
esteem, appears prominently in this material. There are also statements reflecting the lack of trust and acceptance they feel toward adults
both within the family and in the community, particularly the school.
It is clear that with the beginning of a positive relationship to a trust-

worthy and giving adult (the anchor worker), the perception of self and the environment underwent a radical change leading to improved expectations about school, teachers, family, and the girls' own prospects for self-esteem and success.

What is perhaps most striking is that the girls were able to *verbalize* their view of their past and present social experiences, as well as the needs and conflicts they sensed in themselves. This ability supports the idea that the step from anger to verbal communication represents a genuine move toward better ego organization, involving self-observation, a delay of impulse expression, and the capacity to enter into sound relationships that have a strong quality of give-and-take rather than the overwhelming need to be in an egocentric, passive-dependent role.

Current follow-up studies [14] indicate substantial favorable outcome for these girls. Three have gone to college; all have formed warm human relationships and have internalized stable systems of impulse control. Even those who appear to act out, do it in a generally adaptive manner; that is, those who got pregnant as teenagers and kept their children have concentrated on being good parents, and most of them have married the fathers. The status of the families of origin remains a key dimension: unless the family supports the girl's progress, it is difficult for her to sustain it over time. The relationship with the anchor worker remains a sustained supportive interaction, requiring only infrequent contact, but the girls check in with their workers periodically. The workers themselves continue at the job an average of three to five years and do not experience the usual "burnout" phenomenon, wherein street workers tire and leave the job after a year.

ACKNOWLEDGMENT

Much of the material for this essay was shared, developed, and clarified in discussions with Dr. Elizabeth Makkay, Mr. William Monahan, and Ms. Nancy Harkness, all of the Juvenile Delinquency Prevention Project at Tufts–New England Medical Center. Nancy Harkness provided the tape recordings of the girls.

REFERENCES

1. Kaufman I, Makkay ES, Zilbach J: The impact of adolescence on girls with delinquent character formation, *American Journal of Orthopsychiatry* 29 (1):130–143, 1959.
2. Warren MQ: The community treatment project. In *The Sociology of Punishment and Correction.* Edited by Johnson N, Savitz L, Wolfgang ME. New York, Wiley, 1970.
3. Lewis DO: Diagnostic evaluation of the juvenile offender, *Child Psychiatry and Human Development* 6:198–213, 1976.

4. Berman AE: *Delinquency and learning: A neurophychological approach.* Unpublished manuscript from Bradley Howe, 1976.
5. Aichorn A: *Wayward youth.* New York, Vanguard Press, 1956.
6. Eissler K (ed): *Searchlights on delinquency.* New York, International Universities Press, 1955.
7. Redl F: *The Aggresive Child.* Glencoe, Illinois, Free Press, 1957.
8. Rutter M, Tizard J, Whitman K: *Education, health, and behavior.* London, Longmans, 1972.
9. Bandura A: *Aggression: A social learning analysis.* Englewood Cliffs, New Jersey, Prentice-Hall, 1973.
10. Glueck S, Glueck E: *Physique and delinquency.* New York, Harper & Row, 1956.
11. Kety S: Neurochemical aspects of emotional behavior. In *Physiological correlates of emotion.* Edited by Black P. New York, Academic Press, 1970.
12. Miller NE, Dollard R: *Frustration and aggression.* New Haven, Connecticut, Yale University Press, 1948.
13. Hurwitz I, Makkay E, Monahan W, Fisher S, *et al:* Juvenile delinquency—A model for prevention and treatment of acting out youth.
14. Masterson JF: *Treatment of the borderline adolescent: A developmental approach.* New York, Wiley, 1972.

Chapter 8

Childhood and Adolescent Suicidal Behavior with an Emphasis on Girls

Cynthia R. Pfeffer

Disturbances in the processes of development that lead to suicidal behavior among girls have not been systematically studied. The concepts
discussed in this chapter were derived from a literature review and
my many years of experience in treating suicidal latency-age children
and adolescents. A developmental and psychoanalytic framework is
used here to make a comparison of suicidal latency-age and adolescent
girls and of suicidal girls and boys.

Incidence of Suicidal Behavior

Distinctions have been found between suicidal boys and girls and
between suicidal latency-age and adolescent girls in the incidence of
suicidal threats, attempts, and completed suicide. Unfortunately, the
accuracy of such data is questionable for several reasons.

First, social, legal, and religious resistance to reporting death as
suicide may result in an underestimation of incidence. Thus, the cause
of death may be classified as something other than suicide. For example, some deaths in children that are reported as accidents may be
unrecognized suicides.[1] McIntire and Angle,[2] reporting on the notion
that clinicians diagnose serious injury or death as accidental, studied
the charts of 50 children, ages 6–18 years, treated in poison control
centers in Omaha, Nebraska. They found that patient charts documented accidents in 42% of the cases and suicidal behavior in 58% of
the cases. A reassessment of the clinical case histories by the investi-

Cynthia R. Pfeffer, M.D. • Assistant Professor of Psychiatry, Cornell University Medical College; Chief, Child Inpatient Unit, The New York Hospital–Cornell Medical Center, Westchester Division, White Plains, New York.

gators concluded that 4% of the cases were accidents, 70% of the cases were suicidal gestures, 29% of the cases were suicide attempts, 22% of the cases were intoxications, and 2% of the cases were homicides.

Second, the United States Vital Statistics report of the National Center for Health Statistics does not list suicide as a cause of death for children under 10 years old, in part, because suicidal death in young children is considered so rare that it is not worth specifying separately. Also, young children are believed to be incapable of recognizing the life-endangering consequences of their actions because they have not yet attained a full understanding of the finality of death.

Third, because of parents' fear of being blamed and their guilt about being "bad parents," they are often reluctant to discuss openly the events leading to their child's death. Thus, it is very difficult for coroners to perform systematic psychological autopsies in cases where childhood suicide may be suspected.

From 1955 to 1975, there has been a documented increase in completed-suicide rates among children 10–14 years old, from 0.4/100,000 in 1955 to 1.2/100,000 in 1975.[3] The number of deaths for this age group was approximately 170 in 1975.[3] Although in the past, male suicide rates have increased with age, in the last 15 years this trend has reversed, and suicide rates for older males have declined, while the rates for younger males have risen gradually.[4] For females, the age group of 35–64 has the highest rates, while the 5- to 24-year-old group and the 65- to 84-year-old group have the lowest rates.[4] In the last 15 years, the suicide rates for females have increased in all age groups except the 65- to 84-year-old group. The increase was greatest at the younger ages, which include 5- to 14-year-olds, 15- to 24-year-olds, 25- to 34-year-olds, and 35- to 44-year-olds.[4]

Since it is believed that completed suicide for children under 10 years old is rare, definitive statistical data are not available in the United States. Shaffer[5] studied suicide rates for children and adolescents by using psychiatric, medical, educational, and coroners' records in England and Wales, where data are kept for young children. There were 31 children and adolescents who committed suicide between 1962 and 1968. The ratio of boys to girls was 2.3:1. However, none of the youngsters were less than 12 years old. Shaffer thus concluded that completed suicide in latency-age children is a rare phenomenon. However, he noted that 46% of the cases had demonstrated previous suicidal behavior and that his estimates were probably low. Further, he believed that many of these previous attempts and threats had occurred during the latency-age period.

The suicidal behavior of children and adolescents ranges from suicidal ideation, suicidal threats, and suicidal attempts to completed suicide.[6] In the 1960s, it was estimated that 7%–10% of the latency-age children seen in psychiatric outpatient clinics were suicidal.[7] More recently, the incidence of suicidal ideas, threats, and attempts in this age group has been reported to be even higher.[8] In a study of 100 latency-age children referred for psychiatric hospitalization to a large municipal hospital, 33% exhibited suicidal threats and attempts.[8] In the psychiatric outpatient clinic of the same hospital, 33% of the 39 children who were randomly selected for the study demonstrated suicidal behavior.[9]

It has been estimated that 12% of all suicide attempts are made by adolescents and 90% by adolescent girls.[10] In a study of 75 suicidal children and adolescents in which the white and black patients were evenly represented, 73% were girls and 29% were boys, a ratio of 3:1.[11] In a study of 95 hospitalized suicidal adolescents, it was noted that the ratio of suicidal attempts for black girls increased from 11.1% in 1957 to 49.3% in 1970, while there was only a moderate increase for white and Hispanic girls.[12] The findings of this study illustrate that the type of population studied, its geographic location, and its predominant socioeconomic and racial–ethnic class may affect the results of statistical trends. Additional investigations using a broad spectrum of social class and race–ethnic backgrounds are necessary to clarify these factors.

It has been estimated that males predominate over females in suicidal ideas, threats, and attempts in the latency-age group.[13] In a study of 58 psychiatrically hospitalized latency-age children, suicidal boys outnumbered girls, but there was no difference in frequency of either suicidal ideas, threats, or attempts for boys and girls.[6] Other studies disagree and report that among suicidal boys, threats are more common than attempts.[11,14] While it seems apparent that for latency-age suicidal children, boys outnumber girls, it is not clear if there is a sex distribution difference for suicidal ideas, threats, and attempts. Clarification is further hampered because most studies include only small samples of children in this age range.

HYPOTHESES ABOUT SEX DIFFERENCES AND INCIDENCE OF SUICIDAL BEHAVIOR

Distinctions between suicidal rates for young school-age boys and girls may be explained on the basis of physiological maturational variations, degree of neurological development, social interactional patterns, and quality of intrapsychic functioning. Developmental studies point out that girls tend to mature neurologically earlier than boys, and that latency-age girls tend to be less aggressive, impulsive, and intensely reactive and have less frequent emotional disturbances than latency-age boys.[15,16]

Pfeffer et al.,[6] in a study of 58 psychiatrically hospitalized latency-age children, noted that children with deficits in ego functioning were more prone to suicidal behavior. Therefore, it may be that because of developmental differences between boys and girls, ego functions such as impulse control, reality testing, cognitive functioning, and affect regulation may be more advanced in girls than in boys. As a result, girls may be relatively more protected from suicidal acting-out. However, there are no systematic studies that compare the ego functioning of boys and girls in regard to suicidal behavior as a way of testing this hypothesis.

Variations in interactional patterns for the parent and the latency-age child may provide additional clues to an understanding of sex differences in the incidence of suicidal behavior in boys and girls. According to psychoanalytic theory, sexual and aggressive impulses are expressed differently by boys and girls. During early development, girls theoretically turn away from their original love object, the mother, and turn to the father. They are often guilty about this change, and especially about their aggressive wishes toward their mother. However, eventually they are disappointed in their father, and the anger toward the mother subsides.[17] During the latency period, it is common for mothers and daughters to identify with each other and become closer. As a result, mothers believe that their daughters require more protection than their sons, and they may behave differently toward them. One mother stated to me that she did not allow her 10-year-old daughter to walk to school unescorted or to play alone outside because of her fear that the child might be molested by dangerous men. However, she stated that she did not have such fears about her sons "just because they are boys." It may be that this concern of mothers for daughters may have a modifying and deterring influence on the suicidal behavior of latency-age girls. However, systematic studies to test this hypotheses are warranted.

The increased incidence of female adolescent suicidal behavior may be most related to rapid physiological pubertal changes and the resultant disequilibrium in both ego functioning and the parent–child relationship. Intense sexual and aggressive impulses are experienced during this period. Shifts in impulse control, reality testing, and affect regulation occur, and family interactions may become stressful. Intense conflicts about feelings of dependency may become manifest in an increased acting-out behavior,[18] which may include suicidal threats and attempts.

SUICIDAL METHODS

A variety of methods of threatened and attempted suicide in latency-age children have been reported, including "stabbing, cutting, scalding, burning, purposeful running into moving vehicles, and jumping from high buildings." These exceeded "nonviolent" attempts to die by such means as a medication overdose.[19] The use of firearms among suicidal latency-age children appears to be very rare. Bender and Schilder[20] concluded from their case study of 13 hospitalized latency-age children that the majority of suicidal children jumped from high places, "seemingly the simplest way of escape." Similarly, Pfeffer[21] noted that jumping from heights was the predominant method among a large population of hospitalized latency-age suicidal children.

Another parameter in which sexual distinctions have been documented is in the types of suicidal methods utilized. Shaffer,[5] studying completed suicides of children 12–14 years old, found that there were marked sex differences in the methods used, which were similar to the differences noted in older populations. Proportionately more girls took an overdose of drugs, and only boys hanged themselves. Furthermore, a significantly large percentage of the boys (not the girls) used highly lethal methods.

Other reports have also concluded that adolescent girls attempt suicide by ingestion significantly more frequently than boys.[22,23,24] In addition, similar trends in adolescent girls were noted among 66 suicidal hospitalized latency-age children; ingestion was utilized significantly more frequently by the girls than by the boys.[21] In that study, it was observed that jumping from heights was utilized significantly more by boys.

The difference in choice of suicidal method is that girls utilize more passive means, while boys use more aggressive methods. First, conflicts among suicidal girls may involve predominantly oral fixations.[10] As a result, ingestion may be a concrete expression of need satisfaction via oral modes. Second, ingestion may provide a means of producing sleep, which allows for a diminution of painful affects, a state of withdrawal, and a sense of comfort. Because of the increased dependency of girls, sleep may represent both a withdrawal from frustration and also a psychological state of fusion with a wished-for idealized mother.

There have been many clinical case reports describing the variety of suicidal methods employed by girls. Ackerly[14] noted a 9-year-old girl who threatened to kill herself with a knife. According to Ackerly's report, she wrote a note to her mother saying, "I am not going to the hospital to sleep overnight or I will kill myself if you do not stay over with me." Her mother wrote back, "You do not have to stay over-night—we need you." The mother found another letter to the girl's siblings saying good-bye and to be good. Another letter said, "Dear Mommy and Daddy, I would like to be buried next to Zaddy in the same cemetery." Zaddy had been her favorite grandfather. This case is unusual because rarely do suicidal latency-age children write notes.

Another 9-year-old girl screamed at her mother, "You don't love me, you hate me, and I hate you so go ahead and kill me. I don't want to live."[14] Projection of intense anger onto the parent and provocation of punishment are a common fantasy among suicidal latency-age children.

Ackerly[14] described the suicide threats of two girls who wished to kill themselves because they hated to be girls and wanted to be boys. One of these girls threatened to kill herself with a butcher knife because she was "stupid, miserable, and no good." When she got angry, she wanted to jump out a window and drown herself in the river. She believed that then her parents would weep and be sorry and then she would come back to life again. When she came back, she wanted to be a boy.

Among preadolescent girls who attempted suicide, Ackerly[14] noted two who had taken aspirin and one who had attempted to choke herself with a handkerchief on a school bus. Ackerly[14] commented that the two girls who had ingested pills seemed more representative of the adolescent group than of the latency-age group. In fact, they made repeated suicidal gestures in the next five years.

Lukianowicz[7] described a 12-year-old girl who had made a variety of suicide attempts, including lying down in front of traffic and attempting to jump off a bridge. He described another 12-year-old girl who had slashed her wrists. Sabbath[25] poignantly described the sentiments of a 16-year-old girl who overdosed on sleeping pills. She stated, "Why don't I die, there's nothing to live for. I took my father's pills, thirty of them; I have been unhappy since age six when I swallowed half a bottle of aspirin." She continued, "I didn't asked to be born . . . I felt everything was hopeless."

There are many other clinical examples of suicidal ideas, threats, and attempts of latency-age girls and adolescent girls. Such behavior points out the serious life-threatening risk and negates such remarks as that children may have difficulty in effecting a suicide attempt because of lack of size, strength, motor coordination, and ability to obtain the needed materials.[24]

RISK FACTORS IN SUICIDAL BEHAVIOR

The suicidal behavior of children and adolescents is a complex symptom that results from specific effects of intrapsychic and environmental pressures. The types of intrapsychic risk factors in suicidal behavior may include special fantasies and concepts about death, specific affects, and states of ego functioning. Certain types of family interactions may promote a potential for suicidal actions.

In a systematic study of 58 psychiatrically hospitalized latency-age children, two categories of suicidal risk factors were described.[6] Among the factors that significantly correlated with suicidal potential were the wish to die; feelings of hopelessness and worthlessness; sadness; concepts that death is a desired, pleasant state, of temporary duration; and severe depression and suicidal behavior in the parents. Factors associated with severe psychopathology add to the potential suicidal risk. These include severe anxiety, severe aggressive reactions, preoccupations about school failure, learning disabilities, fear of parental punishment, parental separations, abusive home atmosphere, disturbed peer relationships, and multiple deficits in ego functioning. Surprisingly, there have been few systematic studies to evaluate the relative significance of the variables associated with a high risk of suicidal behavior in adolescents. However, many studies of adolescent suicidal behavior stress the importance of depressive affect and intense, long-standing family turmoil.[12,23,25,26]

To augment an understanding of the risk factors of suicidal behavior in children and adolescents, theoretical concepts, information derived from case reports, and data from empirical studies are presented here. There have been no systematic studies to test what risk factors for suicidal behavior are specific to boys and girls. Nevertheless, distinctions in risk factors can be seen.

DEPRESSION. Depression in young children and adolescents has been difficult to diagnose. Questions have been raised as to whether latency-age children can in fact be depressed, since psychic maturity has not occurred; thus, an adultlike depressive clinical picture cannot occur in children.[27] Recently, empirical studies have attempted to evaluate this issue. The criteria that have been used to diagnose depression in these studies have been those used in adult depression. These include the presence of dysphoric mood, poor appetite, weight loss, sleep difficulty, loss of energy, psychomotor agitation or retardation, loss of interest or pleasure, obsessive guilt, poor concentration, and thoughts of death or suicide.[28]

Depressive affect has been considered one of the major contributors to the suicidal behavior of children and adolescents.[6,29] In a study of 581 children and adolescents, it was noted that three months before a suicide attempt, depressive symptoms occurred in 38% of the cases.[30] Another study, of 75 children and adolescents, reported that 40% were depressed one month before being evaluated, as compared with 13% of the 95 nonsuicidal children and adolescents seen in that time period.[11] In a study of 58 psychiatrically hospitalized latency-age children, sadness, withdrawal, the wish to die, and feelings of hopelessness and worthlessness were specifically associated with suicidal behavior.[6]

CONCEPTS OF DEATH. Theoretical constructs maintain that it is not until ages 7–11 that children develop a cognitive awareness that death is final.[31,32] The importance of this awareness in childhood and adolescent suicidal behavior lies in both the deterrent and the facilitating influences of these concepts on suicidal action. If a child cognitively understands that death is irreversible, this knowledge may serve as a deterrent to self-destructive acting-out. Furthermore, certain affective sensations about death, such as that death is pleasant, may serve as a facilitating influence on the potential for suicidal action.

The relationship between the concepts of death of suicidal children and of adolescents has not been sufficiently studied. Suicidal hospitalized latency-age children have been reported to have distinct concepts about death.[6] They believe that death is reversible and that it is associated with feelings of pleasantness. Orbach[33] noted a similar trend and hypothesized that this state of pleasantness is a substitute for the wished-for, idealized, generous and devoted mother.

Adolescents also have varying beliefs about death. McIntire, Angle, and Struempler[34] studied 598 children and adolescents of different religious backgrounds. They found that of the youngsters who were 13–16 years old, 60% believed in a spiritual continuation after death, 20% had doubts about the finality of death, and only 20% believed in a full cessation of life. It was noted that religious training had a marked effect in forming these beliefs. No study has clarified the nature of suicidal adolescents' beliefs about death.

EGO FUNCTIONS. It has been postulated that the suicidal behavior of children and adolescents is associated with severe ego regression and decompensation.[14,35,36] In addition, suicidal risk may be increased by the contributions of constitutional variables that influence the degree of impulse control and the capacity for frustration tolerance.

There have been only a few studies of states of ego functioning in relation to suicidal behavior in youngsters. Suicidal behavior has been observed among children of superior, average, and retarded intellect.[6,37,38] One study reported that an ego regression to a psychotic state had occurred in 31 latency-age children who had attempted suicide.[14] In contrast, other studies have failed to confirm differences in ego functioning between suicidal and nonsuicidal hospitalized latency-age children[6] or between children who have threatened or attempted suicide. In this hospitalized population, deficits in a variety of components of ego functioning were observed, however. The children were mistrustful and felt that the world was a hostile place, and they were subject to extreme states of affect lability. Unfortunately, there have not been reports of systematic investigations comparing the qualities of ego functioning in suicidal and nonsuicidal adolescents.

SUICIDAL MOTIVES. Motivations for suicidal behavior are derived from the fears, wishes, and fantasies especially generated when the child or adolescent is confronted with severe stress. A common wish is to escape from an intolerable situation, such as deprivation of love.[30] The acting out of suicidal impulses may be a form of manipulation, combined with the hope that the parents may respond with added attention and love.[13] It may also be a manipulative form of punishment of the parents. The distress experienced because of a sense of isolation may be overcome by the desire to reunite with an important nurturing person.[11] The distress of psychotic states may be modified by suicidal actions.[13] Finally, suicidal behavior may be a more general "cry for help" to a powerful rescuing force.

Often multiple suicidal motives exist. In a sensitive presentation of an analysis of a 15½-year-old girl, P. Kernberg[39] found suicidal motives occurring at different stages of regression within the transference neurosis. In addition, the changing form of these motives coincided with the degree of resolution of the patient's conflicts about her sexual identity. For example, suicidal impulses were an expression of her attempts to force her therapist to provide unlimited gratification of a need for protection from her own feelings of vulnerability and helplessness, were a means of control over her parents, were an expression of her conflicts about her sexual identity, and were an attempt to return to paradise and ultimate gratification.

The importance of sexual conflicts and fantasies, as a motivating influence on suicidal behavior, for adolescent girls has been illustrated in other case studies. Freud[40] outlined the conscious and unconscious dynamics of an adolescent girl who jumped onto a railroad track. At age 14, the girl felt despondent about the loss of her mother's attention when her mother had a son. In her analysis, the suicidal attempt was seen as a form of self-punishment for her wish to have a child by her father. Zilboorg[41] hypothesized that suicidal behavior in females is related to oral strivings and spite, but that in males, it derives from feelings of loss of love and fantasies of castration from Oedipal wishes. Finally, these hypothesized differences in dynamics have been questioned.

FAMILY INFLUENCES. One of the most important factors influencing suicidal potential is severe family turmoil. Many studies have shown that parental separation due to divorce and death, parental violence, and parental psychopathology increase the risk of childhood mental illness, which may include acting out and suicidal behavior.[6,10,11,19] In one study, 76% of 34 families with a suicidal child or adolescent had a separation from a significant person that precipitated suicidal behavior.[24] In comparison with nonsuicidal adolescents, suicidal adolescents had experienced a significantly greater incidence of parental loss before age 12.[42] There seems to be a greater incidence of suicidal behavior among abused youngsters, in comparison with neglected and normal children and adolescents.[43] It is the child's feelings of worthlessness, badness, and self-hatred resulting from parental harsh punishment that precipitate suicidal behavior. The suicidal behavior of relatives and parents is a very significant specific factor in the suicidal potential of children and adolescents.[6,10] It may be that identification with their parents facilitates the view that one can cope with stress by self-destruction.

Another aspect of family communication is what Sabbath[25] called the "expendable child." In this situation, there is a conscious and unconscious parental wish to get rid of the child. The child perceives this wish and responds to his or her feelings of rejection and self-hatred by suicidal behavior. The mother is often a focus of severe distress leading to suicidal behavior. For adolescents, conflicts with the mother around issues of dependency and rejection are often displaced onto peers. Therefore, while it may often appear that traumatic interactions with the adolescent's peers serve as the precipitant for suicidal behavior, it may be that problem peer interactions actually reflect the effects of serious underlying parent–child difficulties.[10] Aleksandrowicz[44] described the case of a 7½-year-old girl who suffered from a chronic "mismatch" between her temperamental characteristics and her mother's personality. As a result, the child received insufficient nurturing, and the mother received little gratification from the child. Systematic studies are essential to evaluate the relative importance of the types of family influences described.

CASE EXAMPLES

The suicidal behavior of children and adolescents is associated with a wide range of psychiatric diagnoses. Three case examples will provide illustrations of suicidal behavior in a depressed girl, a girl with a behavior disorder and borderline personality organization, and a psychotic girl. It should be noted that children as young as 6 years old attempt suicide, as well as older, latency-age children and adolescents.

Case I: Depression

One evening after Alice, 14 years old, had stopped dating her boyfriend, she expressed a wish to go shopping and talk with her girlfriend. Her grandmother would not permit her to do so. Alice felt angry, lonely, and nervous. She took some pills from the kitchen and aspirin from her blind grandfather's room. After taking 20–25 pills, she went to her room and tried to sleep. Within an hour, she told her grandmother that she had a stomachache. Her grandmother took her to the hospital, and Alice was admitted.

Alice's parents had separated when she was 3 years old. Alice lived with her grandmother because her mother could not care for Alice and her siblings. It was difficult for Alice to talk about her mother's rejection of her, and she rationalized it by saying that she wanted to stay with her grandmother because she was very attached to her.

Alice had been raised in a strict environment. She could not go out alone with her friends until she was 12. She could not go to summer camp, and her grandmother took her to and from school daily. Alice denied being angry about this overprotection even though her younger brothers were allowed to go out alone. Alice justified this discrepancy by saying, "They are boys and can go out alone." The symbiotic relationship with her grandmother was epitomized and perpetuated by her grandmother. Although Alice wished to have her own bedroom, she was not allowed to because her grandmother could not sleep in a bed without Alice.

Alice had several good friends in school. She had told one of them on several occasions that she felt like running away or taking pills. She often stated, "I sometimes feel like crying when I am alone. Also I feel that there is no one who cares for me." Her friend consoled her and Alice felt better.

Alice started going steady with her 16-year-old boyfriend, against her grandmother's wishes. Whenever they went out, they had to take one of Alice's brothers with them.

In this example the characteristics of long-standing family conflicts formed the background for an eventual suicide attempt. Rejected by her mother and raised in a strict and symbiotic family situation, Alice was able to maintain friendships with other girls and develop heterosexual relationships. However, the rage engendered by the restrictions and prohibitions against her desires to separate from the family and to be involved in age-appropriate activities was channeled, via intense guilt, into feelings of chronic depression and self-destructive behavior.

Case II: Behavior Disorder with Borderline Personality Organization

Diane, 6 years old, was admitted to the child psychiatry inpatient unit because of two serious suicide attempts. The first was an attempt to jump out a second-floor window, and the second was an attempt to jump off a bridge. She jumped out the window in response to her mother's refusal to allow her to play outside with her sisters. Without any witnesses, she went to a back room, jumped out the window, and landed in the grass. Miraculously, she was not hurt. She stated that she had thrown herself out "because my mother did not take me outside." She was evaluated medically in a hospital emergency room but unfortunately was released. Subsequently, she was unable to sleep well and wandered around the house. She also became mute and anxious and refused to go to school. During the same week, she attempted to stab her 4-year-old cousin with a small knife. Several days after the first jump, while at a family picnic, she attempted to jump off a bridge. She had been holding her aunt's hand but suddenly broke loose while walking on the bridge and began climbing over the rail. She was retrieved by her aunt.

According to her mother, Diane did not know danger and crossed streets alone, and "the first thing she looks for are windows." Six months before, she had climbed on a closet, jumped off, and cut her leg.

There had been severe parental arguments. One year before, Diane's father had beaten her mother and attempted to cut her face. Physical assault had occurred toward the children, too. Eight months before, the father had beaten Diane because she was jumping.

The mother had gone to court and separated from the father. Diane's father was never heard from after the separation. Diane had frequently asked for him and told her mother, "He is dead and buried." She had told neighbors that the parents fought and that she often dreamed that she was to blame for the things that had happened. She also talked in her sleep and called to her mother. Diane had always sought attention from her mother, who believed that Diane got angry too easily. Her mother believed that Diane had jumped out the window because she was angry.

This example illustrates the serious nature of very young children's suicidal tendencies. Diane was raised in a family in turmoil. The witnessing of dangerous parental battles, as well as the experiencing of physical abuse from her father and the separation of her parents, resulted in heightened anxiety and confusion. Diane identified with her aggressive parents and expressed anger toward her younger sibling. She had an ambivalent relationship with her mother to whom she felt intimately attached, as well as being intensely angry at her. As her anger at her mother intensified, Diane's identification with her punitive, harsh parents resulted in her acting out her own self-punishment in the form of suicide attempts.

Case III: Psychosis

Margaret, age 10 years, was admitted to the child psychiatry inpatient unit after overdosing on her mother's tranquilizers. Margaret said she "felt nervous all day because a boy at school hit me. I took the pills to protect myself from him." Actually, the events were more complex. Margaret was also worried about her mother. That day, when Margaret had returned home from school for lunch, her mother was not there. Frightened that she had been abandoned, Margaret took the pills.

Margaret often heard voices telling her that she should hurt herself, that she should jump out a window, and that she was bad. Her mother blamed her for taking things, and when this happened, Margaret heard voices telling her that she was bad. Margaret had numerous nightmares that her parents were dying. She saw visions of frightening faces and had a fixed belief that someone wanted to kill her.

Margaret's parents had been divorced four years before her suicide attempt because her father had become religious and would spend up to three days at a time praying in his room. About two years before the suicide attempt, Margaret's father had reappeared, had "kidnapped" her, and had kept her for one year. During that time, Margaret's mother had tried to poison herself with pills because Margaret was not with her. Finally her father, coaxed by her relatives, returned Margaret to her mother.

This incident sensitized Margaret to separations from her mother. She spoke about fears that something might happen to her mother because she was alone, for example, that her mother might be killed. Margaret felt that she had to be with her mother to take care of her. While Margaret was in the hospital, she confused her female therapist with her mother. She pleaded with her therapist not to leave her. Margaret heard voices that sounded like her mother's voice.

This example illustrates the confusion and intense anxiety that were precipitated by several family traumas and the child's state of ego disorganization. Margaret's ability to test reality was poor. She confused other people with her mother. She was frightened by the separation from her mother and was sensitized by the unpredictable events she had experienced. The aggression directed toward her by a friend, coupled with her mother's absence when Margaret returned home for lunch, stimulated her fears of harm, abandonment, and confusion. Her suicide attempt was actually an attempt to relieve intense anxiety and her state of disorganization. In death, she believed she would achieve a peaceful pleasant state.

CONCLUSION

The distinctions between males and females with regard to suicidal behavior are found in the techniques utilized and the frequency of threats, attempts, and completed suicides. Some psychodynamic and developmental differences have been noted; however, the contributions of constitutional, social, and intrapsychic variables to the suicidal behavior of females have not been systematically studied and remain a challenging area for research. Such studies will add information about the normal and abnormal processes of the development of women. The factors of risk of suicidal behavior in male and female children and adolescents seem to be remarkably similar. Among these factors, depression and family conflicts have been noted as the most frequent high-risk variables for suicidal behavior in both children and adolescents.

Prevention of and early intervention for the suicidal behavior of children and adolescents are the most pertinent areas in need of development. The treatment must always involve the family as well as the youngster.[45] Treatment may include medical stabilization; psychiatric hospitalization; individual, family, and group therapy; and psychopharmacology.[46] The outcome appears to be good when appropriate treatment and follow-up are offered.[19]

References

1. Connell HM: Attempted suicide in school children, Medical Journal of Australia 1:686–690, 1972.
2. McIntire MS, Angle CR: "Suicide" as seen in poison control centers, Pediatrics 48:914–922, 1971.
3. Fredrick CJ: Current trends in suicidal behavior in the United States, American Journal of Psychotherapy 32:172–200, 1978.
4. Holinger PC: Adolescent suicide: An epidemiological study of recent trends, American Journal of Psychiatry 135:754–756, 1978.
5. Shaffer D: Suicide in childhood and early adolescents. Journal of Child Psychology and Psychiatry and Allied Disciplines 15:275–291, 1974.
6. Pfeffer CR, Conte HR, Plutchik R, Jerrett I: Suicidal behavior in latency age children: An empirical study. Journal of the American Academy of Child Psychiatry 18:679–692, 1979.
7. Lukianowicz N: Attempted suicide in children, Acta Psychiatrica Scandinavica 44:415–535, 1968.
8. Lomonaco S, Pfeffer CR: Suicidal and self-destructive behavior of latency age children. Presented at the annual meeting of the American Academy of Child Psychiatry, San Francisco, Calif., 1974.
9. Pfeffer CR, Conte HR, Plutchik R, Jerrett I: Suicidal behavior in latency age children: An empirical study. II: An outpatient population, Journal of the American Academy of Child Psychiatry 19:703–710, 1980.
10. Teicher JD: Suicide and suicide attempts. In Basic Handbook of Child Psychiatry. EKD/ ited by Noshpitz JD. New York, Basic Books, 1979.
11. Mattsson A, Seese LR, Hawkins JW: Suicidal behavior as a child psychiatric emergency, Archives of General Psychiatry 20:100–109, 1969.
12. Schneer HI, Perlstein A, Brozousky M: Hospitalized suicidal adolescents, Journal of the American Academy of Child Psychiatry 6:242–261, 1975.
13. Toolan JM: Suicide and suicidal attempts in children and adolescents. American Journal of Psychiatry 118:719–724, 1962.
14. Ackerly WC: Latency age children who threaten or attempt to kill themselves, Journal of the American Academy of Child Psychiatry 6:242–261, 1967.
15. Heinicke CM: Development from two and one-half to four years. In Basic handbook of child psychiatry. Edited by Noshpitz MD. New York, Basic Books, 1979.
16. Solnit A, Call JD, Feinstein CB: Psychosexual development: five to ten years. In Basic handbook of child psychiatry. Edited by Noshpitz JD. New York, Basic Books, 1979.
17. Kaplan EB: Manifestations of aggression in latency and preadolescent girls, The Psychoanalytic Study of the Child 31:63–78, 1976.
18. Blos P: On adolescence. Glencoe, Ill., Free Press, 1961.

19. Paulson MJ, Stone D, Sposto R: Suicide potential and behavior in children ages 4 to 12, 8:225–242, 1978.
20. Bender L, Schilder P: Suicidal preoccupations and attempts in childhood, *American Journal of Orthopsychiatry* 7:225–234, 1937.
21. Pfeffer CR: Clinical observations of play of suicidal latency age children, *Suicide and Life Threatening Behavior* 9(4):235–244, Winter 1979.
22. Jacobziner H: Attempted suicides in adolescents, *Journal of the American Medical Association* 191:7–11, 1965.
23. Schrut A: Suicidal adolescents and children, *Journal of the American Medical Association* 188:1102–1107, 1964.
24. Gould RE: Suicide problems in children and adolescents, *American Journal of Psychotherapy* 19:228–246, 1965.
25. Sabbath JC: The suicidal adolescent—The expendable child, *Journal of American Academy of Child Psychiatry* 5:272–289, 1966.
26. Teicher JD, Jacobs J: Adolescents who attempt suicide, *American Journal of Psychiatry* 122:1248–1257, 1966.
27. Rochlin GN: *Grief and discontents: The forces of change.* Boston, Little, Brown, 1965.
28. Puig-Antich J, Blau S, Marx N, Greenhill L, Chambers W: Prepubertal major depressive disorder: A pilot study, *Journal of the American Academy of Child Psychiatry* 17:695–707, 1978.
29. Toolan JM: Depression in children and adolescents, *American Journal of Orthopsychiatry* 32:404–415, 1962.
30. Otto V: Suicidal attempts in adolescence and childhood, *Acta Paedopsychiatrica* 31:397–402, 1964.
31. Nagy M: The child's theories concerning death, *Journal of Genetic Psychology* 73:3–27, 1948.
32. Piaget J: *Language and thought of the child.* London, Routledge, Kegan, Paul, 1923.
33. Orbach I: Unique characteristics in children's suicidal behavior, *Proceedings of the Ninth International Congress in Suicide Prevention and Crisis Intervention,* pp. 382–388, 1977.
34. McIntire MS, Angle CR, Struempler LJ: The concept of death in midwestern children and youth, *American Journal of Diseases of Children* 123:527–532, 1972.
35. Schechter MD: The recognition and treatment of suicide in children. In *Clues to suicide.* Edited by Schneidman ES, Farberow NC. New York, McGraw-Hill, pp. 131–142, 1957.
36. Shaw CR, Schelkum RF: Suicidal behavior in children, *Psychiatry* 28:157–168, 1965.
37. Editorial: Suicide in children, *British Medical Journal* 1:592, 1975.
38. Lawler RH, Nakielny W, Wright NA: Suicidal attempts in children, *Canadian Medical Association Journal* 89:751–754, 1963.
39. Kernberg P: The analysis of a 15½ year old girl with suicidal tendencies. In *The analyst and the adolescent at work.* Edited by Harley M. New York, Quadrangle, New York Times Book Co., pp. 232–268, 1974.
40. Freud S: The psychogenesis of a case of homosexuality in a woman. *The Standard Edition of the Complete Psychological Works of Sigmund Freud,* Vol. 18. London, Hogarth Press, pp. 147–172, 1955.
41. Zilboorg G: Considerations on suicide with particular reference to that of the young, *American Journal of Orthopsychiatry* 7:15–31, 1937.
42. Stanley ES, Barter JT: Adolescent suicidal behavior, *American Journal of Orthopsychiatry* 40:87–96.
43. Green AH: Self-destructive behavior in battered children, *American Journal of Psychiatry* 135:579–582.

44. Aleksandrowicz MK: The biological strangers: An attempted suicide of a 7½ year old girl, *Bulletin of the Menninger Clinic 39*:163–176, 1975.
45. Toolan JM: Suicide in children and adolescents, *American Journal of Psychotherapy 29*:339–344.
46. Pfeffer CR: Hospital treatment of suicidal latency age children, *Suicide and Life Threatening Behavior 8*:150–160, 1978.

PART II

Symptom Formation and Illustrative Symptoms

Chapter 9

The Organic–Functional Controversy

THEODORE NADELSON

INTRODUCTION

The view that mind and body coexist separately was as old as written history and had gone through many shifts before the dichotomy was codified by René Descartes in the seventeenth century. Dualism, or the view that *there is mind* and *there is body,* has been called untenable by many philosophers of science.[1,2,3,4,5] They argue for a holistic or monistic perspective, maintaining that all phenomena described as *either* mind *or* body are one in the same. Despite the lack of strict scientific authenticity, the position held by most of us is that mind *and* body exist as separate entities and that these two forces act "on" us and interact within us. An analogy might lead to more clarity: When seeing a painting, the perspective of the art lover is different from that of a pigment chemist. They both view the same phenomenon evolving out of the materials that give color to the canvas, but the picture, as painted, is to be understood by its own values and rules. For the chemist (who may have little aesthetic concern), the value of the painting resides in the composition of the paint in terms of amounts of cobalt, zinc, lead, titanium, cadmium, etc. The art lover (probably unaware of chemistry) sees the totality of the painting as residing only within the viewer's experience. Neither of these extremes alone encompasses all of reality.

The language and logic to which we are attuned does not permit a simultaneous description of mind and body phenomena. One may shift from one perspective or stance to another, but viewing or describing such phenomena at the same time is as impossible as simultaneously describing paint pigment and aesthetics. Yet, again, dual-

THEODORE NADELSON, M.D. • Department of Psychiatry, Tufts University School of Medicine; Chief of Psychiatry, Boston Veterans Administration Medical Center, Boston, Massachusetts.

ism is the position from which most patient or client complaints initially fledged, and the usual initial questions before any other are "Is it body, or is it mind?"; "Is it organic or functional?"; "Is the complaint the result of a bodily defect or the way the person feels and thinks about his body?"

Such questions are most usual in a routine medical context. For example, "Does this burning, gnawing upper abdominal pain 'mean' active peptic ulcer?" Addressed this way, the pain either is or is not "real"; it is or is not a symptom of organ deficit. Physicians prefer the symptom that turns out to be causally related to a palpable deficit or lesion, because that is the framework within which the doctor is trained. As a result of this preference, most persons in the health care professions are reluctant to give up the exclusive consideration of the "organic etiology" of disease. In practical, clinical, everyday decision-making, the psychological and social factors are most often neglected by the physician in deference to an organic bias within the dualistic framework.

There is another persistent attitude to which physicians adhere. It is part of a general social attitude toward women reinforced by physicians' education. The bias directed toward women and supported by social attitude places them in a position of weakness, firstly physically, and then, in consequence, psychologically and morally. Often, such biases are accepted as truth, without examination, and become a part of a seemingly "scientific" attitude and clinical practice.

In summary, three biases, separable but interrelated, are often found in physicians' practice:

1. A dualistic model of mind and body that tends to obliterate the importance of the multiconvergence of forces in disease, including social and historical forces, in favor of an "either/or" view.
2. A preference for favoring and emphasizing the organic factor exclusively, within the above framework.
3. A view of women as the weaker sex and as subject to the diseases of the weak.

Throughout this chapter, the reader will detect the writer's own bias; the necessity to view factors in illness as the result of *only conceptually separable* elements of anatomy, physiology, psychology, and, most importantly (partly because most often omitted), sociology and history. This position, it is realized, is also a compromise within a proper scientific view. Philosophically, it would be better to argue for a unitary model of feeling, thought, behavior, and physiology—mind and body as one. Such a position is, however, impossible to maintain except as an ideal. The basis for this position is developed in the following sections.

A HISTORY OF THE DUALISTIC APPROACH TO SICKNESS

During the earliest periods of human history, witch doctors and shamans attempted to give patients a revived will to health by the power of suggestion, involving a borrowing of magical power. Such healing practice truly was holistic and proceeded from the view that spirit, matter, and psyche were indivisible.[6] There was also no distinction between the animate and the inanimate.[7] In Western society, physicians, "healers," priests, and priestesses all offered equal chances of surcease from suffering before the last 150 years.

Magical thinking still has currency in the rapidly disappearing Stone Age cultures of the world. Such thinking is also a basic attribute of disordered psychotic thinking in Western culture, and because our culture is so invested with a consciousness of the difference between the subjective and the objective, the real and the unreal, the material and the immaterial, we usually feel that such distinctions are innate and that only those with disordered thinking could perceive things differently from us. Yet, we may reflect on the fact that all of us share "primitive" or paleolithic animistic thinking to a great degree. In our dreams, inanimate objects are often willful, and wishes and fears freely take great liberties with what we ordinarily view as hard, objective fact. Then, too, it is often observed, and yet more surprising to us than it is to a Bushman, that people become well or sicker or die as a result of suggestibility. Suggestion and "influence" (from our view) are the meager entirety of the shaman's repertory; to him or her, they are the essence of medicine and of science.

Descartes is regarded as having most thoroughly influenced modern thinking on the mind and the body, separating them conceptually as to the influence of soul (or mind) over body. After Descartes, matter, finite and substantial, became the proper concern of most thinkers, artists, and scientists. The Cartesian epistemology cleaved the world into either substance or thought and is believed to have initiated the serious study of human psychology by codifying a dualistic interactionist theory.[8] This was a step forward, but the division of the world into "real" and "ideal," into substance and soul, or body and mind, is most obviously a struggle for us today.

The nineteenth-century pathologist Rudolf Virchow radically changed medical thinking, creating a purely materialistic, organic focus on the understanding of disease. From his time on, the perspective of Western medicine was to find the source of the disease within

the body space in the derangement of body organs. It is often a surprise to us that medical thinking was not always so. Virchow (and
Robert Koch) established a limiting structure for diagnosis and subsequent treatment to which most physicians adhere today. Medicine
advanced by keeping within the framework of those two great scientists.

Franz Alexander viewed psychosomatic disease monistically, despite his long association with the term *psychosomatic*. [9] He took the
position that psychic and somatic phenomena are "probably two aspects of the same process" and that psychological phenomena should
be studied with psychological methods, just as the physiological phenomena in their physical causality should be studied by means of
neurophysiology and biochemistry. His work on specificity—viewed
in the 1940s and 1950s as seminal, and still of some importance today—pointed to "vegetative dysfunctions" occurring as a "result of
specific emotional constellations." The specificity of psychosomatic illness is now more widely questioned. *Psychosomatic* may now be characterized more as an approach to patients, rather than being assigned
etiological importance. In such an approach, an either/or dichotomy is
avoided. [10]

Whether it is unitary or monistic, the "correct" scientific or philosophical position is achieved "with effort." [11] Most often, it seems to
be hardly worth the effort. Mind as opposed to body, presented as a
practical clinical problem, is best resolved, we feel, by studiously
avoiding the emphasis on the either/or position. We view factors in
sickness as only conceptually separable. Anatomy, physiology, emotion, and social elements are categories of our own devising rather
than those of nature.

In summary, I have presented the monistic argument while discussing a dualistic view in practical terms—mind and body as conceptually separable elements:

> The dichotomy of body and mind represents a special case of the more
> general division of thing and thought. These dichotomies are misleading
> because they verbally allude to a split which does not correspond to the
> unitary nature of experience and of the living organism. Therefore, the so-
> called "mysterious leap" from the mind to the soma (a phrase used to de-
> scribe "conversion" of unconscious conflicts to somatic symptoms in hys-
> teria) represents an invitation to reunite certain ways of dividing an organ-
> ism which itself was never actually divided. [12]

Mind and body, however, remain separated conceptually because (1)
they are phenomenologically really different; (2) we have different
words for the phenomena; and (3) such terms are not interchange-
able—the term *neural event*, for example, does not refer to an experi-

ence coextensive with, for example, the experience of love, aesthetic pleasure, jealousy, irony, etc. Mind and body are, in Russell's term, then, "different *logical* types" (italics added). And with such statements, one invariably (and unrealistically) hopes to end the dilemma forever.

THE DUALISTIC BIAS IN CLINICAL PRACTICE. Despite our optimistic annihilation of the ancient dualism-versus-monism philosophical quarrel, we still encounter simple dualistic differentiations in the practical, day-to-day problems in the helping professions. We may best use a practical, rational, and comfortable *interactionism* (that is, the idea that mind *influences* body and body influences mind). We may then avoid the common either/or attitude, that a phenomenon is related to mind *or* body phenomena. Such a workable framework is worth the violation of strictly scientific idealism. The usual either/or attitude blurs the reality of multiple causes in the interests of simplicity. In truth, Occam's razor cuts too close for many human affairs. We are, after all, in health or in sickness, embedded in a social framework of family, economics, and history in interaction with a genetic matrix, and we are subject to the accidents of the environment.

For example, disorientation and delirium* frequently occur, particularly among the aged, in patients hospitalized for other illness. Such abnormal states usually lead to continued hospitalization, because of a fear that the disorientation may become worse without professional monitoring and medical intervention. The patient may, intermittently, and in the midst of bizarre delusions, request a return to her or his home, and often, families indicate that they would be willing to try to manage the patient's care at home. Still, physicians are understandably reluctant to sanction discharge; they continue to keep the patient in the hospital for a "few more days" in order to "clear the patient's thinking" and to allow the "organic delirium" to dissipate. Often psychotropic drugs are used to decrease anxiety or to combat delusional thinking. Such medications, unfortunately, distort a clinical picture already complex because of physiological dysfunction. Paradoxically, it is found that sending the patient home often changes the patient's mental state dramatically. It is important to understand that the deterioration of mental functioning associated with aging or disease—even with gross signs of organic, neurological decay—may change in response to environmental influences. Patients are always influenced by the hospital environment; it is unfamiliar and is often perceived as hostile or alien. Many people who have made a reasonable adjustment to an environment that is not demanding are disturbed by the strange-

---

*Defined as a "clouding of consciousness,"[13] often with disorientation.

ness of the institutional environment. Hospitals can, literally, "drive people crazy," particularly those people already in tenuous balance because of disease, pain, age, and attendant metabolic abnormalities. A familiar environment can help restore coping even in the face of "organic" dysfunction.[14] The health care professional, because of a bias for an either/or decision, may not always perceive the importance of environmental influences coexistent with "organic" defect.

POWER AND PREJUDICE

Professionals are often unaware of the powerful influence of their own presence and manner of approach on the patient. They often do not see the patient's reaction as a response to the environment (hospital or office) or to the doctor's own mode of structuring such interactions. Patients or clients tend not to ask questions of the professional. They sometimes present their concerns obliquely, often displaced from the center of their anxiety. There is a built-in attitude toward the professional that places him or her in a position of great power. Often, the disparity between the person seeking help and the care deliverer engenders animosity in the former. It may be the case that professionals unknowingly foster this reaction.

For example, Waitzkin and Stoeckle,[15] in examining physician–patient relations, addressed the manner in which communication about illness is presented to the patient. Their theoretical proposition, supported by others,[16,17] is a sociological examination of the doctors and patients in terms of power interest (largely unconscious) on the part of the doctor: "A physician's ability to preserve his own power over the patient in the doctor–patient relationship depends largely on his ability to control the patient's uncertainty."[16]

The patient's ignorance preserves the privileged position of the dispenser of services. It is pointed out that the poor and the dying may be told more about their disease then the middle-class, relatively healthy patient, since they have no real power and the information is less crucial to their position with regard to the physician.[18] The poor or lower socioeconomic groups also tend to ask fewer questions and rarely actively ask the physician to do anything.

THE SOCIALIZATION OF THE PHYSICIAN

There is a less-than-subtle tendency on the part of some writers on this subject, who are usually nonclinicians, to be sharply critical of doctors, particularly for ineptitude, rigidity, or serious character flaws, and because of a seemingly singular blindness to the psychosocial issues in the treatment of illness. Although the observations may be accurate, there is, on the part of such social observers, often a lack of understanding of the physician's motivation, partly because of the paucity of firsthand knowledge regarding the difficulty of clinical judgment.

In discussing the reasons for this phenomenon,[19] Bergen pointed to the role to which the physician is "socialized" (rather than "trained"). The physician's perceptions are supported by teachers and peers. Like everyone else, she or he develops, with training, a set of assumptions about the world in which she or he lives, as well as assimilating the informational content of courses on diagnosis and treatment.

To recapitulate, the physician's "reality," or better, the physician's assumption regarding sickness, had its historical antecedents crystallized in the latter part of the eighteenth century. Modern medicine (and to a great degree, modern thinking regarding health and disease) emerged when there was a shift from metaphor and the language of imagination to what could be described, seen, and possibly measured. Objectification was emphasized as more important than individual phenomenological experiences. Stated broadly, from that time on, patients' complaints were to be viewed as "subjective symptoms" and achieved the status of "reality" only when the doctor was able to place the cause within the space of the body. Rudolf Virchow, the greatest pathologist of his time, crystallized such thinking later by establishing the idea that if there is disease, there is cellular or tissue pathology.[20] Bergen has pointed to "resistance" on the part of the physician to reeducate himself or herself with regard to these assumptive beliefs.[19]

Physicians are aware (within the usually accepted dualistic-integrationist framework) of the *existence* of psychosocial factors as part of the framework of disease etiology. The difficulty is more than a cognitive one; it is not simply a matter of increased educational opportunity. For example, doctors are often so locked into the dualistic framework of either/or that they are unable in their usual practice to widen their focus to include the social context and themselves.

THE SHIFT TO A PSYCHOSOCIAL FRAMEWORK

It is no longer necessary to emphasize the importance of psychosocial factors only as an abstract verity. There is now a group of psychosomaticists who wish to scrap the concept of psychosomatic disease in order to move toward a more inclusive view of health and disease. Some wish to maintain a psychosomatic focus as a core concept but to be rid of the either/or duality imposed by the nosological concept of psychosomatic disease.[21] The term *psychosomatic* is considered outdated[6,21] in the sense that it implies such a duality. It was useful in the past to oppose the Virchovian mode, which held back the understanding of psychological factors. There is growing evidence that psychological and social variables are etiological factors in *all* illness.[22,23,24] Weiss[21] suggested that the psychosomatic approach is best preserved by relinquishing the nosological term *psychosomatic disease.* He feels that the attributes of the disease category are untested, untestable, and nondiscriminatory. His alternative approach is one that asks, "To what extent is the incidence or course of a given illness a function of psychological variables?" rather than, "What illnesses are psychosomatic?" In a clinical setting, the doctor may ask, "To what extent and in what ways are psychological factors manifested?" as an alternative to "Is this psychosomatic disease? Is this person suffering from 'nerves'?"

What is being suggested here is a shift from a usual orientation for the physician. Illness has its locus not only in the space of the body but in the space of interpersonal relations—a "life space."[9] Many older physicians were not trained to tolerate such ambiguity or to look outside the patient's body for the definition of the illness. Changes are apparent, however, in some young physicians. Continued emphasis on psychosocial factors by their teachers in a clinical setting also influences them. As they become more open to each patient's inviduality, they may learn from the patient also—and that is properly the focus of clinical medicine.

THE ORGANIC BIAS

Although it is acknowledged that the interaction of humans with other humans affects health, at the clinical-pragmatic level some health-care professionals, even younger ones, remain somewhat reluctant to accept even a dualistic position and to identify psychological factors in illness. Such resistance is understandable, and when physicians defend this position, they usually point to the following:

1. The "Type A error," that of missing the diagnosis of physical disease when present, may be of greater danger to the patient than a continued attempt to establish a physical cause when none is actually present.
2. Psychological diagnoses are often not acceptable to patients, particularly when they suffer from symptoms.

The tenaciousness of this position on the part of the doctors is, however, remarkable and is found in sensitive, aware physicians whose views on general social issues outside their clinical interactions might be termed enlightened.

> A 49-year-old woman was seen by an internist in a hospital clinic. According to the information obtained by the receptionist, she was a widow with a principal complaint that her "feet hurt" and "interfered with her job." The patient was noted to have a normal physical exam and was sent to the orthopedic clinic for "corrective" shoes. A liaison psychiatrist, who was reviewing outpatient charts, noted that the physician had made no inquiry about when and under what circumstances the patient had lost her husband. Although the physician had inquired about the patient's work (she had recently taken a job as a waitress), there was no questioning about the relationship between her husband's death and her new job.
>
> The patient did not keep her appointment at the orthopedic clinic and was lost to follow-up.

We cannot be certain about the outcome if an alternative approach had been used. If the physician had asked further questions relevant to the demographic information available at the outset, however, the reasons for the patient's complaint would have been clearer. Certainly, the patient's economic status may have changed after her husband's death and may have necessitated her taking on a new job. Also, it was possible (or probable) that feelings of loss and depression contributed to the patient's somatic predisposition. Patients may recognize loss, depression, relationships, and failing health as the source of the complaint they bring to the doctor but cannot openly acknowledge this. It is as if they have to produce a symptom to communicate their suffering to the physician.

> A 52-year-old married woman came to an outpatient clinic complaining of muscle aches and general malaise, as lingering symptoms of a "cold." She presented her symptoms with force, emphasizing the fact of fever and muscle ache—as if to convince a skeptic. The doctor was compassionate and gentle throughout. Physical examination revealed no signs relevant to the complaint. The patient was subsequently interviewed by a psychiatrist, who asked a few questions about her life.
>
> Her son-in-law had unexpectedly died a year before, and she felt terribly overworked in a marriage that had not been gratifying. Another daughter, her favorite, was about to marry and move away. After hearing this, the psychiatrist suggested that she "might feel burdened." The patient exploded, "Burdened—yes—would you believe I came here wanting them to put me in the hospital?"

Somatic symptoms are often communicators of emotional and interpersonal distress.[29] Although the internist took a careful history, he failed to perceive the pressure behind this patient's complaint and her wish to be relieved of her burden of anger at her husband. Her life was dreary and wearying; she had suffered many life losses; and she could not directly express her anger toward her husband, who, from her point of view, did little for her.

SICKNESS, DISEASE, AND ILLNESS. The terms *sickness, disease,* and *illness* are most often used interchangeably. Even at the risk of making further fine distinctions, I would like to impose more definitions on these often imprecise terms.[25,26] *Disease* refers to organ dysfunction. *Illness* refers to the phenomenological aspect of sickness. Illness is formed by experience and shaped by cultural forces.[26] We invariably feel some portion of it within our bodies. The difference between disease and illness parallels the difference between signs and symptoms, the objective and the subjective. Physicians would prefer, as we have said, to work within the structure presented by Virchow. Most of their training is directed toward it. Yet, estimates of the number of nondisease complaints usually range from 40% to 80% among practitioners.[27] In one study, 50% of visits were for "nonorganic causes."[28] A similar study conducted by one of the writers assessed the percentage of outpatients as slightly higher. Although such patients frequently present with disease, the visit to the physician on that particular day is precipitated by psychological dissonance, by some emotional force that upsets an emotional balance. Nonpsychiatric physicians encountering patients whose complaint is finally diagnosed as being outside the usually acceptable causality (i.e., not within Virchow's model) often designate these patients variously as "hysterical," as psychosomatic, or, less tolerantly, as "crocks." There is usually little rationale to such discrete categorizations except that emotional issues are the leading edge in these patients' complaints.

THE WEAK-WOMAN BIAS

It has been said that in medical practice, an implicit tenet in the treatment of women is that "only men can be healthy."[30] Women's frailty is seen as being derived from her innate qualities. Her relative physical weakness is the base on which a number of other qualities, also deemed natural or biological, are heaped, for example, lack of aggressiveness and a tendency to decompensate under stress and inconstancy. It is only recently that such assumptions have been massively challenged from the social-historical context rather than from within the purely dualistic bias. Such challenge has come almost exclusively from women. Women are still very often viewed, when they seek professional help, in a context that was present at the beginning of this century.

Women, then, are often viewed as sick or defective.[31,32] The organic bias, usually favored within the dualistic framework of medical practice, does not apply as generally to women as it does to men. Functional disease is seen by the public and by doctors as a special weakness and perhaps also as intrinsically feminine. That may be another reason for the reluctance to assign such a diagnosis to a man. The concept of women's inherent weakness has a long tradition in our culture. The legal, social, and religious emphasis on women as physically weak emerges with their legally weak position (as chattel) and with a religious view of women as uniquely inconstant, morally corruptible, and corrupting.

The general tendency, then, to view women as second-class or second-rate, as God's afterthought, most often leads to diagnostic bias. The issue of possible sexual prejudice in the assignment of psychogenic causes to various female disorders (dysmenorrhea, the nausea of pregnancy, and pain in labor) has been addressed.[32]

Many of such attitudes are further underscored by quasi-scientific statements about woman's susceptibility to "endocrine storms." The psychological approach to women presented in gynecology texts and advocated as a proper, scientific attitude in a clinical setting has changed little since Kinsey.[33] Women are still seen, even in eminent journals and texts, from the vantage point of sex-role stereotypes, as anatomically destined to reproduce, nurture, and keep males happy. Such textbooks, it is pointed out, are primary professional socialization agents, and they are usually written by men.

This particular conceptual duality (seeing femaleness as tending toward weakness and seeing maleness as tending toward health) is, then, parallel with the mind and body duality. Diagnoses viewed in this light involve both deductive reasoning and unexamined value judgments.

HYSTERIA AND NEURASTHENIA. A further aspect of the organic-functional controversy can be seen in a historical comparision of hysteria and neurasthenia.[34,35] Neurasthenia became a popular diagnosis in the United States after the Civil War. It was one of the functional diagnoses (along with hysteria and hypochondriasis). It provides a historical illustration of the supposition that disease entities delineated by the medical profession depend on the values and the cultural referents of both doctors and patients.[33] Men were more usually diagnosed as neurasthenic and women as hysterical. The person with neurasthenia was seen as a victim of overwork—as someone who had exhausted his "supply of nervous energy." Neurasthenia, before it passed into oblivion as a diagnosis, had become a national peril. It was seen as a result of social stress, brought on by the forces of industrial change operating within society. There was generally sympathy for the victims, and the treatment was humane caretaking. On the other hand, hysteria, seen as a woman's disease, had its base in her inherent weakness. Moreover, the public and medical attitudes toward the hysteric were more critically judgmental: the hysteric was seen as perverse.[34]

FUNCTIONAL DIAGNOSES FOR WOMEN. Women, more than men, have functional diagnoses ranging through the diagnostic spectrum from psychoneurosis through psychosomatic illness to psychosis.[29,30] This actuarial fact also influences clinical diagnosis. The practitioner, for that reason alone, may tend to diagnose women as having functional disorders. There are, then, in summary, two related social and historical reasons for such diagnoses: the physician's value system relative to women and the self-perpetuating nature of clinical diagnoses.

WOMEN'S ATTITUDES TOWARD THEMSELVES IN THE MATRIX OF "FUNCTIONAL" DISEASE

Yet, the most important factor probably has to do with women themselves: an etiology unexamined from within the medical dichotomization. Women have been taught that submissiveness is both a sign of maturity and a manifestation of their femininity.[30] Among the factors leading to psychological symptoms is "learning."[36] Sickness often is a way of avoiding a terrifying sense of alienation deriving from personal incongruities within a larger social network.[24] Incongruities are often "built into" women's lives as social "fact," to which they must submit. Aspirations and ambitions, if not set aside, can potentially disbar a woman from genuine femaleness, not just for others but as a self-perception.

Sickness limits and restores a woman to submissiveness and can indirectly express anger toward those who are responsible. Taking on an acceptable role as a sick or fragile person permanently sets limits on capacities. The price paid for such comfort is often depression.

This simple statement hardly encompasses the totality of the etiologies of psychological dysfunction. It only underscores an important psychosocial dimension. It is opposite to the position that views women as biologically and psychologically weak. There has never been any genuine evidence of such a position, despite a usual implicit acceptance within medicine.

REFERENCES

1. Cobb S: Monism and psychosomatic medicine, *Psychosomatic Medicine* 19:77, 1957.
2. Cobb S: Neurology. In *American handbook of psychiatry*. Edited by Arieti S. New York, Basic Books, p. 1639, 1966.

3. Cobb S: In *On the mysterious leap from the mind to the body*. Edited by Deutsch F. New York, International Universities Press, pp. 11–13, 1969.
4. Cohen H: Monism, *Philosophy 21*:1, 1952.
5. von Bertalanffy L: General systems theory. In *American handbook of psychiatry*, Vol. 3. Edited by Arieti S. New York, Basic Books, pp. 705–721, 1966.
6. Kaplan H: History of psychophysiological medicine. In *Textbook of psychiatry*. Edited by Freedman A, Kaplan H, Saddock B. Baltimore, Williams & Wilkins, p. 1624, 1975.
7. Modell A: *Object love and reality*. New York, International Universities Press, 1968.
8. Nagler S: The mind-body problem. In *Comprehensive textbook of psychiatry*. Edited by Freedman A, Kaplan H. Baltimore, Williams & Wilkins, p. 1037, 1967.
9. Alexander F: Fundamental concepts of psychosomatic research: Psychogenesis, conversion, specificity, *Psychosomatic Medicine 5*:205–218, 1943.
10. Wise T: Pain: The most common psychosomatic disorder, *Medical Clinics of North America 61*:771–788, 1977.
11. Knapp P: In *On the mysterious leap from the mind to the body*. Edited by Deutsch F. New York, International Universities Press, p. 19, 1969.
12. Fox H: In *On the mysterious leap from the mind to the body*. Edited by Deutsch F. New York, International Universities Press, p. 14, 1969.
13. Lipowski Z: Delirium, clouding of consciousness and confusion, *Journal of Nervous and Mental Diseases 145*:227–235, 1967.
14. Nadelson T: Sending the patient home, *Psychotherapy and Psychosomatics 30*:68–75, 1978.
15. Waitzkin F, Stoeckle J: The communication of information about illness, Clinical sociological and methodological consideration. In *Advances in psychosomatic medicine: Psychosocial aspects of physical illness*, Vol. 8. Basel, S. Karger, pp. 180–211, 1972.
16. Moore W, Tunin: Some social functions of ignorance, *American Sociological Review 14*:787–795, 1949.
17. Parsons T: *Social structure and personality*. New York, Free Press, 1964.
18. Glazer B, Strauss A: *Awareness of dying*. Chicago, Aldine, 1965.
19. Bergen B: Psychosomatic knowledge and the role of the physician: A sociological view. *International Journal of Psychiatry in Medicine 5*:431–442, 1974.
20. Alexander F, Selesnick S: *The history of psychiatry*. New York, Harper & Row, 1966.
21. Weiss J: The current state of the concept of psychosomatic disorder, *International Journal of Psychiatry in Medicine 5*:473–482, 1974.
22. Lipowski Z: Introduction. In *Advances in psychosomatic medicine*. Volume 8. *Psychosocial aspects of physical illness*. Edited by Lipowski Z. Basel, S. Karger, 1972.
23. Lipowski Z: Physical illness and psychopathology. *International Journal of Psychiatry in Medicine, 5*:483–495, 1974.
24. Moss G: Biosocial resonation: A conceptual model of the links between social behavior and physical illness. *International Journal of Psychiatry in Medicine 5*:401–410, 1974.
25. Reading A: Illness and disease, *Medical Clinics of North America 61*:703–710, 1977.
26. Kleinman A, Eisenberg L, Good B: Culture, illness and care: Clinical lessons from anthropological and cross-cultural research. *Annals of Internal Medicine 88*:251–258, 1978.
27. Roberts B: The prevalence of psychiatric illness in a medical outpatient clinic, *New England Journal of Medicine 245*:82–86, 1952.
28. Stoeckle J, Zola I, Davidson G: The quantity and significance of psychological distress in medical patients, *Journal of Chronic Diseases 17*:959–970, 1964.

29. Fishman G, Nadelson T: Crisis intervention. In *The psychosomatic approach to medical practice.* Edited by Wittkower E, Warmes H. pp. 15–29, 1976.
30. Chesler P: *Women and madness.* New York, Doubleday, 1972.
31. Ehrenreich B, English D: *Complaints and disorders.* New York, Feminist Press, 1973.
32. Lennane J, Lennane R: Alleged psychogenic disorders in women: A possible manifestation of sexual prejudice, *New England Journal of Medicine* 288–292, 1973.
33. Sully D, Bart P: A funny thing happened on the way to the orifice: Women in gynecology textbooks, *American Journal of Sociology* 78:1045–1050, 1973.
34. Sicherman B: The uses of a diagnosis: doctors, patients and neurasthenia, *Journal of the History of Medicine and Allied Sciences,* 32(1):33–54, 1977.
35. Smith-Rosenberg C: Some reflections on sex roles and role conflict in 19th century America. *Social Research,* 39:652–678, 1972.
36. Knapp P: Current theoretical concepts of psychophysiological medicine. In *Comprehensive textbook of psychiatry.* Edited by Freedman A, Kaplan H, Saddock B. Baltimore, Williams & Wilkins, p. 1631, 1975.

Chapter 10

The Painful Woman: Complaints, Symptoms, and Illness

Don R. Lipsitt

> [Women] *take a heavy, unhealthy pleasure in suffering; it subtly pleases them to be hard put upon; they like to picture themselves as slaughtered saints. Thus they always find something to complain of; the very conditions of domestic life give them a superabundance of clinical material.* [1]

These words by the satirist H. L. Mencken were no less inflammatory in 1922 than they are today. They were the product not only of a curmudgeonly journalist but also of the social climate in which they were written. The suggestion that women often were complainers racked with pain was abundantly promoted from the stage by playwrights of the day. Today, more modern versions of the same theme, that women are the "weaker (and sicker) sex," find their way into cartoons, medical advertisements, and other media.

Thoughtful concern and a sense of fairness prompt one to dispute such sentiments. Nonetheless, statistics do record higher rates of hospital admission, utilization of clinics, visits to doctors, and use of drugs by women.[2] Still, in the face of such incontrovertible data, it is no myth that women live longer than men.[3] Even Mencken, elsewhere in his book, acknowledged, "I am convinced that the average woman, whatever her deficiencies, is greatly superior to the average man."

What are we to make of these seemingly paradoxical observations? Is it possible that women are sicker than men, experience more pain and complain more, and receive better medical care? Or do they merely complain more of somatic distress although they are not "really sick"? Is it conceivable that there can be a salutary relationship between complaining, doctoring, pill taking, and longevity?

Behavioral and social differences between men and women in the

Don R. Lipsitt, M.D. ● Departments of Psychiatry, Harvard Medical School and Mount Auburn Hospital, Cambridge, Massachusetts.

ways they deal with issues of dependency, passivity, and denial may help to account for some of those disparities; women may find it easier to acknowledge disease or symptoms, to turn to others for help, and to be more receptive to helpful remedies.

This chapter explores how the woman in pain complains of her symptoms and how this process affects how she is treated medically. To understand the complexities of this process, it is necessary to consider definitions of illness and disease; the general process of symptom formation and somatization; and the specific relationship of female psychology, physiology, and anatomy to manifestations of painful experience. The medical encounter for women must also take account of illness behavior, sociocultural influences on the expression of pain, and the process of labeling in medical practice.

ILLNESS AND DISEASE

The invention and use of the word *disease* suggest that illness and disease are not necessarily the same, and several writers have attempted to bring some precision of meaning to these words.[4,5,6,7,8] There is some agreement that while the expression of both illness and disease may be colored by social, cultural, and psychological factors, illness is more experiential and subjective, while disease is more structural, corporeal, and objectifiable. Illness most often is what one feels as a result of a disease process, but each may occur without the other. It is *illness* rather than *disease* of which the patient most often complains and that generally produces symptoms. In our discussion of symptoms and complaints, we should take note of Reading's observation that "Illness that does not result from disease is simply not as respectable in our society as is illness that does."[4]

The dualism of medicine that separates illness and disease also splits dysfunction into psyche and soma, symptoms and signs, empirical (anecdotal) and scientific, nonverbal and verbal, unverifiable and verifiable. In responding to a patient's "disturbance," the physician generally relies on history to focus on the first of the pair, physical examination to focus on the second. In a sense, the signs and corporeal soma of disease are the physician's province, and the symptoms and the personal psychological meaning of the experience of illness are the patient's province. The way in which these two systems interact constitutes the doctor–patient encounter and ultimately determines the outcome for both. Sociologists have studied and described these interactions as "illness behavior" and "sick role."[9,10,11]

Even as refinements in definition evolve, the ideology and vocabulary of illness and disease change. Some "conditions" (e.g., homosexuality) once regarded as illness are declared "normal variants" in response to social and political pressures. Some writers insist that all mental illness is a myth, while others stridently decry the medicalization of a broad spectrum of what they regard as otherwise normal human behavior.[12,13,14] Still others have insisted that much of what has been labeled illness or symptomatology in the past is merely the product of sexism, racism, and the domination of American medicine by male physicians.[15]

This ferment has lent credence to the recurrent observation that medicine, and perhaps more especially psychiatry, is once again undergoing an "identity crisis,"[16] but it probably does little to make less murky the current sociopolitical morass of medicine. What is clear, however, is that one cannot discuss sickness, symptoms, or illness behavior without acknowledging their social context. In a penetrating analysis of attitudes and treatment related to tuberculosis and cancer, Sontag[17] has recently described how "illness as metaphor" is intricately interwoven with our language, our expectations, our biases and knowledge, all in a time-related social context.

COMPLAINING

The time and social context in which a physician's education takes place clearly have an impact on that physician's attitudes and beliefs. The approach to history taking, however, seems to remain timeless; eliciting symptoms and complaints continues to be the touchstone of medical diagnosis and treatment. The medical student is taught that every patient's record begins with a "chief complaint," which is then elaborated upon through a medical history of the present and the past, a family and social history, and a review of the body's systems intended to ensure that no symptom or complaint will be overlooked or forgotten. In theory, the physical examination is essentially an opportunity to test out hypotheses formulated during an exhaustive history-taking. It is a way to examine the soma for signs that will objectively confirm or deny the patient's subjective "story" of the symptoms and illness felt.

Most medical students and physicians learn to abhor illness unaccompanied by disease. Though the physician is taught to ritually coax every complaint of pain and discomfort from the patient, vagueness of complaints that defies diagnosis is often a disappointment to the physician and ultimately a frustration for the patient. Clearly defined disease, with or without illness, is the physician's preference and is generally assured the best treatment. Anything else runs a serious risk of inappropriate labeling, misunderstanding, inadequate treatment, and rejection of the patient. We shall return to this theme again in a discussion of hypochondriasis, labeling, and the "problem (or painful) patient."

"Complaining" is universal, part of the human condition, even unrelated to medical encounters. The very first cry of the newborn is generally interpreted as a sign of distress. Until the evolution of language in the developing child provides a clearer means of communication, unpleasant utterances in the nonverbal mode are generally interpreted as signs of discomfort (complaints). But during that developmental phase, the responses elicited in others by the nonverbal cry will have shaped much interpersonal behavior and will have lent form to a characterological style of complaining.[18] Complaining implies an actual or wished-for interaction with another person, with the expectation that the act of complaining will evoke some means of alleviating the underlying distress. The distress may be physical or emotional, conscious or unconscious. Complaining in the absence of distress or disease is considered malingering.

Complaining may become a way of relating, a defense against improvement, a coping activity, a gratification in itself or for what it evokes in others, or a means of avoiding responsibility. How the process of complaining is woven into the tapestry of one's life is not well understood, but clearly, learning from early life plays an important role. The rewards and punishments for behavior and communications, the development of intrapsychic defense mechanisms (e.g., denial, rationalization, identification, projection), the perception of one's body, the relation between internal and external milieus, deprivations, entitlement, and masochism all contribute to the ways in which discomfort is expressed. Character structure and personality styles thus influence symptom and complaint (whether or not disease is present).

For example, one's early deprivations may leave a lifelong sense of neediness, emptiness, or entitlement expressed through complaining of a "painful body" in later years. The nurturance evoked by complaining may temporarily soothe the pain, diminish feelings of deprivation, and appear to compensate for previous losses. Or a person who has experienced caretaking, love, and attention in the context of previous illness or pain may unconsciously (and sometimes even wittingly) seek the painful state that can recall previous gratifications.

Hence, at the extremes, one may seek medical intervention for "insignificant troubles," or one may uncomplainingly ignore the early signs of serious disease and consult a physician only when the disease process has blatantly declared itself. Some may consistently report *physical* distress, while others perceive *emotional* repercussions for every kind of stress.

We may speculate to what extent the earliest responses of the parent to a child's distress tend to fix a preferential way of looking at and complaining about distress: almost all parents offer some sort of *physical* remedy for a nonverbal outburst of anguish—a glass of milk or water, a pacifier, a trip to the bathroom, a change of environment, or a lamp turned on. Perhaps out of such early experience, a preference is shaped, in patients and physicians alike, for somatic rather than psychological explanations of discomfort and distress.

The patient's conscious and unconscious motives for complaining need to be understood by the physician. The language of the whiny complaint as an expression of hostility must be distinguishable from the complaint of pain due to physical trauma or a deteriorative lesion if doctor and patient are to communicate meaningfully with one another in a beneficial relationship. Some people have no other mechanism available to them to "compute" their experience, except through the language of physical discomfort.

SYMPTOMS

It is perhaps from such early cultural and interpersonal learning that most symptoms are experienced as unpleasant sensations and events in the body.[19,20] When the illness (or distress) is related to organic physical disease, there is often greater congruence between the felt sensation and the bodily event than when the symptom is psychologically determined. In the latter instance, the symptom is more difficult to define, to verify, to measure, to test. It is experienced by the person as often not belonging to himself or herself, as ego-alien. When it is attributed to a body part, though undiseased, it is more tangible and therefore more believable for both patient and physician; such attribution is called *somatization.*

It is common for essentially affective or psychological distress (illness) to be "somatized," to be perceived and described as emanating from a body part, and thereby to be denied as a conscious subjective experience.

Clearly, what and how disequilibrium of any kind is translated into symptoms (and complaints) depends on one's sense of self, a perception that is filtered through a complex screen of attitudes, experiences, beliefs, defenses, culture, and personality structure. Different observers have noted the remarkable variation in response to trauma in children and adults, apparently related to the individual "interpretation" (meaning) of pain. For example, soldiers in battle in World War II seemed to tolerate tissue deterioration with less complaint of pain than men sustaining similar damage in other settings not imbued with the special meanings, fantasies, rewards, pride, heroism, etc., of the battlefield.[21] Similarly, Anna Freud commented on the "tough" child who "does not mind pain," because of differences in unconscious fantasies connected with the pain.[19]

One of the commonest symptoms—pain—has been convincingly shown to respond sensitively to cultural differences alone.[22,23,24] In the sense that males and females have been reared in different sociocultural environments, it is to be expected that the experience of illness and the nature of symptom reporting and complaining will show sexual differences.

SYMPTOM FORMATION

All symptom formation is multidetermined by both internal and external factors. Infection, for example, is the result of pathogenic forces interacting with host elements such as susceptibility, resistance, and tissue integrity. As we have noted, disease may exist without symptoms (e.g., latent diabetes or hypertension), just as symptoms may be present without disease (e.g., conversion hysteria). Complaints may arise in the presence or absence of either or both. In those instances where material or physical change cannot be defined, detected, or demonstrated by inspection or technological measurement, symptoms become more subjective, elusive, and difficult to explain.

Sigmund Freud's studies of patients with "unfounded symptoms" were instrumental in the development of his theories of symptom formation. Prior to the establishment of psychoanalytic or psychodynamic explanations, all such "baseless" symptomatology was generally referred to as *functional* or *hypochondriacal* (in many cases, the implication was that the disease, if not the illness, was imaginary, "all in the patient's mind").

In psychiatry, the conceptualization of the mechanism and process of somatization replaced more negative ways of looking at non-physically based symptoms. Symptoms of both physical and emotional illness share the characterization of the individual's (organism's) response to circumstances (stimuli) that threaten physical or mental intactness and well-being. The defenses that are mobilized to protect the body against experiencing pain or other distress generally check the symptoms, whether through the aggregation of leukocytes (e.g.) to fight off an infection, or through mobilization of denial (e.g.) to reduce the ego's awareness or to enhance the mastery of anxiety or depression. To the extent that the system's defenses are ineffective or inefficient, the symptoms of illness–disease become more perceptible. In this sense, all symptoms represent compromise formations, a lesser condition (e.g., swelling and redness, or anxiety) to ward off a more destructive condition (e.g., systemic infection, or psychosis). The term *compromise formation*, however, is more at home in psychoanalysis than in physical medicine, having first been conceptualized by Freud in his theories of dreaming.[25] Nonetheless, since "symptoms may be viewed from the outside in clinical, descriptive terms, or from the inside, as the consequence of causally related psychological forces,"[26] it becomes the physician's (whether psychiatrist, gynecologist, or internist) task to decipher the symptom by attempting to define the several vectors of which it is a compromise expression.

SOMATIZATION

Somatization, therefore, both as a defense and as a symptom, presents one of the most exacting challenges to the physician, since there is usually a paucity of verbal, reflective, introspective material produced by the patient to assist in the diagnostic and therapeutic process.

Somatizing has its psychogenetic roots variously in the fears generated by previous (and since treated) physical disease or illness in oneself, in members of the family, or in other close individuals with whom the patient identifies; an unconsciously mimicked style of family communication; in interpersonal conflicts only partially or not at all perceived; or in acculturated "habits" normative in one's environment of origin.[27]

Hysterical conversion represents a special type of somatization in which the physical manifestation psychologically (symbolically) represents a deep-seated conflict (often sexual) previously accompanied by a profound emotion that was not sufficiently expressed at the time of the earlier event.[28]

Complicating the physician's task of interpreting a patient's somatized presentation of illness are her or his cumulative knowledge, experience, definitions, and biases about what constitutes illness, as well as the kinds of unconscious mechanisms at work in the physician's own psyche. Though psychoanalysis has shed some scientific light on the intrapsychic mechanism of symptom formation, our language, our culture, and our attitudes have been powerful determinants of the *social* response to disease, symptoms, and complaints. The physician's traditional education exposes him or her to very little psychoanalytic knowledge and does little to modify the inherent social set with which every student embarks on the medical education process. Therefore, since the vagaries of disease, or symptom naming, are as fluid as social and political pressures, the task of defining what does or does not constitute illness or "justified" symptomatology becomes enormously complex.

Body Awareness and Expression of Symptoms

The experience of the body, as mentioned, begins early in life, although there is no way to know what it means to an infant or what is actually felt. Freud[29] regarded the formation of the ego as having its beginnings in the "body ego." Brenner[28] described Freud's belief that "our bodies occupy a very special place in our psychic lives as long as we are alive and . . . they begin to occupy that special place very early in infancy." It has been emphasized that cumulative body experience influences the expression of physical as well as psychological distress.[29,30,31] Body awareness, which is greater for women than for men,[32] evolves out of physiological function, which is then invested with personal meaning. Emotional states thus interact with, influence, and are influenced by the physiological process. Awareness of body form and function is a composite of self-perception and others' perceptions of oneself. The character of identifications with others of the same and opposite sexes affects one's own self-image. Psychiatrists working with obstetric-gynecological patients and physicians have noted the highly charged meaning invested in body parts such as the breast, uterus, and ovaries that is often mobilized in the face of threatened or actual surgery.[33,34,35]

That girls and boys very early in life realize basic (especially genital) anatomical differences cannot be an insignificant contributor to one's ultimate self-image or body experience. Though Freud has been widely criticized for the notion that "anatomy is destiny," the forceful role of body experience and self-esteem in the quality and meaning of life lends credence to this idea; one must be careful, however, to define the limits and nature of any inferred causality. Much of the ferment around this expression arises from a misinterpretation of the concept. Clearly, one's biology and anatomy are powerful influences on one's life. The reproductive function is unassailably part of femaleness, but it must not be misconstrued to automatically prescribe or circumscribe the social roles and the behavioral dimensions of life.

Psychoanalytic theory has been considered by some to be doctrinaire on this point, but the following quote illustrates the influence of social climate on theory:

> As to the origins of the adult feminine character, particularly the capacity for adequate mothering, Blum believes they cannot be derived in the main from masochism and penis envy, although the latter is an impor-

tant influence. The equation of femininity with passivity, along with their linked definitions, has to be re-examined so that the various expressions of ego activity and strivings for mastery in the woman, as well as in the man, may be taken into account. The complexities of development cannot be described in terms of early models or an anticipated reductionism. Among the many new concepts considered in the course of the recent re-evaluation of the psychoanalytic psychology of women are the preoedipal formation of gender identity and female self-representation. Conscious and unconscious parental attitudes and rearing may supersede the formative influence of biology and anatomy. While there is undoubtedly a biological female bedrock which may also confer an inherent rhythmicity upon female experience, cultural influences as well as biological development must be included in a broad psychoanalytic perspective.[36]

The contribution of anatomy to destiny is further underscored by one's perception of one's internal organs; the impact of early (probably post-oedipal) learning is suggested in Kumin's poem "Body and Soul: A Meditation."[38]

Body and Soul: A Meditation

Body, Old Paint, Old Partner,
I ought to have paid closer
attention when Miss Bloomberg
shepherded the entire fifth grade
into the Walk-Through Woman.
I remember going
up three steps, all right,
to enter the left auricle.
I remember the violet light
which made it churchly
and the heartbeat amplified
to echo from chamber to chamber
like God speaking unto Moses.

But there was nothing about the soul,
that miners' canary flitting
around the open spaces;
no diagram in which
the little ball-bearing soul
bumbled her way downhill
in the pinball machine
on the interior, clicking
against the sternum,
the rib cage, the pelvis.
The Walk-Through Woman ceased
Shortly below the waist.
Her genitals were off limits.

Once again, this is different for females than for males, since the onset of puberty brings menarche and endocrinological changes, which vividly influence body configuration and awareness. The impact of anatomy on one's destiny need not be limited to sexual characteristics, since tallness, shortness, thinness, fatness, and other attributes can all modify perception of self.

THE REPRODUCTIVE SYSTEM. Few adolescent girls have an accurate picture of the internal aspects of their own genital anatomy,[37] but there is a beginning preoccupation with the regularity and duration of menstrual flow, the pain resulting from menstrual cramps, a periodicity of other physical and emotional variations, and new concerns about odors, cleanliness, and illness as the young female enters puberty. New interest emerges as the adolescent girl anticipates the physical aspects of sexuality, pregnancy, parturition, and breast-feeding and the implications these have for body configuration, change, and attractiveness.

The fantasies accompanying such new perceptions include fears of loss of control implied by processes that are preordained, fears about physical inadequacy and damage resulting from pregnancy, and developing concerns about the relation of potential motherhood to future career choice and lifestyle. While good statistics are not available relating the number of complaints and symptoms referable to reproductive organs, there has been some historical linkage of symptoms (and complaints) in women with "women's troubles."[39,40,41] (In men, perhaps only "prostate trouble" is comparable, but that is more often related to a later stage of life than to ongoing experience.) Bardwick,[42] noting the great variability, frequency, and range of dysfunctions related to the female reproductive system, stated that

> Because the reproductive system is so salient it can become for some women the most logical and obvious vehicle for the expression of aggression, anxiety and desire—especially relating to their sexual feelings, their maternal longings, and their relationship with themselves and with the important people in their lives. Symptoms often express a strong conflict that cannot be revealed more directly, resolved more efficiently, or sublimated healthily.

Many physiological changes, both normal and abnormal, seem associated with the marked alternations in endocrine balance throughout the menstrual cycle. There is some controversy about whether the mood shifts observed in women correlate with the peaks of the menstrual cycle, in large part determined by endocrine levels.[42,43,44,45] Though sex-role expectations and cultural attitudes about menstrual cramps, illness, and depression may influence symptom expression, many good studies have demonstrated the interrelation of cycle phase, endocrine shifts, and emotional state in women.[46,47,48]

Some researchers have suggested that depression occurs premenstrually ("premenstrual tension") and abates with the onset of menses, thought by some to be a response to estrogen–progesterone levels.

Thus, Gottschalk *et al.*[50] and Ivey and Bardwick[47] demonstrated lower levels of anxiety, hostility, and depression at midcycle (during ovulation) and during menses, when estrogen is relatively high, than at other phases of the cycle. Such findings support the now disputed belief that depression, anxiety, and irritability are highest in the woman at the three times when estrogen production is at low ebb, namely, before menstruation, just after childbirth, and during menopause.[41] Although concomitant biochemical changes clearly are affected by the menstrual cycle—including water and sodium retention, variations in blood glucose levels, fluctuations in antidiuretic hormone, and the altered production of aldosterone and other corticoids—such correlations cannot be accepted as fact without considering the social, behavioral, and political aspects of such research. The intensity, meaning, and "coloration" of any symptom, no matter what its biochemical correlates, depend on individual attributions, personality structure, and the degree of underlying psychopathology.[43,44,50,51]

PELVIC PAIN. The complaint of pain, for women, very often is experienced in the reproductive system and therefore often comes to the attention of the organ-oriented obstetrician-gynecologist as much as to the internist or the generalist. Castelnuovo-Tedesco and Krout pointed out[53] that although several psychiatric researchers[53,54,55,56] have stressed the entity of psychogenic pain, most gynecological writers appear to regard (pelvic) pain as being a result of disease or physical malfunctioning of the pelvic organs. Castelnuovo-Tedesco and Krout demonstrated that patients with chronic pelvic pain, regardless of the presence or absence of physical pathology, showed a high degree of psychopathology, by both psychiatric interview and psychological testing. It was found that patients with pain, with or without active pathology, tended to score higher on the Hypochondriasis and Hysteria Scales of the MMPI than patients without pain, while those without pain, in spite of active physical pathology, scored higher on the Depression than the Hypochondriasis or Hysteria Scales; psychiatric interviews bore out the findings on the psychological tests.

The former patients were said to employ the defense mechanisms of denial, somatization, and repression to a greater extent than the latter. These findings were regarded by Sternbach as supporting the suggestion of Pilling *et al.* that pain may represent a symptom substitution for otherwise distressing affects such as depression.[58] To properly assess the significance of such findings, however, negative correlations must also be acknowledged. Sternbach *et al.*[59] did not find significant differences in Depression Scale scores for low-back-pain patients with or without physical pathology. While their study is representative of others,[59] Sternbach nonetheless concluded that "people with psychogenic pain tend to be neurotic, and in this respect do not differ much from those with chronic pain of organic origin."

While studies using statistical methods and rating scales are of some interest, the elucidation of the mechanisms by which psychological conflict is translated into pain comes primarily from psychoanalytic data; clarification depends on examining in great detail the unique characteristics of the individual's developmental processes and patterns of response to psychological stress, both internal and external.

Castelnuovo-Tedesco and Krout have combined statistical methods with a psychodynamic exploration of patients' associations to their pain. Their findings have practical relevance to gynecological management: psychiatric assessment is useful even when a patient's pain seems validated by organic findings, since there is poor congruence or implication of causality between the degree or kind of physical pathology and the presence or absence of pain. It is simply not true that finding any organic lesion in the pelvis necessarily explains the pain, and indeed, many "physical findings" may well be artifactual. According to these researchers,

> Chronic pelvic pain, even in the presence of definite organic pathology, is "more" than pelvic disease. It is a complex psychosomatic entity, variable in its make-up, involving with considerable regularity and to an impressive degree the emotional status and total functioning of the patient and, in particular, her outlook toward sexuality and her capacity for human relatedness.[53]

DEPRESSION AND WOMEN

Depression may appear as a mood state, a symptom, or a syndrome. The precipitants are complex and the manifestations are varied. The affective state of depression may go unrecognized when it is experienced primarily as somatic distress or pain in one or another body part. If the person presents with these pains to a physician who does not discover the related emotional problem, the depression may remain untreated indefinitely. Thus, the process of somatization adds a special element of risk and delay in obtaining proper health care.

Weissman and Klerman[46] have recently urged a clearer distinction between the physiological precursors of depression and the psychological factors implicit in broad stereotypical terms like *empty-nest syndrome* or *housewife syndrome*. These authors indicated that dualistic approaches to the problem have flourished since at least the nineteenth century and have generated theories to support either biological or psychological determinants. Current data, however, they believe, is too scanty to fully support the conventionally espoused endocrinological basis for observed differences. Whether supportive or not of Freud's psychoanalytic theories of female psychological development, findings suggest that early learning and assigned social roles heighten the vulnerability of women to low self-esteem, masochism, dependency, narcissism, and repressed hostility, creating susceptibility to depression.

DOCTOR–PATIENT INTERACTIONS AND LABELING

Whether or not a physican regards a patient as a hypochondriac often revolves around the degree of "realness" that the physician assigns to the patient's complaint, usually of pain. Pain is the most common distress for which patients visit physicians; both patient and physician seek an explanation, which is translated—by attribution by the patient and by diagnosis by the physician—into a label.

When physicians are baffled in their attempts to establish a diagnosis or a pseudodiagnostic label, they sometimes regard complaints and symptoms as "trivial" or "nonexistent." Persistence on the patient's part to clarify the problem frequently results in frustration, anger, or discharge or referral by the vexed physician. Since women exceed men in the numbers of visits they make to physicians' offices, they are clearly more at risk of being pejoratively labeled.

Hypochondriasis is one of the most commonly misapplied pseudodiagnostic labels. Interestingly, hypochondriasis was originally considered an affliction primarily of men, but in the nineteenth century, the term began to be more commonly assigned to women, perhaps, in part, as a result of social and attitudinal changes and, in part, as a reflection of a new definition of *hysteria,* which demanded more specificity than the "wandering uterus" of that term's earlier origins.[65]

It is important to understand the psychodynamics and sociodynamics by which the respectably solicited chief complaint of the well-ordered history-taking comes to connote an abrasive, objectionable utterance translated into pseudoobjective labels like *demanding patient, chronic complainer, problem patient, hypochondriac,* or *crock.*[60] Such terms usually reveal the physician's frustrated efforts to understand or treat, suggest a sense of loss of control when complaints arc generated without being elicited by the physician, and reflect the doctor's penchant for seeing these patients as dependent, neurotic women who "over-utilize services." These patients are ultimately classified as individuals who do not fit the institutionalized practice of medicine and who arouse in others the socially enforced statement that "Nobody likes a whiner."

Sometimes subtle nuance in the quality of interaction between patient and physician characterizes the process by which the patient slips from the designation "good patient" to "chronic complainer." Though the literature contains some helpful suggestions for understanding and "treating" such people,[61,63,83] the prevailing medical attitude is that they "clog the system" or "have nothing the matter with them" and "merely waste the doctor's time."

There may be some credence in the view that both the woman's mode of presenting herself and the doctor's (usually male) response are encrusted with sex-role stereotypes, discriminatory learning, and social determinants of self-regard.[10] Nonetheless, large numbers of patients seeking "primary care" present in this way, and any health system that purports to be fair and effective must take account of this fact.

In describing the process by which the individual attaches meaning to any alien sensations, Ladee[65] described this preoccupation with one's bodily feeings as

> . . . a growing awareness, experienced by the patient, of the *concretization of the process of becoming affected.* The patient of course tries to combat this, either by means of outside help or by mobilizing his or her own resources. The patient is continually trying to put the process of becoming affected into words; but this attempt is never successful, even though the patient does pigeonhole it under a particular disease, giving it a concrete name; for even though the hypochondriac patient may be convinced that he is suffering from a particular complaint, he can be observed trying to pin it down ever more closely. The preoccupation, and self-observation, as a particular form thereof, are thus being kept alive, the more so when strong variations in the patient's bodily awareness accentuate his failure to pinpoint what is wrong with him.

PAIN, DEPRESSION, AND HYPOCHONDRIACS

Pain very frequently accompanies depression or, in the case of somatization, often presents in place of the more familiar vegetative signs of depression. Although some psychoanalytic and psychiatric writers[66] have referred to pain (and other behaviors) as "depressive equivalents," depression is often excluded from the physician's differential diagnosis when the patient presents primarily with a complaint of pain in some body part.

A number of writers have commented on the association of pain and depression,[67,68] although most reports are of uncontrolled studies and do not necessarily confirm a greater association of pain with depression than with anxiety, or, for that matter, with physical illness.[69] Nonetheless, large numbers of people consult physicians primarily for pain, and of those who have psychiatric conditions, the greatest percentage are depressed.

Sternbach, on the subject of pain, suggested that "the complaint of pain occurs in slightly more than half the general medical and psychiatric populations, and in psychiatric populations the presence of a pain complaint is about equally likely to predict a diagnosis of anxiety hysteria or reactive depression."[71] He believes that when patients present to their physicians with pain or some other somatic complaints, these may mask depression and result in the underdiagnosing of depressive illness. I would suggest that the process is more complex, that the physician *prefers* working with somatic complaints and therefore, in a sense, "conspires" with the patient's own unconscious to ignore the psychological reality of the patient's presenting problem (pain). The idea that the somatic complaint "masks" the affective disorder also charitably assumes that the problem would be correctly diagnosed if the physical complaint were not present.

While there is, to my knowledge, no study that examines the correlative incidence of pain, depression, and a "diagnosis" of hypochondriasis, clinical anecdote, experience, and observation suggest that this triad is not uncommon. Scientific evidence supports the relationship of at least the first two parameters, wherein treatment with antidepressant drugs resulted in either increased tolerance to or complete alleviation of pain concomitant with relief from depression.[52,70]

The notion that pain may be substituted for unpleasant feelings of anxiety or depression is a psychodynamically supportable hypothesis,[71] which nonetheless remains essentially unconfirmed by well-controlled studies. The absence of such studies, unfortunately, is used by some to perpetuate a belief in "imaginary pain." The study by Pilling et al.[58] examined data from 562 patients seen in psychiatric consultation at the Mayo Clinic. Patients were separated into two groups, one with "presumed psychiatric pain" and the other with "presumed psychosomatic conditions" (i.e., presenting physical symptoms other than pain), and they were studied with clinical interviews, a symptom checklist, and the Minnesota Multiphasic Personality Inventory. These authors noted that there were fewer signs of depression in patients with pain than in those without and concluded, rather subjectively, that pain is less distressing than anxiety or depression and therefore presents as a substitute for these affects.

THE PAIN-PRONE PATIENT AND UNNECESSARY TREATMENT

As suggested earlier, the expression of pain is a complex manifestation of multiple determinants. Attempts to understand pain and its relationship to experience and individual development have been the catalyst for the formulation of a number of theories of personality. One of Freud's basic hypotheses was the pleasure principle, considered a guiding measure and determinant of the ego's capacity to master anxiety. In simplistic terms, Freud hypothesized that the mind attempted at all cost to avoid experience that caused "unpleasure" (*Unlust*), a concept including but extending beyond physical pain. Stated in more positive terms, the ego seeks for itself the sensation of pleasure, by developing techniques (mental mechanisms) for reducing tension and avoiding anxiety and other painful experiences.[29]

More complex modifications of this simple "pleasure–pain" principle are necessary to explain how the ego could actually seek out and accept one form of pain to avoid a more threatening (or "forbidden") one; for example, a self-inflicted painful wound could conceivably reduce the tension (anxiety, unpleasure) caused by frightening (painful) sexual or aggressive thoughts.

Extensions of this concept shed light on seemingly paradoxical clinical phenomena like "preferring" pain, failure, suffering, or hardship, to other conflict-ridden (and therefore presumably *more* painful) circumstances. It is thus not uncommon to find in the literature references to the long-suffering,[73] masochistic,[74] "pain-prone"[55] individuals who seem to prefer illness to wellness,[25] are refractory to all treatment methods,[76] are unwilling or unable to get well,[77] and "need" to be sick. Such patients are especially troublesome to physicians who are taught to ameliorate pain under all circumstances. The zealous physician who would cure the patient whose pain pays some psychodynamic debt can expect to encounter the most massive resistance to treatment. Sternbach has written of "pain patients,"

> The fact that there are millions of unfortunate persons who persist in seeking relief from pain, which is not forthcoming, suggests that the problem is not so simple, and that understanding pain may not be sufficient for treating pain patients.[70]

Engel[56] described the "pain-prone patient"; Szasz[79] wrote of the patient who engages in "painmanship" as a mode of interaction with physicians; Lipsitt[80] has defined the "rotating patient," patients who are "masochistically depressed characters" with a medical history of "doctor-shopping"; and several authors have provided medical, psychological, phenomenological, or behavioral descriptions of those individuals pejoratively referred to as crocks.[60,62,80,81] All reporters have made a number of similar observations: these patients have been characterized as long-suffering and appear to have pain that serves symbolically as retribution or punishment for some guilt-ridden conscious or unconscious transgression. They engage in complex sadomasochistic relationships (replicated in the doctor–patient interaction) that provide some kind of gratification and intimacy but ultimately are self-defeating, and they manifest a seeming intolerance of comfort, good fortune, success, praise, or well-being.

It is often difficult to elicit developmental histories from patients with an intense fixation on the here-and-now experience of pain. The data that are available suggest that these patients were reared in families where illness was prevalent, where overt or covert aggression abounded, and where interest, love, and intimacy revolved around physical disability or distress. The pattern was well-learned and, of course, is repeated chronically later in life and acutely around important critical developmental phases like separation, courting, marriage, pregnancy, childbirth, and child rearing. The pain itself sometimes serves the purpose of preventing separation from persons and experiences of an earlier existence, through either identifications or enforced caretaking by others. The intervals of time during which essential others are unavailable or are present but uncaring are marked by self-caring, self-mothering, or hypochondriacal preoccupations with one's own body as an ambivalently held love object. The driving determination of these people to relate to others through their suffering and pain causes them to be described as demanding, controlling, manipulative, vengeful, or hostile, as though such behavior were conscious. The countertransference hate,[82] the physician's inappropriate hostile response to his or her own helpless feelings, engenders considerable confusion about whether the symptoms serve the function of "primary gain" (i.e., a resolution of intrapsychic conflict through symptom formation) or "secondary gain" (e.g., "just trying to get attention"). Whatever the language used to describe the behavior, it has been observed that the nature of such interactions frequently leads to sometimes risky medical workups or even surgery.[83,84,85,86] Castelnuovo-Tedesco and Krout[53] reported in their study a strikingly large number of women with chronic pelvic pain who showed an eagerness to be operated on and to undergo hysterectomy. An index of their eagerness was their failure to inquire about or inform themselves of such matters as the degree of risk entailed, the incidence of surgical failure, or the probability of complications. "It was clear," the authors stated, "that they regarded surgery not only as a solution to their pelvic pain but also to their multiple life problems which characteristically they ascribed to the presence of pain."

Perhaps equally impressive is the willingness of physicians, in the face of their own sense of helpless frustration, to accede to the requests. Because of the facility with which the demanding pain-racked patient, interacting with the physician trained to cure, can so readily lead to unnecessary surgical intervention, the need for the physician to be knowledgable about the psychodynamic aspects of pain is all the more striking.

The same interpersonal process between patient and physician that leads to labeling probably also leads to unnecessary medical and surgical treatment. Complicating the picture, as noted by Castelnuovo-Tedesco and Krout, is the fact that

> Patients who have chronic pain and are insistent that something be done to relieve it, often do not *seem* in pain, so that their manner and appearance frequently are out of keeping with their stated complaint and, presumably, with their inner perception of it.

Of even more concern is the observation[86] that following a possible pain-free interval after surgery, there may occur a substitution of other psychological symptoms or a return of pain and renewed demands for further surgery.

The recent burgeoning of multidisciplinary "pain clinics" is a hopeful sign. Their growth suggests that there is increasing awareness of the complexities of chronic pain, that many modalities are essential to treatment, and that sometimes the experience of pain is irremediable, although the adaptation to stress may respond positively to acceptance, support, and continuity of care offered in nonjudgmental settings.

SEX ROLE, SOCIETY, AND SYMPTOMS: A SUMMATION

Many of the controversies surrounding sex-role stereotyping converge in the area of health care. Ehrenreich and English wrote that "Medicine stands between biology and social policy."[15] Paradigms of male–female relations can certainly be found in doctor–patient interactions, especially where the patient is a woman. Indeed, psychiatrists and psychoanalysts can observe the transferential reflections of the family romance, early object relations, and attitudes toward self replicated in the therapeutic encounter.

To what extent illness and the illness behavior of female patients are compliance with medical expectation and to what extent medicine has responded to the perceived needs of women begs the chicken-and-egg analogy.

Of what can we be certain? Beyond question, since at least the nineteenth century, women have been greater users of virtually all types of health care services: short-stay hospitalization, surgical procedures, visits to physicians' offices, ambulatory clinics, nursing homes, and prescriptions of all kinds.[87,88] Available data from the National Center for Health Statistics indicate that beginning before birth, males have a higher mortality than females, but morbidity and disability are generally greater for females than males.[87] Some investigators[89,90] have suggested that except for diseases that are related to the reproductive function, sex differences in illness *behavior* are due to the influence of family, society, and culture rather than greater susceptibility to disease. Weissman and Klerman[46] concluded that there is strong evidence to suggest that the learned helplessness of and the social discrimination against women account for some apparent differences in women's rates of illness compared with those of men. While definitive evidence of the influence of behavior on health statistics is elusive, clinical observation suggests that the trend toward sexual equality is accompanied by an elimination of sex-related differences in the incidence of disease in some conditions. The prevalence of smoking and alcohol abuse, for example, has begun to equalize, and certain diseases like anorexia nervosa, at one time considered almost entirely a female condition, have begun to be reported in greater numbers of young males; again, one must take into account possible modifications of the description of the disease and of the approved methods of diagnosis before assuming that the observed changes are entirely related to changing sex roles.

Changes in the incidence of alcoholism are believed to reflect social change. But even with an absolute increase in alcoholism among women, certain differences continue to be observed. Generally, women become aware of their problem earlier than men, seek help sooner, and move through the treatment process more quickly. They also use more drugs in addition to alcohol. Alcoholism in women is more commonly associated with affective disorder, with drinking in relation to life stress, and with more suicide attempts, more isolated drinking, and more broken marriages than in men.[91,92] Which of these differences can be attributed to sex-linked (biological) differences and which to social factors is virtually impossible to say. Many believe that even with a new acceptance of social equality, there is a differential response to men and women. There is speculation that the negative reaction of society to female alcoholism acts as a brake on its rampant spread. There is also a suggestion that a genetic relationship exists between affective disorder and alcoholism in women, though Weissman and Klerman believe that this, too, may be artifactually related to socially learned ways of expressing depression.

Suicide, as an index of illness, has also traditionally shown marked sex differences, with a greater incidence of attempts in women and more successful suicides in men. The method chosen appears to be related to sex role, for example, passive (pills) for women and aggressive (guns or hanging) for men. It will be of considerable interest to observe whether, as the suicide rates for women increase, the means will also change.

As women compete with men in more areas, it is believed that not only will they manifest a greater incidence of lung cancer and heart disease, but they will also "choose" psychosomatic diseases like peptic ulcer, thought in the past to be related to stress in male-dominated occupations.

Whatever the trends, difficulties remain in relating sex-related, biological, hormonal, or behavioral patterns to disease entity or to morbidity and mortality data. Measuring the complex interactions of psyche, soma, learning, and social force has always presented methodological problems. But some sociological observations are of interest and are of probable relevance to the *use* of health care services, if not to the *incidence* of illness. For example, marriage appears to protect both males and females against admission to long-term psychiatric facilities,[87] although "the data suggest that marriage has protective effect for males but a detrimental effect for women."[45] Gove and Tudor[95] reported data that underscore the possible relevance of psychosocial factors, at least to the incidence of mental illness. They found that tightly structured, stable, family-oriented communities isolated for cultural influences have lower rates of mental illness.

There can be no doubt that illness behavior, like other behaviors, is strongly influenced by social learning, in the response to the effects of society and the destiny of anatomy. Lewis and Lewis[88] stated that

> Children are engaged early in life in social learning about their future roles as consumers of health services in society. At an early age girls acquire orientations associated with the tendency to seek care for many kinds of complaints, where boys learn to disregard pain and avoid demonstrating "sissy-like" behavior (that is, acting like girls).

Paradoxically, boys more than girls are more frequently taken to doctors by their mothers and admitted to hospitals, but when permitted to determine their own help-seeking behavior, girls visit physicians more often.[95]

The expectations arising from beliefs and attitudes about health "are reinforced by providers who treat patients as they expect them to want to be treated," and "this attitude helps to maintain the differences in the roles of women and men in society related to health and illness";[88] nonetheless, Lewis and Lewis do not accept the accusation that institutional medicine or male physicians are the sole villains in determining the health status of women.

One might speculate about the impact that women have had and continue to have on the use of health care services and health policy itself. Interestingly, this influence would seem to occur through the

illness behavior of women as a group rather than through their eleva-
tion in the medical hierarchy to positions of power and importance.
This social restriction to the consumer rather than the provider role
perhaps, in part, accounts for the rate of utilization of health care services by women and their status of "brokers" for their children and
husbands. Whether as consumers or providers, however, women's potential power in the health delivery field is unmistakable; which caretaking role society permits them to fulfill will probably determine how
they influence their family's health and illness behavior as well as that
of society at large. This influence, in turn, may well determine the
future ways in which complaints are reported and perceived, pain is
experienced and described, and diagnosis and treatment are negotiated.

CONCLUSION

We can expect the controversies over nature versus nurture, mind
versus body, biology versus society, and sex stereotyping versus sex
differences to continue. It is our purpose not to adopt an adversary
position but to note that the women's movement has, in the field of
medicine as in other vocational and avocational areas, promoted a
greater awareness of possible relationships that were little noted previously. Medical literature has been markedly deficient in reporting
sex-related differences in illness. Learning, sex-role stereotyping, and
physiological factors and illness behavior have all taken on greater
meaning. Even if the quest for sexual equality results in equity in male
and female mortality and morbidity, women's social status cannot be
ignored as an important vector in illness, disease, and health-care
seeking.

In the meantime, physicians must continue to inquire into the
meaning of a patient's presenting complaint, attempting always to
unearth the complex determinants of the symptom, while assessing
the patient's and their own behavior as part and parcel of the illness,
the diagnosis, and the treatment.

When all physicians, male and female, can accept symptoms as
compromise formations with multiple determinants, having both conscious and unconscious elements, terms like *crock, problem patient,* and
hypochondriac will find less expression in medical lexicography, and
painful patients will experience better treatment and care.

REFERENCES

1. Mencken HL: *In defense of women.* New York, Knopf, 1922.
2. National Center for Health Statistics, 1975.

3. The Statistical Bulletin of the Metropolitan Life Insurance Company, August 1974.
4. Reading A: Illness and disease, *Medical Clinics of North America* 61:703–710, 1977.
5. Cassell EJ: *Illness and disease. The healer's art: A new approach to the doctor-patient relationship.* New York, Lippincott, 1976.
6. Morgan WL, Engel GL: *The clinical approach to the patient.* Philadelphia, Saunders, 1969.
7. Feinstein AR: *Clinical judgment.* Baltimore, Williams & Wilkins, 1967.
8. Spiro HM: The tools of our trade: Some comments on disease and disorder, *New England Journal of Medicine* 292:575, 1975.
9. Mechanic D: Social psychologic factors affecting the presentation of bodily complaints, *New England Journal of Medicine* 286:1132–1139, 1972.
10. Parsons T: *The structure of social action.* Glencoe, Ill., Free Press, 1949.
11. Friedson E: Dilemmas in the doctor-patient relationship. In *Human behavior and social process.* Edited by Rose A. Boston, Houghton Mifflin, 1962.
12. Szasz T: *The myth of mental illness.* New York, Harper & Row, 1961.
13. Torrey EF: *The death of psychiatry.* Radnor' Pa., Chilton Book, 1974.
14. Illich I: *Medical nemesis.* London, Calder and Boyars, 1975.
15. Ehrenreich B, English D: *Complaints or disorders: The sexual politics of sickness.* New York, Feminist Press, 1973.
16. Levitt M, Langsley DG: The education of psychiatrists, *Change* 6:30–35, 1974.
17. Sontag S: *Illness as metaphor.* New York, Farrar, Straus & Giroux, 1978.
18. Szasz T: The communication of distress between child and parent, *British Journal of Medical Psychology* 32:161–170, 1959.
19. Freud A: The role of bodily illness in the mental life of children, *Psychoanalytical Study of the Child* 7:69–81, 1952.
20. Fabrega H: The study of disease in relation to culture, *Behavior Science* 17:183, 1972.
21. Beecher HK: *Measurement of subjective responses: Quantitative effects of drugs.* New York, Oxford University Press, 1959.
22. Zola IK: Culture and symptoms—An analysis of patients' presenting complaints, *American Sociological Review* 31:615–630, 1966.
23. Zbrowski M: Cultural components in response to pain, *Journal of Social Issues* 8:16, 1952.
24. Wolff, BD, Langley S: Cultural factors and the response to pain: A review, *American Anthropologist* 70:494–501, 1968.
25. Freud S: *New introductory lectures on psychoanalysis.* New York, Norton, 1933.
26. Nemiah JC: *Foundations of psychopathology.* New York, Oxford University Press, p. 121, 1961.
27. Schur M: Comments on the metapsychology of somatization, *Psychoanalytical Study of the Child* 10:119, 1955.
28. Brenner C: *An elementary textbook of psychoanalysis.* New York, Doubleday Anchor, p. 43, 1957.
29. Freud S: *The ego and the id.* Translated by J. Riviera. London, Hogarth Press, 1927.
30. Lipowski ZJ: The importance of body experience for psychiatry. *Comprehensive Psychiatry* 18:473–479, 1977.
31. Schilder P: *Image and appearance of the human body.* New York, International Universities Press, 1950.
32. Shontz FC: Body image and its disorders. In *Psychosomatic medicine.* Edited by Lipowski ZJ, Lipsitt DR, Whybrow PC. New York, Oxford University Press, 1977.
33. Fisher S: *Body consciousness.* New York, Aronson, p. 50, 1974.
34. Nadelson CR, Notman MT: Emotional aspects of the symptoms, functions and disorders of women. In *Psychiatric medicine.* Edited by Usdin G. New York, Brunner/Mazel, 1977.

35. Asken MJ: Psychoemotional aspects of mastectomy: A review of recent literature. *American Journal of Psychiatry* 132:56–59, 1975.
36. Polivz J: Psychological reactions to hysterectomy: A critical review. *American Journal of Obstetrics-Gynecology* 118:417–426, 1974.
37. Galenson E: Report of Proceedings of Panel on Psychology of Women, Chairman HP Blum, American Psychoanalytic Association, New York City, December 1975. *Journal of American Psychoanalytic Association* 26:163–177, 1978.
38. Kumin M: *The retrieval system.* New York, Viking, 1978.
39. Rosenbaum MB: *The changing body image of the female adolescent.* Presented at the 30th Annual Meeting of the American Psychiatric Association, Miami, May 4, 1977.
40. Ehrenreich B, English D: *Complaints and disorders: The sexual politics of sickness.* New York, Feminist Press, 1973.
41. Lennane KJ, Lennane RJ: Alleged psychogenic disorders in women: A possible manifestation of sexual prejudice, *NEJM* 288:288–292, 1973.
42. Bardwick JM: *Psychology of women: A study of biocultural conflicts.* New York, Harper & Row, p. 72, 1971.
43. Sommer B: Menstruation and behavior: A review, *Psychosomatic Medicine* 35:515–533, 1973.
44. Seiden AM: Overview: Research on the psychology of women, I and II. *American Journal of Psychiatry* 133:995–1007, 1111–1123, 1976.
45. Parlee M: *Psychological aspects of menstruation, childbirth and menopause: An overview with suggestions for further research.* Presented at the Conference on New Directions for Research on Women, Madison, Wis. May 31–June 2, 1975.
46. Weissman MM, Klerman GL: Sex differences and the epidemiology of depression, *Archives of General Psychiatry* 34:98–111, 1977.
47. Ivey ME, Bardwick JM: Patterns of affective fluctuation in the menstrual cycle, *Psychosomatic Medicine* 30:336–345, 1968.
48. Dalton K: *The premenstrual syndrome.* Springfield, Ill., Charles C Thomas, 1964.
49. Koeske RD: Premenstrual emotionality: Is biology destiny? *Women and Health* 1:11–14, 1976.
50. Gottschalk LA, Kaplan S, Gleser GD, Winget CM: Variations in the magnitude of emotion: A method applied to anxiety and hostility during phases of the menstrual cycle, *Psychosomatic Medicine* 24:300–311, 1962.
51. Sommer B: Menstrual cycle changes and intellectual performance, *Psychosomatic Medicine* 31:263–269, 1972.
52. Paige K: Women learn to sing the premenstrual blues, *Psychology Today* 7:41–46, 1973.
53. Castelnuovo-Tedesco P, Krout BM: Psychoanalytic aspects of chronic pelvic pain, *International Journal of Psychiatry in Medicine* 1:109–126, 1970.
54. Bradley JJ: Severe localized pain associated with the depressive syndrome, *British Journal of Psychiatry* 109:741–745, 1963.
55. Rangell L: Psychiatric aspects of pain, *Psychosomatic Medicine* 15:22–37, 1953.
56. Engel GC: "Psychogenic" pain and the pain-prone patient, *American Journal of Medicine* 26:899–918, 1959.
57. Walters A: Psychogenic regional pain alias hysterical pain, *Brain* 84:1–18, 1961.
58. Pilling LF, Brannick TL, Swenson WM: Psychologic characteristics of psychiatric patients having pain as a presenting symptom, *Canadian Medical Association Journal* 97:387–394, 1967.
59. Sternbach RA, Wolf SR, Murphy RW, Akeson WM: Aspects of chronic low back pain, *Psychosomatics* 14:52–56, 1973.
60. Woodforde JM, Merskey H: Personality traits of patients with chronic pain, *Journal of Psychosomatic Research* 16:167–172, 1972.

61. Lipsitt DR: Medical and psychological characteristics of "crocks," *International Journal of Psychiatry in Medicine* 1:15–25, 1970.
62. Pilowsky I: The response to treatment in hypochondriacal disorders, *Australian and New Zealand Journal of Psychiatry* 2:88–94, 1968.
63. Wahl CW: Unconscious factors in the psychodynamics of the hypochondriacal patient, *Psychosomatics* 4:9–14, 1963.
64. Mead BT: Management of hypochondriacal patients. *Journal of the American Medical Association* 192:119–121, 1965.
65. Ladee GA: *Hypochondriacal syndromes.* Amsterdam, Elsevier, 1966.
66. Lipsitt DR: Psychodynamic considerations of hypochondriasis, *Psychotherapy and Psychosomatics* 23:123–141, 1974.
67. Fenichel O: *The psychoanalytic theory of neurosis.* New York, Norton, 1945.
68. Lesse S: The multivariant masks of depression, *American Journal of Psychiatry* 124:35–40, 1968.
69. Diamond S: Depressive headaches, *Headache* 4:255–258, 1964.
70. Cassidy WL, Flanagan NB, Spelling BA, Cohen ME: Clinical observations in manic-depressive disease: A quantitative study of one hundred manic-depressive patients and fifty medically sick controls, *Journal of the American Medical Association* 164:1535–1546, 1957.
71. Sternbach R: *Pain patients: Traits and treatment.* New York, Academic Press, p. 42, 1974.
72. Merskey H, Hester RN: The treatment of chronic pain with psychotropic drugs, *Postgraduate Medical Journal* 48:594–598, 1972.
73. Reider N: Symptom substitution, *Bulletin of the Menninger Clinic* 40:629–640, 1976.
74. Kahana RJ, Bibring GL: Personality types in medical management. In *Psychiatry and medical practice in a general hospital.* Edited by Zinberg N. New York, International Universities Press, 1964.
75. Brenner C: The masochistic character, *Journal of the American Psychoanalytic Association* 7:197, 1959.
76. Lipsitt DR: *Geriatric patients who cannot afford to be well.* Presented at the 21st Annual Meeting of the Gerontological Society, Denver, November 1, 1968.
77. Riviere J: A contribution to the analysis of the negative therapeutic reaction, *International Journal of Psychoanalysis* 17:3104, 1936.
78. Hackett TP: The patient who doesn't want to get well, *Medical Economics,* March 7, 1977.
79. Szasz T: The psychology of persistent pain: A portrait of l'homme douloureux. In *Pain.* Edited by Soulairic A, Cahn J, Charpentier J. New York, Academic Press, 1968.
80. Lipsitt DR: The "rotating" patient: Challenge to psychiatrists, *Journal of Geriatric Psychiatry* 2:51–61, 1968.
81. von Mering O: The diffuse health aberration syndrome: A bio-behavioral study of the perennial outpatient. *Psychosomatics* 13:293–303, 1972.
82. Meyersburg HA, Boggs ST, Richmond MB: *The crock: A study of dysfunctional doctor-patient relationship in chronic illness.* Unpublished manuscript.
83. Groves JE: Taking care of the hateful patient, *New England Journal of Medicine* 298:883–887, 1978.
84. Chertok L: Mania operativa: Surgical addiction, *Psychiatry in Medicine* 3:105–107, 1972.
85. Menninger K: Polysurgery and polysurgical addiction, *Psychoanalytical Quarterly* 3:173–199, 1934.
86. Merskey H, Spear FG: Pain, *Psychol and Psychiat Res* 1:239–245, 1962.
87. Munro A, Neal CD: Psychiatric patients who undergo unnecessary operations, *International Mental Health Research Newsletter* 11:2–3, 1969.

88. Lewis CD, Lewis, MA: The potential impact of sexual equality on health, *New England Journal of Medicine* 297:863–870, 1977.
89. Vobecky J, Kelly A, Munan L: Population health care practices: An epidemiological study of physician visits, hospital admissions and drug consumption, *Canadian Journal of Public Health* 63:304–310, 1972.
90. Hinkle LE, Redmont R, Plummer N: An examination of the relation between symptoms, disability and serious illness in two homogeneous groups of men and women, *American Journal of Public Health* 50:1327–1336, 1960.
91. Enterline PE: Sick absence for men and women by marital status, *Archives of Environmental Health* 8:466–470, 1964.
92. Shuckit MA: The alcoholic woman: A literature review, *Psychiatry in Medicine* 3:37–43, 1972.
93. Winokur G, Clayton P: Family history studies: II. Sex differences and alcoholism in primary affective illness, *British Journal of Psychiatry* 113:973–979, 1967.
94. Gove WR: The relationship between sex roles, marital status and mental illness. *Social Forces* 51:34–44, 1972.
95. Gove WR, Tudor JF: Adult sex roles and mental illness. *American Journal of Sociology* 78:812–835, 1973.
96. Mechanic D: The influence of mothers on their children's health attitudes and behavior, *Pediatrics* 33:444–453, 1964.

Chapter 11

Emotional Reactions to the Miscarriage of a Consciously Desired Pregnancy

ROCHELLE FRIEDMAN AND KAREN A. COHEN

INTRODUCTION

Miscarriage* is a commonly occurring event. Any pregnancy that terminates spontaneously before the fetus reaches viability may be correctly termed a miscarriage. The majority of reported miscarriages occur in the second or third month of gestation. Early miscarriages, those occurring in the first month or so of pregnancy, often go unrecognized or are noted only as a delayed and perhaps heavier-than-usual menstrual period. Taking this into account, the actual incidence of miscarriage is probably considerably higher than statistics indicate. A conservative estimate is that between 14% and 18% of all pregnancies end in miscarriage.

In our culture, miscarriage is a death that goes unacknowledged by social ritual. It is celebrated in the tears of women, while its true significance is denied in the world of men. Although the loss of an

---

*The authors recognize that *spontaneous abortion* is the accepted medical term for a miscarriage. The word *abortion* has, however, a very different meaning for nonmedical people. Our subject is the emotional consequences of miscarriage for the women experiencing it. The perspective is the patient's, and so the term we use is hers.

ROCHELLE FRIEDMAN, M.D. • Psychiatrist, Massachusetts Institute of Technology, Cambridge; Clinical Associate in Psychiatry, Massachusetts General Hospital, Boston; Clinical Instructor in Psychiatry, Harvard University School of Medicine, Boston, Massachusetts. KAREN A. COHEN, M.A. • Program Coordinator for Health Education, Capital Area Community Health Plan, Albany, New York.

undesired pregnancy may be met with relief, the miscarriage of a consciously desired pregnancy is often experienced by the woman as a loss of major proportions. Her reaction to this loss may vary from mild depression to a pathological grief state.[1]

Physicians tend to regard miscarriage as an obstetrical crisis—a physiological event that rids the body of nonviable fetal material. For the most part, medical curiosity about the interplay between the emotions and miscarriage has been limited to speculation about the intrapsychic determinants of miscarriage[2,3,4,5,6,7,8]; at the same time, the often-encountered and frequently significant emotional sequelae of miscarriage have been largely ignored.

In our work as psychiatrists in a university-based practice and as a health educator involved in prenatal education, we have worked with people for whom the spontaneous abortion of a consciously desired pregnancy constituted a major life crisis. In this chapter, we describe the pattern of emotional and social reactions commonly experienced after the miscarriage of a consciously desired pregnancy. We also share our understanding of why the loss is traumatic and suggest some ways in which care for this population can be improved. The material presented has been drawn from several years of clinical work with women who have miscarried, including women seen in brief psychotherapy following a miscarriage (35 cases); women seen in long-term psychotherapy (8 cases); and a group of 5 women who participated in a time-limited postmiscarriage psychotherapy group.[15] In 5 cases, the husband and wife were seen jointly. Although the population with whom we have worked is small, we believe that attention to their experience is warranted. We share our findings in the belief that one must begin somewhere, and that a phenomenological description is an essential first step toward understanding the experience of miscarriage from the patient's perspective.

EMOTIONAL REACTIONS TO MISCARRIAGE

THE PREGNANCY AND ITS LOSS A pregnant woman's attachment to her future child begins well before birth. The strength and quality of this attachment seem to be a function of several factors: the woman's own mothering experience; the nature of her identification with her own mother; her acceptance of the mothering role for herself; her capacity to have positive feelings about herself and by extension about her child; and her ability to form a relationship with another person. What part, if any, maternal instinct and hormonally induced receptive tendencies play in promoting the mother's attachment to her child has been speculated on but remains unknown.[9]

Commonly, the pregnant woman forms a fantasy image of—as well as an attachment to—her future child early in the pregnancy. As the pregnancy progresses, the child's movements enhance the mother's real knowledge of it and also help her to experience it as separate from herself. Throughout pregnancy, the child may be experienced by the mother both as a part of the self and as a separate being who is loved.

A woman's ego structure appears to influence her capacity for a relationship with her unborn child in much the same way as it does other relationships in her life: If a pregnant woman forms an attachment to her child, its loss by miscarriage has a significant psychological impact on her, however early in the pregnancy the loss actually occurs. We see a woman's ability to mourn the child she has lost through miscarriage as evidence of her capacity for relatedness, and not a "neurotic" overreaction, as is commonly thought.

MISCARRIAGE: THEORETICAL CONSIDERATIONS The spectrum of emotional reactions to miscarriage is wide. The miscarriage of an unwanted pregnancy tends to bring relief, while the loss of a much desired pregnancy often causes sadness and disappointment. Grief and mourning are appropriate emotional responses to the loss of a significant object and are considered pathological only if any of the symptoms are excessively intense, or if the process of mourning is unduly long. An inability to mourn a loss may also be pathological. The usual mourning period following miscarriage is several weeks to several months in duration; however, mourning of a year or more is not unusual.

The way in which an individual copes with miscarriage appears to be a function of those same factors that determine how she deals with the psychobiological crises of pregnancy. Bibring enumerated what she felt to be the critical determinants of a pregnant woman's ability to cope: her individual personality structure, her prepregnancy adjustment and coping mechanisms, and her life setting and family constellation.[10,11]

It is common for the pregnant woman to develop a strong attachment to her future child very early in the pregnancy. That this attachment is to an "other" known only through physical sensation, or by fantasy alone, does not seem to make the attachment any the less intense. However early in the pregnancy the miscarriage occurs, and whether or not what is lost is a blighted ovum, the feelings of grief that accompany the loss can be considerable.

When miscarriage occurs, the woman suffers many losses: narcissistic injury, object loss (albeit the loss of a fantasized object), and other losses that are derivatives of these. While most women experience the loss of the child as the single most significant issue, the loss of "being pregnant" and the loss of the fantasy of the self as the mothering person are also important issues for many. Derivative losses that tend to be significant are the loss of being special and the loss of being cared for in special ways by husband and family, and, not insignificantly, by the medical establishment.

When a woman gives birth, she experiences the loss of the child that was part of her, while gaining an outside child. The woman who has miscarried suffers a double sense of emptiness.

Mourning someone who is not physically present is known to be difficult. The woman who has miscarried has no tangible outside child to mourn. In addition, she has no memories and no shared life experiences to facilitate mourning.

The miscarried fetus is an internally experienced child to the mother, and perhaps to a few people close to her; to the rest of the world, a miscarried fetus is someone who did not exist. This discrepancy between a woman's internal life experience and social reality complicates the already difficult task of mourning. In our culture, miscarriage is a nonevent. Our discomfort with death, our lack of ritual, and our failure to appreciate a woman's internal life experiences all discourage acknowledgment that something of significance has occurred, thereby hindering the mourning process.

GRIEF AND MOURNING. The individual who has lost a beloved person often goes through a grief process that consists of several stages. We have found that women who have miscarried a consciously desired pregnancy commonly experience a grief process that parallels that described by Lindemann.[12] The women in our sample commonly had feelings of disbelief and experienced an emotional numbness on first learning that miscarriage was inevitable. For many, these feelings were most pronounced in the period before the miscarriage actually occurred. Two women who knew that they were carrying nonviable fetal material for several weeks before they finally miscarried reported recurrent feelings of disbelief during this period: Only after they finally miscarried did the numbness give way to feelings of anguish and despair.

In the initial stage of the grief process, denial is often utilized as a means of coping with an overwhelming loss. Through denial, the acute emotional impact is diminished and the individual gains an opportunity to mobilize her resources and to come to terms with her loss. The passage of time, a supportive environment, accurate information about what has happened, and opportunities to ventilate and to share grief all seem to aid the bereaved woman in accepting her loss.

The second phase of acute mourning is characterized by an increased acceptance of death. During this period, the bereaved woman tends to be preoccupied with thoughts of the lost child, to feel somatic distress, to cry easily, and to feel depressed and inadequate. Guilt, anger, blame, and jealousy are also commonly experienced during this stage.

In our sample, the majority of women experienced some guilt following miscarriage, although all of the pregnancies were consciously desired and none of the women had made attempts to induce abortion. Many of the women shared fantasies that their thoughts or actions had caused the death. Connections were frequently made between the subsequent miscarriage and particular events, such as traveling, sexual intercourse, or physical exertion. Others denied any feeling of responsibility but experienced a vague sense of guilt nonetheless. Folklore about miscarriage usually served to reinforce this guilt, since most of the myths imply a causal relationship between something the woman has done, or has failed to do, and a miscarriage: "You shouldn't have had intercourse at the time of month when your menstrual period would have been due"; "You shouldn't have moved that heavy furniture"; "You shouldn't have waited so long to have a child"; etc.

The near universality with which our sample of otherwise "healthy" women expressed some feelings of guilt raises some interesting and still unanswered questions. Is the guilt a woman feels following miscarriage a consequence of prior ambivalence toward the pregnancy, an internalization of society's ideas about cause and effect, or a manifestation of her feelings about not being in control of her bodily processes and of having failed as a woman? Unfortunately, most of our psychotherapeutic interventions were not extensive enough to provide answers to these questions.

Anger and blame were often directed outward as well as at the self. Anger was aroused in response to feelings of helplessness, as a reaction to the deprivation that the woman had experienced, and in relation to whatever or whoever she felt had let her down: God, her husband, her obstetrician, or Fate. In those cases where a husband or an obstetrician was the recipient of the anger, a displacement of anger from the dead fetus for dying to a third party sometimes appeared to be present.

The reported frequency with which women switch from one obstetrician to another after a miscarriage appears to be one indication of the intensity of this anger. In all likelihood, anger at the obstetrician is not only a displacement but also a response to the physician's failure to be sufficiently supportive during the mourning process.

Almost all of the women with whom we spoke reported some feelings of jealousy. Although the strongest feelings of jealousy were usually experienced toward pregnant friends or relatives, it was not unusual for women to report experiencing jealousy in response to women whom they did not know, but who were pregnant or the mothers of infants. During the period of acute grief, social confrontations that either stimulated feelings of jealousy or brought the women into direct confrontation with their loss were generally avoided.

The woman who has had a miscarriage is especially vulnerable to feelings of inadequacy. She may feel diffuse anxiety about the functioning of her biological processes, or concern that she is "damaged" in some way. It is not uncommon for a woman with underlying concerns or conflicts about her femininity, her reproductive adequacy, or her ability to mother to experience a miscarriage as evidence of her own failure in one or several of these areas. Anxiety about the capacity to achieve and sustain a pregnancy appears to be only one expression of these more general concerns. This anxiety has been observed in women who in the past had never encountered any difficulty in becoming pregnant, as well as in those who had:

> "I am still (four months later) experiencing the mental pain, especially as this is when it was due. I am bottled up with fear of not becoming pregnant again—I've had a lot of female problems in the past. My parents, brother, and husband cannot understand why I'm not over this, and I therefore cannot discuss my innermost feelings with them. My doctor suggested a psychologist—my husband doesn't think I need one. The only thing I need is a baby and that's the one thing I haven't been able to acquire."

Anxiety about one's ability to produce a normal child is also frequently experienced. The woman who learns that she was carrying a "blighted ovum" may have concerns about being defective and about producing defective children. Similar concerns are often experienced by women who have miscarried genetically defective fetal tissue. The woman who learns that no evidence of fetal material was found on pathological study may feel that she has been dealt a double blow. What pleasure she may have taken in her ability to conceive a pregnancy may be eroded if she interprets the report as casting doubt on whether she had ever really been pregnant: "If they couldn't find anything, maybe I was never pregnant."

Most women welcome the arrival of the first menstrual period, postmiscarriage, as an indication that a new pregnancy can soon be attempted. Subsequent menstrual periods are experienced as failure and are usually accompanied by feelings of sadness and disappointment. The menses are often experienced as painful evidence of the nonpregnant state and are unconsciously associated with the miscarriage.

It is not infrequent for a woman's feelings of inferiority and worthlessness to spread beyond the biological; when this occurs, more generalized feelings of self-doubt and low self-esteem result.

According to classical psychoanalytic theory, the more intensely ambivalent a woman is about a given pregnancy, the more likely she is to experience a severe depressive reaction after a miscarriage.[3,9] It is our impression that the presence of unconscious ambivalence toward the pregnancy is only one of several factors that might influence a woman's reaction to its loss. Since some degree of ambivalence must be quite common—if Bibring's view of pregnancy as a time of intense psychological upheaval is correct[10,11,13]—it is difficult to determine what effect, if any, it has on the grief process. Several factors that clearly seem to create a predisposition to intense mourning are a history of multiple miscarriages; marginal fertility; advanced age; unusual vulnerability to loss or a compromised ability to cope; and miscarriage late in the pregnancy.

Miscarriage as a Life Crisis

The woman who has miscarried is often deprived of ongoing services at a time when her need for care is great. Traditionally, obstetrical services have been oriented toward maintaining the physical health and well-being of the mother–fetus unit; when this relationship is prematurely disrupted by miscarriage, obstetrical care is most often terminated. Similarly, few supportive social services are available to help the woman deal with her loss.* The helping professions, too, have failed to recognize the needs of the majority of women who have miscarried.

It is not clear why a life crisis that affects so many people has received so little attention from the medical and social community. Is it because the physician views miscarriage solely as a benevolent physiological mechanism that rids the body of nonviable fetal material? Is it because miscarriage is seen as a medical and emotional problem that affects only women, so that, like other difficulties peculiar to women, it has been trivialized and ignored? Is it because the mourning period postmiscarriage is thought to be self-limited and easily remedied by a new pregnancy? Is it because a physician, in part, experiences miscarriage as his or her own failure? Or is it that our society

*In a few cities, organizations exist that offer services to women following miscarriage. Examples of these organizations are SHARE, Resolve, AMEND, and The Compassionate Friends (see Appendix).

has systematically avoided confronting intense emotional responses evoked by such life crises as irrevocable loss, fatal illness, death, and miscarriage?

Miscarriage is a life crisis for the woman, for the father-to-be, and for any existing children. Like pregnancy, miscarriage is a life crisis for which modern Western society makes few allowances. In a discussion of the psychological processes in pregnancy, Grete Bibring wrote,

> What was once a crisis with carefully worked out traditional customs of giving support to the woman passing through this crisis period, has become at this time a crisis with no mechanisms within the society for helping the woman involved in this profound change of conflict solutions and adjustive tasks.[13]

Nor are there mechanisms for helping the woman through the trauma of miscarriage. The loss of the fetus is a death without a ritual, a life crisis that goes virtually unacknowledged by society.

The following comment illustrates the postmiscarriage woman's reaction:

> "One minute I was pregnant, and the next I wasn't—I was told that I would have an operation in a few hours and could go to work on Monday, like nothing happened—my whole life changed in a couple of minutes. Something that was a part of me was gone all of a sudden—like losing a limb. The doctor doesn't think about all that, because he is thinking about saving your life—while you are thinking of months of your life, and your dreams shot to hell."

EFFECTS OF MISCARRIAGE ON THE FAMILY. Family, friends, and medical practitioners shared a common tendency to avoid the mourner's painful feelings. The net effect of this avoidance is often to leave the woman feeling isolated in her grief. Even when a husband shares in the grief, the woman is apt to resent him for escaping the full emotional burden of the loss. Most men develop an attachment to the future child later on in the pregnancy and less intensely than their wives. While it is not unusual for a woman to experience grief in response to a miscarriage occurring during the earliest stages of pregnancy, in our experience most men either were unable to cathect (develop an attachment to) the child during pregnancy or were able to do so only after they could observe tangible evidence of its existence. Once the child was cathected, its loss by miscarriage was apt to be experienced as a significant loss and was reacted to by the men with disappointment and sadness.

Miscarriage reactions among husbands were reported by all of the women we saw. Disappointment and depression, concern about real or imagined responsibility for the miscarriage, and feelings of helplessness were common reactions. Other responses of the husband included blaming and feeling blamed, and anger at the woman's depressive withdrawal and/or her failure to respond to his ministrations.

Cain et al. reviewed the reverberations of miscarriage throughout the family in their study of "Children's Disturbed Reactions to Their Mother's Miscarriage."[14] Typically, a child's initial reaction to miscarriage is one of puzzlement and confusion about exactly what happened and why. This response is often compounded by the parents' tendency to deny their children's awareness of and reactions to the miscarriage.

The child's own reactions to miscarriage seem to be determined by the child's personality structure, by his or her level of development, by the concepts and understanding of pregnancy and miscarriage available to him or her at this level of development, by the child's own wishes for the unborn child, by what the child sees of the miscarriage or is told about it, and by the parents' responses to the miscarriage.

Miscarriage reactions in children may range from disturbances of a minimal and transient nature to those that have significant and far-reaching effects on the child and secondarily on his or her family. Children's overt and immediate symptomatic responses to the miscarriage may include anger, aggression, depression, phobic behavior, nightmares, and anxiety. Children may blame the mother for destroying the unborn baby; they may experience disappointment and anger at the loss of the expected sibling; or they may feel guilt about causing the miscarriage through destructive, jealous anger at the expected rival or through what they perceive to have been their own destructive behavior.[14]

Cain also described enduring psychopathology discernible in adults who, as children, experienced their mothers' miscarriages. The residual effects varied from isolated fantasies, which minimally affected the individual's basic personality structure, to critical and pervasive effects on character structure. It seems that to appreciate the full impact of miscarriage, one must assess not only its immediate physical and emotional impact on the mother, but also its many and varied effects on other family members.

LIFE PLANNING AND SCHEDULING ISSUES. Pregnancy, in general—and miscarriage, especially—raises many of the questions asked when one is planning one's life. Among them: In what order do a man and woman married to one another study, pursue careers, relocate, acquire property, travel, and start or continue to have children? A woman who miscarries finds herself in limbo—faced with figuring out what the next step is when the previous step didn't work out. Decisions about whether to change jobs, move, buy a house, or go back to school may have been based on the pregnancy and future parenthood. After a miscarriage, life-planning decisions must be made without knowing when or if the woman will conceive again.

MEDICAL CARE AND MISCARRIAGE

HOW THE SYSTEM OPERATES. For many healthy women, a miscarriage may be the first substantial contact, apart from routine checkups, with the medical care system. Until a miscarriage occurs or threatens to occur, a pregnant woman has generally been seen on a regular basis and has been monitored for a variety of signs of well-being. The transition from being a well pregnant woman anticipating a healthy baby to being a patient who is in danger of losing, or who has already lost, the pregnancy may be sudden and difficult to cope with. As a patient, the woman who miscarries frequently takes away from the experience negative impressions of the medical care system. These impressions are based on the quality of her experiences with her physician, with other care givers, and with the hospital where she receives care.

Physicians and Nurses. Women in our sample based their assessment of the quality of care they had received both on their physician's ability to deal with the physical aspects of the miscarriage process and on his or her capacity to be empathetic and supportive. None of them had significant complaints about the quality of the medical care that they had received, despite the loss of the pregnancy in all cases. However, almost all had significant reservations about the way in which their own physicians had related to them during the miscarriage and its aftermath. They experienced their physicians variously as distant and inaccessible, as uncaring, and as tending to avoid emotionally charged confrontations. This impression probably stems from a difference in perspective. Although most physicians regard the loss of a desired pregnancy as an unfortunate occurrence, their responses are likely to be influenced by several factors: (1) the knowledge that in 50%–75% of cases, what is lost is a blighted ovum; (2) their failure to appreciate the extent of their patient's attachment to the imagined–real child she was carrying; (3) their belief that the loss is replaceable; and (4) their greater emotional distance from the loss. Nurses and nurse–midwives were generally perceived as more empathetic, caring, and responsive to their patients' needs than physicians, largely because of their willingness to extend physical and emotional comfort and support, as well as their greater ability to tolerate expressions of grief.

Hospitalization. Since the majority of miscarriages occur in the early months of pregnancy—75% in the first trimester, 25% in the second— it is unlikely that either member of a couple, particularly if it is their first child, has ever been inside the hospital where the woman is to deliver. At a time then of unanticipated stress, the couple must cope with an unfamiliar hospital and its personnel, facilities, procedures, and rules.

Unfortunately, the trauma of unanticipated hospitalization is all too frequently increased by rooming arrangements that may compound a woman's pain. It is fairly common practice to hospitalize women who have miscarried on obstetrical floors, or on wards with women having elective abortions. The obstetrical floor presents the woman who has miscarried with an unavoidable reminder of what she has lost, while hospitalization on wards with women having elective abortions confronts her with a painful paradox. The latter arrangement also increases the likelihood that she may have to deal with hospital staff members who mistakenly believe that she has elected an abortion. Separating the woman from her spouse for all procedures is another hospital practice that tends to increase anxiety for the couple.

> "At admission, I asked if I could possibly be placed in a room other than on the maternity floor. I was told that there was only one room available in the entire hospital and that was on the maternity floor. I can accept that all patients of an OB-GYN type would better be housed on the same floor in order for the best nursing care to be given to the patients. I then asked (in tears, even) if I could possibly use the stairs to get to this room so that I would not have to pass by the nursery. I was told that this was not allowed, but that I could be taken by a route that did not pass by the nursery. When the aide came to take me to the room, I again made the same request to her and received the same answers.
>
> "When I got off the elevator, there was the nursery right in front of me. Although the drapes were closed, I could hear the cries of the babies. To a woman who is carrying in her body the dead baby she has so long desired, this amounts to torture of the most inhumane and cruel kind."

IMPROVING CARE. There are a number of ways in which the existing medical care system could be altered to deal more effectively with miscarriage.

The Need for Information. The women in our sample were unanimous in their desire for more information from the obstetrician at all stages of the pregnancy and miscarriage.

Obstetricians rarely inform pregnant women of the possibility of miscarriage, although there is at least a 1 in 6 chance that any given pregnancy will not be successful. It is a commonly held belief that presenting the newly pregnant woman with this information would make her unnecessarily anxious. None of the women with whom we worked knew how common miscarriage was until after they had miscarried; the majority felt that their experience was unique and that they had been singled out. They felt that even though previous knowl-

edge about the actual incidence of miscarriage would not have miti-
gated the grief they experienced, it might have allowed them to cope
with their loss in a more realistic manner.

At the time when miscarriage is a possibility or an inevitability,
the knowledge women want is very specific: what to look for, what to
do and when, what to expect, what not to do, and what they can anticipate in the way of hospital and medical procedures.

After the miscarriage, the woman and the couple want to know:
What happened and why? Did they do anything to bring on the miscarriage? Could they have done anything to prevent it? They want to
know the results of laboratory tests, and they want clear and detailed
information about any findings that might affect subsequent pregnancies. They also want to know how long to wait before trying to conceive again.

When specific information is not available, it is still helpful to
address the patient's concerns and to provide information about what
is generally known. If this is not done, many patients hold themselves
responsible, blame others, or resort to magical thinking in an effort to
establish causation. A patient's limited capacity to utilize factual information during the period of acute grief, when the emotions have
primacy, should not be interpreted as a reason to withhold information. While knowledge of what occurred will probably not erase the
grief, it does provide a framework for ordering the experience and
making it more comprehensible.

Providing Support. Many women felt that the same physician, who
had been warm and supportive during the pregnancy, was cool and
unavailable at the time of miscarriage: "He never once looked at me;
it was as if all of a sudden I had become a nonperson"; "I was told
not to worry and then left completely alone"; "I was crying, and he
kept telling me that it was all for the best." Our patients often interpreted the physician's apparent aloofness as criticism or lack of concern. The physician who already has a relationship with his or her
patient is in a unique position to help her cope with the crisis of miscarriage. In order to do so, however, the physician must first be aware
of the patient's need for emotional support. The physician can provide
support and facilitate mourning by helping the patient to digest the
loss and to make it real; by encouraging her to review the pregnancy
and the events leading up to the miscarriage; and by helping her to
ventilate her feelings. Most helpful is the physician's ability to understand the woman's emotional reaction and to respond empathetically
to the loss she has suffered.

Although the reactions of the husbands in our sample differed
from those of their wives, they, too, had a great many emotions to
cope with: anger, guilt, disappointment, sadness. A sensitivity on the

part of the obstetrician to the man's reactions and a practice of including the man in discussions pre- and postmiscarriage would enhance the ability of both partners to cope effectively. Physicians and nurse–midwives also need to know what counseling resources are available in their community, and they need to establish links with the mental health professions. We feel that information about the availability of counseling services should be provided routinely to every woman who miscarries, whether or not she specifically requests it.

Children, too, may react to a miscarriage in the family. Many parents tend to avoid the issue with their children, thereby leaving them to deal, unaided, with their fantasies, guilt, fears, and sadness. The physician is in a good position to encourage parents to deal with this issue and to help them give clear and honest explanations. Even with clarification, it is difficult for children to grasp the loss of something that never quite existed for them.

Extending the Time of Obstetric Care. We found that just at the time when the woman was most in need of medical support, that support was cut off. The only standard postmiscarriage care is a checkup, usually four to six weeks after the miscarriage. We would recommend that care be extended and more frequent during the postmiscarriage period.

Modifying Hospital Procedures. Current hospital practices need to be modified so that they are more responsive to the special needs of the woman who has miscarried. First, all personnel should be informed about the patient's situation so as to avoid causing needless grief and embarrassment. Medical, nursery, and administrative staff need help in recognizing the emotional consequences of miscarriage, and they need to reflect this awareness in their behavior.

Ideally, a patient's preferences about a private or shared room should be elicited, and if at all possible honored. When possible, patients should be given the option of hospitalization either on the maternity floor or elsewhere in the hospital if they prefer.

During the miscarriage process the patient needs good medical care; equally important is her need for support and comfort from those who are close to her. As far as is possible, visiting hours should be flexible and tailored to the needs of the individual couple. If the couple wish to be together during procedures, and there is no medical counterindication, this should be permitted whenever possible.

Counseling. A range of counseling services needs to be developed to meet varied needs. Although the majority of individuals who suffer miscarriage do not develop a gross psychological disturbance, many might benefit from counseling. Education, support, and insight oriented therapy, singly or in combination, can be successfully utilized to treat individuals or couples. The mode of treatment should, as in all therapy, be tailored to the specific needs of the individual or couple.

CONCLUSION

Miscarriage is common and is, for the vast majority of women who experience it, traumatic. A woman who has lost a consciously desired pregnancy through miscarriage is like to experience what appears to be a fairly classical mourning reaction, usually of several weeks' to several months' duration. During that period, she is apt to feel unusually vulnerable, to cry easily, and to see the world, intermittently, as disappointing and frustrating. For some women, miscarriage is the first experience of loss; for others, the experience may reopen issues of previous loss. Most women experience the loss as specific and irreplaceable. The loss is painful regardless of when in the pregnancy the miscarriage occurs and regardless of the cause. While each woman's response to miscarriage is in part a reflection of her own unique past history, her current environment, and her particular coping abilities, there are many shared elements in the miscarriage experience. It is a sad and trying time for a woman and for a couple: dreams are shattered, life plans are interfered with, and painful losses are sustained.

Miscarriage represents a death or loss for which society has no ritual, no traditional form of acknowledgment. Neither obstetrics nor psychiatry has dealt effectively with this particular life crisis. Obstetrics has concentrated on the medical management and ignored the emotional consequences. Psychiatry has dealt only with extreme reactions to miscarriage and has not provided preventive or life-crisis intervention. Support from friends and relatives and from medical caregivers is vital to the well-being of the patient and her spouse who have suffered a miscarriage, but it is not enough.

With the help of women (and their spouses) who have experienced miscarriage, we have been able to identify some of the problems that face the woman who has miscarried. It is our hope that observations such as ours will help both potential patients and health workers to think about the issues that miscarriage raises for the people experiencing it, and to deal with this life crisis more effectively.

APPENDIX

AMEND   Moreen Conley
                               4324 Berrwick Terrace
                               St. Louis, Missouri 63128
                               (314) 487-7582

SHARE

National Headquarters
800 East Carpenter
Springfield, Illinois 62769
(217) 544-6464

Resolve, Inc.

P.O. Box 474
Belmont, Massachusetts 02178
(617) 484-2424

The Compassionate Friends

National Headquarters
P.O. Box 1347
Oak Brook, Illinois 60521
(312) 323-5010

REFERENCES

1. Corney RT, Horton FT, Jr: Pathological grief following spontaneous abortion, *American Journal of Psychiatry* 131(7):825–827, July 1974.
2. Grimm ER: Psychological investigation of habitual abortion, *Psychosomatic Medicine* 24:369, 1962.
3. Deutsch H: *The psychology of women.* Volume 2. *Motherhood.* New York, Grune & Stratton, 1945.
4. Tupper C, *et al*: The problem of spontaneous abortion, *American Journal of Obstetrics and Gynecology* 73:2, 313, 1957.
5. Michel-Wolfromm H: The psychological factor in spontaneous abortion, *Journal of Psychosomatic Research* 12:67–71, 1968.
6. Malmquist A, Kaij L, Nilsson A: Psychiatric aspects of spontaneous abortion, I, *Journal of Psychosomatic Research* 13:45–51, 1969.
7. Kaij L, Malmquist A, Nilsson A: Psychiatric aspects of spontaneous abortion, II, *Journal of Psychosomatic Research* 13:45–51, 1969.
8 .Simon NM, Rothman P, Goff JT, *et al*: Psychological factors related to spontaneous and therapeutic abortion, *American Journal of Obstetrics and Gynecology* 104:799–806, 1969.
9. Benedek T: The psychobiology of pregnancy. Boston, Little, Brown, 1970.
10. Bibring GL, Dwyer TF, Huntington DS, Valenstein AF: A study of the psychological processes in pregnancy and of the earliest mother-child relationship: I. Some propositions and comments. *Psychoanalytic study of the child*, Vol. 16. New York, International University Press, 1961.
11. Bibring GL, Dwyer TF, Huntington DS, Valenstein AF: A study of the psychological processes in pregnancy and of the earliest mother-child relationship: II. Methodological considerations. *Psychoanalytic study of the child,* Vol. 16. New York, International University Press, 1961.
12. Lindemann E: Symptomatology and management of acute grief. *American Journal of Psychiatry,* 101, 1944.
13. Bibring GL: *Some considerations of the psychological processes in pregnancy,* Vol. 14. New York, International University Press, 1959.
14. Cain AC, Erikson ME, Fast I, Vaughan RA: Children's disturbed reactions to their mother's miscarriage, *Psychosomatic Medicine* 24(1):58–66, January–February, 1964.
15. Friedmann RR, Cohen K: The peer support group: A model for dealing with the emotional aspects of miscarriage, *GROUP* 4:42–48, 1980.

Chapter 12

Depression in Women: Epidemiology, Explanations, and Impact on the Family

Myrna M. Weissman and Gerald L. Klerman

Depression is a disorder of special importance when one is considering the health of women. A review of the epidemiological literature finds few exceptions to the observation that clinical depression is more common in women than in men.[1] Moreover, its incidence may be increasing, and it is no longer confined to the middle-aged, the elderly, or the hospitalized. Today, the typically depressed patient is apt to be a young woman in her reproductive years, often married, living at home, and rearing children. The illness has a serious impact on her capacity to enjoy life.

This chapter describes the nature and epidemiology of depression and the various explanations for the increased predominance of depression among women, and it concludes with a description of the impact of maternal depression on family life and children.

Depression: A Mood, a Symptom, a Syndrome

The term *depression* covers a broad spectrum of moods and behavior, which range from the disappointments and sadness of normal life to the suicidal acts of severe melancholics. There are at least three

Myrna M. Weissman, Ph.D. • Professor of Psychiatry and Epidemiology; Director, Depression Research Unit, Yale University School of Medicine, Department of Psychiatry, Connecticut Mental Health Center, New Haven, Connecticut.   Gerald L. Klerman, M.D. • Professor of Psychiatry, Harvard Medical School, Massachusetts General Hospital, Boston.

meanings of the term; depression is a mood, a symptom, and a syndrome. Depression as a normal mood is a universal phenomenon that no one escapes. It can be produced by situations of loss and is a signal that something is wrong in one's life.

Depression as a symptom, or an abnormal mood, is also common. There is an indistinct line between what is normal and what is pathological. Depression of mood that is unduly persistent, pervasive, or inappropriate to circumstances is generally considered pathological. The symptom of depression is, again, a common one experienced by most psychiatric patients, including many who may not be regarded as suffering primarily from depression but may be alcoholic, schizophrenic, etc.

Beyond the symptom, there is a more specific and limited psychiatric phenomenon, the syndrome. The term *syndrome* refers to a cluster of symptoms, usually having a common mechanism but a variety of causes. This is clinical depression as most psychiatrists are concerned with it, and as it will be described here.

THE SYNDROME OF CLINICAL DEPRESSION

Depressive mood is described as feeling sad, blue, and unable to experience pleasure and is often accompanied by crying and a sense of fear and anxiety. These are typical features of the depressive syndrome. There are many additional disturbances, the most characteristic of which are feelings described as helplessness, hopelessness, and worthlessness, ranging from a vague sense of lowered self-esteem and denigration of accomplishments to intense feelings of failure. Closely allied may be thoughts of suicide, ranging from the feeling that life is not worth living, to wishing one were dead, to thoughts of taking one's life, to unsuccessful or successful suicide. The helplessness of depression takes different forms. Besides the feeling of being helpless, useless, and unable to function, actual activities might be impaired. Apathy, poor concentration, neglect of personal grooming, and difficulty in completing work may occur. Many depressives show psychomotor retardation—a slowing in the speed of thoughts, speech, and movement—which, in the rare case, may extend to virtual immobility and absence of speech. The opposite state, overactivity or agitation, may also occur. Sleep disturbances usually occur and include difficulty getting to sleep on retiring, disturbed sleep with troubled dreams, or waking very early in the morning. Occasionally, patients sleep excessively. Likewise, appetite disturbance is common, usually loss of appetite and weight loss, but at times, appetite may be increased. There are many other symptoms, and not all depressed patients show all of these features. Because of the diversity of symptoms, numerous attempts are being made to define subtypes of depression with specific symptomatology, age of onset, and family pattern. While these classification schemes are of considerable research interest, none, as yet, is completely satisfactory.

Epidemiology

The epidemiology of depression (its prevalence and its sex and age distribution) highlights its significance to women.

Prevalence. Regardless of how the figures are calculated, there is little doubt that depression is a common disorder. The lifetime expectancy of developing a depressive illness of any type ranges from 8.5% to 17.7%. These figures are based on several Scandinavian studies and include a broad range of disorders.[2] A recent community survey in New Haven, Connecticut, conducted by Myers and Weissman, showed that approximately 4.5% of women had a diagnosis of major depressive disorder at the time of the interview.[3] The figures were twice those of the men interviewed.

Hospital admissions reflect rates for the most severely ill—usually those classified as manic or psychotic depressives—as well as the availability of treatment facilities and the utilization practices in the community. In the United States, the most recent figure for the annual rate of first admissions to psychiatric facilities for the treatment of depressive disorders is about 11 per 100,000 population.

Outpatient figures reflect the rate for the mildly to moderately ill. A recent report from the National Institute of Mental Health noted that depression is one of the leading diagnoses for persons seeking outpatient treatment in the United States.[4]

Untreated depression is considerably more common. It is believed that most individuals with depressive illness never see a physician. Two independent studies estimated that only 20% of depressed persons received treatment.[5]

Sex Ratio. Although there is considerable debate about the reasons, there are few exceptions to the observation that depressions are considerably more common in women than in men. This is true regardless of the time period, the country, or the method of ascertainment.[1] Moreover, the age of greatest risk for depression in women coincides with the reproductive years, age 25–44. Therefore, depression can have an impact on family life.

A number of explanations for the female predominance have been offered. One set of explanations questions whether the findings are "real" and hypothesizes that they are more likely an artifact accounted for by women's perceptions of stress, their coping responses and willingness to express affective symptoms, and the high frequency with which they seek medical help. Alternately, the finding is considered a real phenomenon and attributed to female biological susceptibility, genetic or endocrine, or to social causes.*

THE ARTIFACT HYPOTHESIS ABOUT THE SEX DIFFERENCE

The artifact hypothesis proposes that women perceive, acknowledge, report, and seek help for stress and symptoms differently than men and that these factors account for the sex ratio findings. Put another way, the artifact hypothesis holds that response set and labeling processes serve to overestimate the female depressives. Also included under the artifact hypothesis is the observation that alcohol use and abuse are considerably more common in men. It has been hypothesized that depression and alcoholism are different but equivalent disorders. Women get depressed. Men are reluctant to admit being depressed or to seek treatment, and they mitigate their symptoms by drinking. Men self-prescribe alcohol as a psychopharmacological treatment for depression.

In most industrial nations, women clients predominate in the health care system and men clients in the law enforcement system and correctional institutions. It is hypothesized, therefore, that depressed men may show up in the courts rather than in the clinics; for example, a depressed man may get drunk, get into a fight, and end up in court. Our review of evidence for the artifact hypothesis has led us to conclude that the sex differences are not an artifact; they are real.

A recent review by Weissman and Klerman[1] found that women do not report more stressful life events than men and do not judge life events as more stressful. While women acknowledge having symptoms and affective distress more frequently than men, it does not seem to be because they feel less stigma or because they wish to win approval. Women and men have different help-seeking patterns. However, increased female utilization of health care would not account for the preponderance of depressed women in community surveys, since most survey "cases" were not in psychiatric treatment either at the time of the interview or in the past.

There is no question that more males than females have alcohol

*For a full discussion of the evidence for these hypotheses, see Weissman and Klerman.[1]

abuse problems, so that some unknown proportion of depressed men appears in the alcoholism rates and is not identified as depressed. There could be debate, however, about whether these men are really depressed. Accurate diagnostic assessments are required to determine the morbid risk of depression and the time sequence of onset in relationship to alcoholism. Similar considerations apply to the possibility that the depressed men are to be found in the law enforcement system. Pending future research to test this possibility, it remains an interesting but unproven hypothesis. When all these possibilities are considered, our conclusion is that the female proponderance is not an artifact.

EXPLANATIONS FOR A REAL DIFFERENCE

We regard the sex differences as real findings and have examined the possible explanations. These include hypotheses involving biological susceptibility and others involving social discrimination and its psychological consequences. Among the biological hypotheses, possible genetic transmission and female endocrine physiological processes have been investigated.

GENETIC TRANSMISSION. The possibility of a genetic factor in the etiology of depression has regularly attracted attention. There are mainly four sources of evidence for the genetic hypothesis: family aggregation studies, which compare illness rates within and between the generations of a particular family, based on the fact that members of the same family share the same genes to varying degrees; studies of twins comparing illness rates in fraternal with those in identical twins; cross-rearing studies*; and studies in which known biological genetic markers are used to follow other traits through several generations or in siblings. The majority of genetic studies in depression are concerned with evidence from the first two types of studies.

The available evidence summarized by several investigators shows an increased morbid risk of affective disorder in the first-degree relatives of diagnosed patients as compared with the general population and a higher rate for affective disorders in identical than in fraternal twins. Taking all of the studies, there is reasonable evidence of a genetic factor operating in the more severe types of depressive illness.

A greater frequency of a disorder in one sex is a genetically interesting phenomenon. One possible explanation is X linkage, that is,

---

*Cross-rearing studies examine the rates of psychiatric illness in children with a psychiatrically ill biological parent who are reared from birth by nonbiological parents who are not psychiatrically ill.

the location of the relevant locus on the X chromosome. Another possible explanation of the different incidences in the two sexes is a differential interaction of genotype and environment, depending on sex.

At this stage, the findings are in need of further examination. The samples studied are small, and family data on depressives who are not severely depressed are not available. There is still insufficient evidence from genetic studies to draw conclusions about the modes of transmission or to explain the sex differences.

FEMALE ENDOCRINE PHYSIOLOGY AND DEPRESSION. Interest in the possible relationship between female sex hormones and affective states derives from observations that clinical depression tends to occur in association with events in the reproductive cycle. Included are the menstrual cycle, the use of contraceptive drugs, the postpartum period, and the menopause. Four questions are raised for each event: (1) Are depressive symptoms more likely to be associated with these events? (2) Do they occur with sufficient frequency to account for the excess of depressed women? (3) Is there a specific clinical syndrome associated with the event? (4) Is any specific female hormone implicated as mediating the depression?

Our review of this evidence leads us to conclude that the pattern of the relationship of endocrine to clinical states is inconsistent. There is good evidence that premenstrual tension and the use of oral contraceptives have an effect, but the effect is probably of small magnitude. There is excellent evidence that the postpartum period does induce an increase in depression. Contrary to widely held views, there is good evidence that the menopause does not increase rates of depression.

There is little evidence to relate these mood changes and clinical states to altered endocrine balance or to specific hormones. However, it must be emphasized that no study could be located that utilized modern endocrinological methods or sensitive quantitative hormonal assays to correlate clinical state with female endocrines. Here is an area for fruitful collaboration between endocrinology and psychiatry. While some portion of the sex differences in depression, probably during the child-rearing years, may be explained endocrinologically, this factor is not sufficient to account for the large differences.

PSYCHOSOCIAL EXPLANATIONS. Sociologists, psychologists, feminists, and others concerned with women have become increasingly concerned about explaining why more women become depressed. The conventional wisdom is that the long-standing disadvantaged social status of women has psychological consequences that are depressing, and the persistence of social status discrimination is proposed to explain the long-term female predominance in depression.

Various hypotheses have been proposed specifying the pathways whereby women's disadvantaged status might contribute to clinical depression. Our review of these hypotheses indicates two main proposed pathways. One emphasizes the low social status of women and the legal and economic discrimination against them; the other emphasizes women's internalization of role expectations, which results in a state of learned helplessness.

The first pathway, which we call the *social status hypothesis,* has been widely accepted in the recent discussions of social discrimination against women. Many women find their situation depressing since the real social discriminations make it difficult for them to achieve mastery by direct action and self-assertion, further contributing to their psychological distress. Applied to depression, it is hypothesized that these inequities lead to legal and economic helplessness, dependency on others, chronically low self-esteem, low aspirations, and, ultimately, clinical depression.

The second pathway, which we call the *learned-helplessness hypothesis,* proposes that socially conditioned, stereotypical images produce in women a cognitive set against assertion, which is reinforced by societal expectations. In this hypothesis, the classic "femininity" values are redefined as a variant of "learned helplessness," characteristic of depression. Young girls learn to be helpless during their socialization and thus develop a limited response repertoire when under stress. These self-images and expectations are internalized in childhood, so that the young girl comes to believe that the stereotype of femininity is expected, valued, and normative.

In the few attempts to test this hypothesis that the high rates of depression are related to the disadvantages of the woman's social status, particular attention has been given to differential rates of mental illness among married and unmarried women. If this hypothesis is correct, marriage should be of greater disadvantage to the woman than to the man, since married women are likely to embody the traditional stereotyped role and should therefore have higher rates of depression. Gove and Tudor[6] in particular, have focused their research on examining rates of mental illness among married women as compared with other women and married men. They found that the higher overall rates of many mental illnesses for females are largely accounted for by higher rates for married women. In each marital status category, single, divorced, and widowed women have lower rates of mental illness than men. Gove and Tudor concluded that being married has a protective effect on males, but a detrimental effect on females. Similar conclusions were reached by Radloff,[7] using data from a community survey of depressive symptoms conducted in Kansas City, Missouri, and in Washington County, Maryland; by Porter in a study of depressive illness in a Surrey, England, general practice; by a National Health Survey of psychological distress; and by Manheimer, Mellinger, and Balter in a California survey of factors related to psychotropic drug use.[8]

The most convincing evidence that social role plays an important part in the vulnerability of women to depression is the data that suggest that marriage has a protective effect for males but a detrimental effect on women. This finding supports the view that elements of the traditional female role may contribute to depression. Social stress and its interactions with components of the female vulnerability in the traditional role offer a promising area of research. This research would need to take into account intervening variables, such as women's employment and the quality of the marriage. Any comprehensive theories, including the biological ones proposed to account for the predominance of depression among women, must explain both long-term rates and recent changes in rates.

Conclusions about the Sex Difference

Our conclusion is that the male–female differences in rates of depression are real. The evidence in support of these differential rates is best established in Western industrialized societies. Further studies in non-Western countries, particularly in Africa and Asia, are necessary before any conclusions can be drawn about the universality of these differential rates.

It is highly unlikely that any one of the explanations offered describes the sole factor accounting for the phenomenon nor that all types of depressions are associated with the same risk factors. The explanations cross such a wide variety of disciplines that rarely are all interactions considered by any one group of investigators. There has been an unfortunate tendency toward fragmentation, so that the investigators in genetics, social psychology, or endocrinology are not specifically aware of attempts by their colleagues to deal with similar phenomena.

Impact of Maternal Depression

This review of the reasons for the increase in depression among women would be of only academic interest if not for the fact that most depressives are married women with children, and that the symptoms of depression have an impact on being a parent. For example, the typically depressed person is sad, apathetic, and listless. Juxtapose these symptoms with the demands of parenthood, which requires energy, interest, emotional involvement, and affection. As one might expect, acutely depressed parents have considerable difficulties with their children. In a comparison study of 40 acutely depressed women and their normal neighbors, we found that depressed women were quite impaired as parents.[9] They were only moderately involved in their children's lives, had difficulty communicating with the children, and expressed a loss of affection for and considerable anger at the children. The mothers were guilty about their inadequacy but were unable to control these feelings or to change their behavior, and there was anger and resentment at the entire family for making what were interpreted as unfair demands.

We have identified at least four areas of parental dysfunctioning in depression: emotional involvement; communication; affection; and hostility.

INVOLVEMENT AND INTEREST. Acute depression impaired the parents' ability to be involved in their children's lives. For younger children, this included involvement in their play and physical care. For older children, it included interest and involvement in school progress, social activities, friends, and the dispensing of discipline.

Irritability, self-preoccupation, and lack of energy prevented the parents from meeting their children's normal demands for attention. Involvement was limited by the emotional or physical distancing of the parent or by overcontrol. For example, one mother left the house so that she would not have to answer the children's questions. Another took to her room when the children came home from school. A third regimented household activities, allowing the children only specified times for snacks, meals, and homework, and any deviation from the schedule was met by her harsh reprisal.

In some families, especially where there were young children, household chaos became the norm. The younger children looked physically uncared for and suffered more than the usual accidents as a result of parental inattentiveness and lack of interest.

COMMUNICATION. Children became less inclined to talk over daily events or deeper feelings and problems with the depressed parent, whose troubled affect and self-preoccupation conveyed lack of interest and an unwillingness and inability to listen.

Parent–child relations became disengaged, and the children either took their problems elsewhere or allowed them to build up. One 13-year-old youngster abruptly stopped attending school during the height of her mother's illness. She had been having academic difficulties, felt that her teacher was unsympathetic to her, and was embarrassed by her own poor performance in the class. She had not discussed the problem at home as she didn't wish to overburden her mother and didn't feel she would understand. The mother was totally perplexed by the girl's sudden refusal to attend school.

Affection. Depressed parents reported a lack of affection for their children, which produced feelings of guilt and inadequacy. This was particularly true of the mother of small children and infants, who worried about not being able to love their children or to feel warm emotions spontaneously. Some mothers worried about doing psychological harm, and others became frightened about their hostile feelings toward all their children or, sometimes, toward one child who was singled out.

Hostility. Contrary to older writings on depression, we have found that acutely depressed patients show increased rather than decreased hostility. This hostility is directed primarily toward intimate family members (the spouse and especially the children), and somewhat less toward casual acquaintances or the professionals to whom the depressives have gone for treatment. The compliant and obsequious patient in the office can be quite hostile at home. The discrepancy in the patient's affect at home and with strangers may account for the discrepancy in the literature regarding hostility and depression.

While most of the hostility toward the children in our study took the form of irritability, at times overt and intense conflicts and physical violence were reported. Conflicts with an adolescent child could become quite serious, especially if the child exploited the parent's helpless state and became rebellious and demanding. A substantial minority of adolescent children developed problems in school, with friends, or with the law or had an intensification of ongoing problems in association with the parent's depression. We also observed children who became withdrawn and sad. For example, one 14-year-old boy was afraid to make any comments or requests that would disturb his mother. She had spoken so openly of the hopelessness of her life that he was afraid she might kill herself.

At times, the depressed parent's intense rage toward her children was frightening to both the parent and the child:

> When Ms. W came for her weekly appointment she could barely speak. With a trembling voice she described an incident the evening before. Her daughter had been deliberately defiant and challenging, and the mother couldn't take it any longer. In a fit of rage, she held a knife to her daughter's throat, and when she considered the impact of what she had done, the mother felt weak, terrified, and full of remorse.

In general terms, the acute symptoms of depression conflicted with the demands of being a parent. Depression has been described as a signal for nurturance, assistance, and succor.[10] These are the very demands made on parents by their children. At the simplest level, the apathetic, sad, and anergic depressed mother is put in the untenable position of having demands made on her by her children for the help, care, and affection that she herself requires. Moreover, if her husband is unsupportive, unhelpful, or hostile, her problem is further compounded.

The impact of paternal depression can be just as serious, depending on the amount of direct care the father gives the children or the extent to which his depression impedes the mother.

Clinical Implications

There is little doubt that depression can have a serious impact on the health of individuals and families. This is particularly true because of its tendency to occur in young women. Considerable progress has been made in therapeutics. There are now available effective treatments, both pharmacotherapy and psychotherapy, for relieving the acute symptoms and for reducing the chance of their return. Moreover, there are a number of simple screening techniques for early detection. There is an air of optimism about the ability to control, if not the causes, at least the consequences of depression. However, the information and tools that are available are not always widely used, nor have health care programs been planned that take into account the clinical course of depression.

It is generally agreed that acute depression carries a good prognosis, that the chance of recovery is excellent, and that social functioning between episodes is unimpaired. Formerly depressed patients resume their work, child care, and social life. However, data on the long-term course of depression suggest that depressions are less benign than commonly believed. While most acute symptoms resolve rapidly, especially with modern treatment, there is a tendency for them to recur. We have found that only 30% of the women we treat who initially recover from an acute depression remain completely asymptomatic over the following two years; 10% are chronically symptomatic; and the majority, nearly 60%, have mild recurring symptoms, including disturbances of mood, sleep, and appetite. These periods of symptom recurrence are usually accompanied by difficulties in participating fully in care-taking roles. There is also evidence from several studies that an important minority of patients, about 10%–15%, remain chronically symptomatic two to five years after a depressive episode. These findings document the intermittent and chronic nature of depressive disorders and emphasize that persons who have had an acute depressive episode have a reasonably high likelihood of recurrence accompanied by impairment in social functioning. These findings on the clinical course of depression make early detection important.

Early detection will be accelerated if education programs for social workers, nurses, and all medical and professional nonmedical personnel who work with families are trained to recognize the symptoms of depression in adults; the consequences in children; and the persons and periods of high risk. This information should be included as part of the professional education, as well as the in-service training, of these workers. All clinicians who deal with women should also be alert to the detection, treatment, and consequences of depressive disorders.

REFERENCES

1. Weissman MM, Klerman GL: Sex differences and the epidemiology of depression, *Archives of General Psychiatry 34*:98–111, 1977.
2. Silverman C: *The epidemiology of depression.* Baltimore, Johns Hopkins University Press, 1968.
3. Weissman MM, Myers JK: *The New Haven community survey 1967–75: Depressive symptoms and diagnosis.* Presented at the Society for Life History Study of Psychopathology Meeting, Fort Worth, Texas, October 6–8, 1976.
4. Lehman HE: The epidemiology of depressive disorders. In *Depression in the 70's.* Edited by Fieve RR. The Hague, Excerpta Medica, 1971.
5. Klerman GL, Barrett JE: The affective disorders: Clinical and epidemiological aspects. In *Lithium: Its role in psychiatric research and treatment.* Edited by Gershon S, Shopsin B. New York, Plenum Press, 1973.
6. Gove WR, Tudor JF: Adult sex roles and mental illness, *American Journal of Sociology. 78*:812–835, 1973.
7. Radloff L: Sex differences in depression: The effects of occupation and marital status, *Sex Roles 1*:249–269, 1975.
8. Bachrach L: *Marital status and mental disorders: An analytical review,* Publication (ADM) 75–217. U.S. Department of Health, Education, and Welfare, 1975.
9. Weissman MM, Paykel ES: *The depressed woman: A study of social relationships.* Chicago, University of Chicago Press, 1974.
10. Klerman GL: Depression and adaptation. In *The psychology of depression: Contemporary theory and research.* Edited by Friedman R, Katz M. Washington, D.C., V. H. Winston and Sons, 1974.

Chapter 13

The Myofascial Pain Dysfunction Syndrome: An Unheeded Neuromuscular Disorder

Berit Helöe and Astrid Nøklebye Heiberg

> *If you listen carefully, you hear their discomfort outside of the soma and stoma.* [1]

Characteristics of the Myofascial Pain Dysfunction

Myofascial pain dysfunction (MPD) is characterized by repeated masticatory muscle pain alternating with a feeling of stiffness or fatigue in these muscles and limitation of function. Clicking or popping of the temporomandibular joint often is a precursor to the disorder or may be an accompanying symptom. There are no clinically, radiographically, or biochemically detectable changes in the passive parts of the masticatory system (i.e., the jaw bones, teeth, joints, or ligaments).[2,3] The pain is localized to the ear, temple, or temporomandibular joint region. It usually lasts for weeks or months. It may vary but often becomes gradually worse. Some patients report that it may be difficult to open their mouths in the mornings and that they cannot easily eat breakfast. Others find that their problems become worse in the evenings. As a rule, there is a diurnal variation of symptoms. A few patients report diffuse, constant, aching pain. However it is not so severe that it interferes with sleep.

During the twentieth century, this condition has been the subject of increasing attention in the dental literature in the industrialized so-

Berit Helöe, D.D.S. • Department of Oral Surgery and Oral Medicine, University of Oslo, Norway.   Astrid Nøklebye Heiberg, M.D. • Associate Professor, Psychiatric Institute, University of Oslo, Norway.

cieties (the Western countries and Japan). The demand for treatment is also gradually increasing in these countries.

The Dental Profession and Response to Treatment Demand

The dental profession is a young profession derived from medicine during the last hundred years. Its history is characterized primarily by a surgical and technical orientation. Knowledge from medicine has been transformed and applied, and dentistry has been placed somewhere between health care and a business as far as adult patients are concerned. Dental care is something one buys. This means that regular dental treatment has been primarily used by middle- and upper-class people.

A characteristic feature of middle-class culture in the industrialized societies is confidence and belief in specializing and specialists. This attitude among those who regularly seek treatment strongly affects dentists' attitudes toward their profession, supporting the popular viewpoint that dentistry and dental science represent a highly technically oriented discipline. To push this view to an extreme, one might say that dentistry has been concerned with hard tissue and hard data. How, then, does such a profession respond to an increasing demand for the treatment of a disorder in which no detectable somatic changes are present except for muscles painful to palpation? The most "orthodox" dental approach implies that the etiology of dental disorders and the focus of treatment are in the teeth, and particularly in the morphology and the configuration of the bite. Thus, teeth are often ground and shaped in order to fit better. If one focuses on the problems in the temporomandibular joint, the treatment usually is to use injections varying from local anesthetics to corticosteroids. With the increasing interest in psychological issues, more attention has been paid to the neuromuscular system and psychological functioning. Several studies of this problem have been undertaken, most of them utilizing psychological inventories, which are valuable and provide information but are also mostly "hard-data"-oriented tools. Electromyographic studies are also characterized by some clinical distance from the patient.

The mouth as a communicative apparatus has to a great extent been overlooked. Its smiling, laughing, sucking, sighing, spitting, weeping, singing, talking, and chatting functions have been neglected in dental research, which thus has missed a valuable aspect of the multifaceted symbolic language of the oral neuromuscular system. Comprehensive clinical examinations of MPD-patients' psychological, neuromuscular, and social functioning have not been described.

RESEARCH ON MPD

Psychological studies are unclear and contradictory regarding the personality traits of MPD patients. The Minnesota Multiphasic Personality Inventory and the Eysenck Personality Inventory have been the instruments most frequently used.[4,5,6,7,8] Some investigators have examined control groups;[5,6,8,9,10] some have not. Some have studied only groups resistant to therapy.[11,12] The study groups have varied numerically from 28 to 176 subjects. Conclusions vary from "no common personality traits or patterns of MPD-patients"[8] to "MPD-patients are overgenerous, autocratic, narcissistic, sadistic, dominant, hypernormal, responsible and managerial"[5] and "hypochondriac, hysterical, depressive."[12]

Psychiatric interviews have been performed to a limited extent. Moulton[11] examined 25 therapy-resistant patients and noted two groups: (1) a "hostile, angry, and dependent" group and (2) a "perfectionistic, obsessive, demanding and highly efficient" group; 20 patients were anxious and tense, and 11 were psychotic or prepsychotic. Fine[9] examined 50 consecutively referred patients and 50 controls and found depression and anxiety as outstanding features of MPD patients.

Neurophysiological studies conclude that hyperactivity of the muscles closing the jaw originates in the central nervous system, that such centrally induced activity may be sufficient to lead to disturbed function, to local pain, and to pain referred to adjacent structures.[13] A study of neuromuscular problems among patients with temporomandibular joint disorders documents a strong correlation with pains in the back, shoulders, and neck.[14] Our data corroborate these observations.[15] Recurrent headache and MPD have also been found to be strongly correlated.[16] Berry[17] stated that there is a high incidence of chronic minor illnesses among MPD patients.

The social characteristics of MPD patients generally indicate that they are skilled, self-employed women, aged 20–40.[18,19] Epidemiological investigations, however, have revealed that symptoms of MPD are more equally distributed among women and among upper- and lower-class people than the clinical data have indicated.[20,21]

TREATMENT RESULTS

Few follow-up studies have been reported; however, most of the available data conclude that 70%–80% of MPD patients have been treated successfully, regardless of the treatment used.[22,23,24,25,26] The possible role of occlusal dysharmonies has been raised, but disagreement on this issue prevails at present.

HOW THE PRESENT AUTHORS CAME TO BE INTERESTED

The dentist (Berit Helöe): In practice, I was confronted with a patient who had presenting complaints that had not been very common during my time as a student, 12 years earlier. Since I was the only female dentist on the ward and most of the patients were women who did not need surgery, I soon found that I was the one who took care of these patients. I started to listen to them and became aware that social issues were important in their histories. To my surprise, I often recognized problems that were similar to those of other women I knew. My interest in these problems seemed relevant to me, but often a bit confusing to the patients, who, after all, had come to see a dentist. Emotional reactions varying from weeping and explosive bitter comments on family members to withdrawal or anger were frequent. Furthermore, the physiotherapist who treated some of the patients reported that (1) their muscular tension was not localized only in the masticatory muscles; (2) some patients displayed emotional reactions after treatment; and (3) most of them showed improvement in jaw function after a particular treatment that involved the freeing of respiratory functions.

After a few years, I began to assess my clinical experience with these patients. The following were my findings:

1. Most MPD patients were middle- and upper-socioeconomic-class women of reproductive age.

2. The majority had some, but not an overwhelming number of, minor illnesses, mainly recurrent headache.

3. Most of the patients responded to conservative, nonsurgical treatment.

4. The physiotherapist reported that those patients whom she had treated generally had tense musculature in the masticatory system as well as in the neck, back, shoulders, and upper parts of the arms. They also had restricted respiratory function before treatment. After general physiotherapy emphasizing the freeing of respiratory muscles, their jaw problems diminished, together with the other neuromuscular complaints.

5. The dental status of MPD patients, broadly speaking, was good.

6. The symptom history of the patients seemed to be filled with symbolic material related to their life situation.

The psychiatrist (Astrid N. Heiberg) describes her experience with the syndrome: Since my professional interest was in psychoanalytically oriented psychotherapy and also in the psychosomatic aspects of disease, the offer from the Department of Oral Surgery of Oslo University to cooperate with them in trying to understand MPD came as a gift to me. My interest was in trying to learn more about how and why these patients presented with this type of symptom.

Another aspect of this new situation was to find myself collaborating on a scientific project with a woman of my own age and with a lifestyle similar to mine. Previously, the milieu in which I worked professionally had consisted exclusively of men, and I had not consciously missed female company. To my joy and amazement, I found that the growing personal involvement was fruitful and provided personal expansion.

In addition, the patients' symptoms and complaints shed a new light on the origins of Norwegian psychiatry, which stemmed from Wilhem Reich, who lived in Norway for six years in the 1930s. His concepts of human energy were taken up and used by Norwegian psychoanalysts, who worked out a system of treatment based on clinical observations of bodily reactions to palpation and physiotherapy. The diagnostic assessments that are part of this system are mainly based on 'the observation of respiration, of body posture and resistance to passive movements.' The basic theory is that through the freeing of respiration and through muscular relaxation, the patient has access to the emotions that have been repressed. The patient may then become aware of the bodily defense system that reacts in a parallel way to his or her psychological defenses. This treatment is called *psychomotoric therapy* and has become accepted as a specialty of physiotherapy in Norway. Thus, unlike in America, the physiotherapist and the psychiatrist have a common theoretical base, although the emphasis of physiotherapy is nonverbal, and that of psychotherapy is verbal communication.

THE STUDY

In 1976, a team consisting of the authors and the physiotherapist initiated a research project that included all patients applying for the treatment of temporomandibular joint disorders at the Department of Oral Surgery and Oral Medicine at the University of Oslo during a period of three months.

All patients were examined by the dentist, who based her diagnoses on past symptom history and clinical and radiographic examination. When there were "subjective" symptoms, patients were encouraged to tell her about these in their own words. Information concerning social background, present life situation, and perceived stress was recorded from a semistructured interview opening with the question, "Do you feel stressed?" This question was followed by additional questions pertaining to work situation, economics, and family responsibilities. Since great wealth is rare in Norway, educational level was used as a means of social classification. A three-graded scale, which had been used in Sweden for some years, was used. It had to be modified to fit a female population, since women commonly have been classified in accordance with their husband's or father's social class. In this system, the middle and upper classes consist of people who are in administration, education, and trade, while the lower-class category consists mainly of workers in industry, small farms, fishing, etc. A psychiatric, semistructured interview was conducted, lasting for one to two hours. Data were collected on family history, sexual and marital life, health history, previous psychiatric problems, personality traits, and possible stress factors occurring within the previous two years. The patients were grouped into one of the following three broad categories according to a common psychiatric diagnostic system:

1. *Healthy:* flexible and balanced; good capacity for interpersonal contact; no major disturbances.
2. *Mild psychological disturbances:* emotionally restricted; tense control of emotions and lack of self-realization, or frank symptoms of anxiety or depression.
3. *Severe psychological disturbances:* psychotic or borderline psychotic with confusion, delusions or lack of reality sense; inability to form stable relationships and/or hypochondriac preoccupation; psychopathic, with inability to control emotions and drives, and in constant conflicts with family or society.

The physiotherapist's examination included body posture, respiration, muscular tension, resistance to passive movements, and reaction to palpation.

All of the examinations were performed "blindly"; that is, the members of the team did not have access to the others' findings before they saw the patient, and until a treatment plan was formulated. A control group consisting of patients referred because of well-defined diagnoses was selected and examined. This group was matched with the MPD patients according to sex, age, and social class.

Both groups were examined by the dentist and the psychiatrist and were treated by physiotherapy.

FOLLOW-UP. One year later the MPD patients were contacted by letter and/or telephone and interviewed. They were asked about their present situation and their response to treatment.

THE CLINICAL PICTURE. Of the total number of 134 MPD patients, 85% were women, who ranged in age from 18 to 59 years (60% were aged 20–40 years). Most were of the middle or upper social class, were married, and had one or two children. They were employed, in typically feminine, "subordinate" jobs. They were generally in good health except for a high incidence of neuromuscular complaints. Their sexual functioning was reported to be good.

More of the MPD patients than of the control patients reported an early break in contact with one parent, mainly the father, because of divorce, death, or longstanding illness. Also, a demanding style and lack of solidarity in the childhood home were prominent findings in this group.

Compared with the control group, the MPD patients in general were characterized by a tendency toward emotional control, especially of aggressive feeling. They also demonstrated an attention-seeking style of relating. Their body posture and respiratory pattern indicated an underlying aggressive state. Tense muscles were found in the total "stretching system" of the body. Although they were able to relax when lying down, those patients who were most restrained were also found, on neuromuscular examination, to be most tense. The reported stress factors were equally distributed among MPD patients and control patients. However, there was a marked distinction in the way these stress factors were weighed and presented to those who saw them. The MPD women told the dentist of stressful working conditions and concern about family illness. The psychiatrist learned other aspects of their histories, which are elucidated in the case histories that follow.

The MPD group was a heterogeneous group, according to psychiatric diagnostic categories. They fell roughly into two subgroups: (1) "the typical MPD-patients," encompassing the healthy and the mildly disturbed patients (90% of the total); and (2) "multiproblem patients," encompassing the severely disturbed and/or elderly patients (10% of the total).

The major complaints of the MPD patients were clicking of the temporomandibular joint, pain when they moved the jaw, limitation in jaw mobility, and fear of throwing the jaw out of joint. The multiproblem patients described diffuse, constant, dull, aching pain and/or a feeling of being "homeless in their own mouth" or having no resting position for their jaw. Their symptoms and appearances were very much like those of patients with the atypical facial pain described by Lesse[27] and Lefer.[28]

REACTIONS TO THE EXAMINATIONS. Of the study group, 40% said that they liked the psychiatric interview and that it had been useful to them. They felt good because other aspects of their lives, not only their teeth, were being considered. Another 30% were indifferent, and the remaining 30% reported embarrassment. After the physiotherapist's examination, 80% felt that it had been good and useful to them, 10% were indifferent, and 10% felt embarrassment. All of the patients reported that the dental examination had been good and useful to them, ten per cent were indifferent, ten per cent felt embarrassment. The latter reports, however, were biased by the fact that the patients had sought a dental clinic, and the dentist was the one who interviewed them concerning their primary complaint. This made it more difficult to express displeasure.

The following three case histories are presented to illustrate differences in symptoms, personality traits, life situations, and responses to treatment.

>Solveig was an immature, healthy woman who wept and swept her symptoms away. She was 24 years old and had been brought up in a religious milieu, the younger of two sisters. She was referred because of limitation of jaw mobility, as well as pain when chewing or laughing, of four months' duration. For the past four years, she had been employed in a bank as a typist. There was great performance pressure at her job. She was married to a student, who was always occupied with his work and had little time for her.

>One year before, she had had an abortion because her husband thought it was too early to think of children. A few weeks later, her father died. At the same time, she fell "helplessly" in love with a former schoolmate. Her husband, knowing nothing of the affair, was now "happily" finishing his exams, and they were supposed to move to another part of the country. At the time of consultation, she felt conflict about her situation. She had kept her mouth "locked." She had not told her mother of her "sinful" abortion (which was the first thing she mentioned), nor had she told her husband of her love affair. Further, she had not told her lover that she was supposed to move. She had not permitted herself to grieve over her father, who, she thought, might have died of shame if he knew of her behavior. She also did not complain about her job or try to leave it.

>She told the dentist of her stressful working conditions, but the rest of the story was told to the psychiatrist, between outbursts of tears. The physiotherapist found that she had tense muscles, which were painful to palpation, in the neck, the shoulders, the upper arms, and the masticatory system.

>She called twice during the following month to "talk things over." One year later, she happily reported from another part of the country that she was living with her husband, she was pregnant, and she had decided that her mother did not need to know about her abortion, since it would hurt her and, "after all," it was between her and her husband. She expressed gratitude that she had had the opportunity to talk during her "dark period." With laughter, she said that she had had a relapse of MPD symptoms during her second month of pregnancy and had "exercised it away." Afterward, she thought of the possibility that it might have something to do with her memory of her abortion.

Ingrid was a controlled, idyllizing, and neurotic woman who was tongue-tied but had a slip of the tongue.

A beautiful, expensively dressed woman of 39, Ingrid was referred because of pain on chewing and yawning and difficulties in eating breakfast and brushing her teeth for the previous year. She was the only daughter of a whaler. This implied that she had stayed alone with her mother from November till May every year during her childhood. She had an elementary-school education. For the past 20 years, she had been a housewife, married to an officer, who was now of high rank. She had two children. She was worried about her pain and the possibility of "something evil" (i.e., a tumor) inside her head. To the dentist's questions, she responded in a reserved manner, saying that she led the most wonderful life with her "charming, outstanding" husband, her "nice" son of 19, her "angel" daughter (aged 12), and her "marvelous" mother-in-law. She said she lived in the "nicest" of houses, which was her husband's parents' home. After a while she admitted, sitting on the edge of a chair and twisting her gloves, that something in her life situation worried her. Her husband, who was becoming more and more important, often had to see foreign officers and their wives as guests in their home. When this happened, she became tongue-tied and felt ill at ease.

The psychiatrist, who was five minutes late to the appointment, was reproachfully met by the patient, who stated that she and her husband regarded it as the most important virtue to be precisely on time. The interview thus started with a bit of difficulty. However, it was not long before the picture of a scared little girl with the exterior of a grown-up woman and a set of rigid rules of life emerged. Her mother, obviously a socially ambitious and bitter woman, had wanted her daughter to marry well. The means to achieve this, she believed, were to be nice, to be good-looking, to be orderly, and to be a woman (i.e., fertile). After the patient began to talk about this, the "tap was turned on." Bitter feelings welled up, and a story of three dramatic spontaneous abortions occurring in different military camps after the birth of the son, were revealed. All of them occurred during her husband's absences on distant military maneuvers, in wintertime. All had had to be concealed from her husband and his family, or minimized, in accordance with her mother's advice. When she became pregnant the fifth time, her mother stayed with her for seven months and kept her in bed. The result was the "darling daughter." At that time, her husband was promoted, thus increasing the social distance from her mother.

Two years previously she had moved to Oslo to live with her mother-in-law. It was not easy. Her son was not good at school and could not become a dentist as her husband wished. Her daughter was a kind girl, but she was obese. Her mother called every day complaining of loneliness and illnesses. Her mother-in-law constantly hinted that her mother did not fit very well into their present circles of acquaintance, and that it was not strange that the son was a failure at school when he had such an uneducated mother. She also hinted that the daughter would not have the slightest hope of getting married because of the way she looked, and that obesity obviously was inherited from Ingrid's father.

The patient told of her struggle to make her son keep up with his schoolwork and to keep the house and garden in order, her mother at a distance, and her daughter from eating. Then she suddenly burst out, "Why doesn't she ever mention the holy fat pig in a frame that she herself nailed to the wall of our living room? My husband's father obviously wasn't too slim." After this, she literally locked her mouth.

While there were many rumors of her husband's flirtatiousness and his extramarital affairs, she did not mention these. She was alert when the psychiatrist mentioned the term *psychological functioning*; she pulled herself together, reminded the psychiatrist of her duty as a civil official, asked once if it was definite that she had no signs of something malignant, and rejected all sorts of treatment offers. She said she would rather use her spare time for English lessons and piano playing.

When she was asked about her reactions to the types of examinations she had had, she said that she had never liked "soul doctors." The physiotherapist's examination had been OK, she said, but she did not think such therapy would do her any good.

One year later, she wanted a new radiographic checkup. When she was told that there were no signs of pathological changes, she minimized her symptoms but reported that several of her clubmates had jaw problems and that *they* really were nervous.

Dagmar was an elderly woman with massive family problems whose only pathway to peace was pain. She was an unmarried 54-year-old woman who came to the clinic because of long-standing, dull, aching pains in her jaws and a constant headache. Twice a week, she was forced to stay in bed in a dark room because of her headaches. She answered the dentist's opening question about stress by saying that pain was her only stressor. Concerning her working situation, she explained that three years before, she had had to quit her job in a baker's shop because of her parents' bad health. She volunteered no feelings about that, but at the same time, she revealed a certain envy of people who had a job to go to and an income of their own. Her father had died of a heart attack one year previously, and she was now left with an 83-year-old mother who suffered from diabetes.

To the psychiatrist, she hesitatingly gave the additional information that her younger brother had epilepsy and lived with them in a small apartment. She said that he "sort of dominated" her and her mother, so that no friends were allowed to visit. He had the idea that no "alien" should enter their home after the father had been carried out. She also admitted that some neighbors hinted that they thought her brother was "crazy." She described her situation as one in which there was "nothing one could do, that's only how things are." Her voice and face, however, told of anger toward her neighbors, "who ought to mind their own business"; of feeling anger mixed with shame regarding her brother; and of mourning for her beloved father, who had been "the only kind person she had ever known." She was not able to describe her emotions as such, and she denied being angry at or sorry for anything or anybody. The only thing she could express herself about was her pain. She did not agree with the psychiatrist's assessment that she had a family problem and that she was depressed.

When she was asked about her reactions to the examinations, she answered that she had always regarded it a virtue and a pleasant duty to support medical research, and that she therefore had agreed to participation. However, if this lady who talked nonsense was representative of Norwegian research, she had to revise her thinking. Physiotherapists, on the other hand, had always been good people.

She was treated with a soft, acrylic, self-administrable bite splint and physiotherapy once a week. After four weeks, the physiotherapist felt that the muscles of her neck were less tense. The day after this, however, the patient called to say that her headache was worse than ever, and that she had nausea. Three months later, she said she would try again, but the same pattern was repeated after two sessions of physiotherapy.

One year later, she reported that her mother had died. She was now left with her brother. She had tried, but failed, to get her job back. Her symptoms were constant, although she had seen a neurologist, a rheumatologist, and an otorhinolaryngologist. She had also seen the endocrinologist who had treated her mother's diabetes. None of these doctors had helped. She then saw a gynecologist because of pain in her abdomen, and fibroids in her uterus had been removed. Then, with some aggression, she gave the information that she would try acupuncture.

FACTORS THAT MAKE AN INDIVIDUAL AN MPD PATIENT. In principle, the shift from having symptoms to having a wish for treatment is a three-step process. The first step is to have a disorder. The second step is to recognize the symptoms. The third step is to prepare for and seek treatment. All these steps are influenced by an individual's (1) personality structure, including psychological and somatic vulnerability; (2) present life situation, including possible intolerable and threatening factors; and (3) sociocultural factors, including traditions, experiences, and expectations of possible gains from the symptoms.

MPD patients are individuals who have passed through the three phases described above. They have a disorder, they have recognized the symptoms, and they have sought treatment for them. They have defined themselves as patients. MPD patients give a clinical picture that is characterized by the following features. They are adult women of middle or upper class in their reproductive years, and they generally have good general and dental health. They do not tend to have a large number of symptoms or to demonstrate sick-role behavior. They do not like to take drugs. However, they all control emotions, especially aggression. They have taken traditional feminine roles and do the best they can in domestic and in other conventional work. They have frequently experienced early loss of contact with one parent, primarily their fathers. They are somatically oriented regarding disease, and they believe in the value of professional expertise. Those who report stress emphasize more stressing factors when talking to someone whom they see as a "somatically" oriented health professional than they do when talking to a "psychologically" oriented professional.

What possible connections are there among these factors? Since the era of industrialization and commercial and geographical expansion, middle- and upper-class men have stayed physically and mentally at a distance from active involvement in domestic areas. The transition from a barter economy to a money economy, with its bureaucratic, technical orientation, together with a general rise in educational level and an orientation toward the privatization of family life, has been the pathway that the societies of northern Europe have more-or-less followed. In this social system, upper-class men have mainly been in the positions of control and power. Women and middle-class men have enthusiastically shared the materialistic advantages; however, they have been exposed to the disadvantages, especially the profound role conflicts that have occurred.

Concomitant with these changes was the systematized institutionalization of health care. Female social circles had always existed within the framework of family life. These included grandmothers, aunts, mothers, sisters, female servants, and governesses. Thus, young girls had close female models and the chance to identify with more than one person. Specific feminine stages of life, such as pregnancy, delivery, and early childrearing, were taken care of at critical phases by the family physician, who was often close to the family. The institutionalization of the physician as a reserve symbolic father with great authority soon began to have a life of its own, growing rapidly along with medical and technical progress and becoming integrated into a health care system representing great power. In a parallel way, a rapid centralizing of societal functions, such as industry, business, health care, and administration, has taken place. Consequently, domestic life has been further segregated into a nuclear family system, with the health care system further specialized into a separate sphere, quite apart from domestic life and maintaining special tasks, skills, and diagnostic systems.

For middle- and upper-class women, this development has implied a dispersing of informal female social groups and a consequent orientation toward health service personnel in situations involving personal conflict. Moreover, the superficial maintenance of a facade is supported by the mass media, which demand ladylike (i.e., controlled) manners, cleanliness, good looks, and an appearance of satisfaction and contentment. This demand is not limited to the middle-class woman; her children as well are supposed to reflect the values of their mothers and share the same restrictions.

The maintenance of a facade is dependent on a continual denial of what is behind it, not only not expressing it, but also often not being aware of those feelings. Those who have not learned to see reality are likely to be unaware of the extent of the facade and the amount of effort required for its maintenance.

> If one does not know greed, one cannot be really generous.
> If one does not know hatred, one cannot be really kind.

> If one does not know sorrow, one cannot be really glad.
> What if one does not know anger?

Low self-esteem, passivity, dependence, self-sacrifice, regression, and lack of orientation to reality represent the seamy side of the "happy" facade of many middle-class women. The keeping of a crack-free facade covering realities of this kind requires considerable control, mental effort, and actual muscular work as well.

The present life situation of the MPD patient is influenced by the sociocultural patterns described. The mother–daughter relationship has been intensified by the physical absence of the patient's father during long periods of her childhood. These patients control their health, keep their teeth in order, manage their domestic living, and limit their extradomestic lives. Being sick conflicts with their need to be in control, but when they have been exposed to long-standing stress and have struggled to maintain a facade, they do unconsciously develop somatic symptoms, as an admission ticket to health service.

The dentist is a convenient representative of the health system for several reasons. He or she is technically and somatically oriented and, it is presumed, will not examine the patient in such a way as to evoke threatening self-insight. It is socially safe, secure, and nonstigmatizing to see a dentist. He or she does not have the power to hospitalize the patient and thus deprive her of her control. Finally, he or she is occupied with an important part of the facade, since the teeth represent an important part of the smile.

The typical MPD patient has lived through early childhood without gross trauma. However, it seems reasonable to assume that her emotional exploration and aggression have been subdued, punished, or simply not approved of at a stage of development that is too early for recollection. Aggression and exploration in a wide context have been perceived as threatening and anxiety-provoking. In order to secure safety and gratification, the patient restrains herself, makes as little noise as possible, breathes noiselessly, and does not cry or laugh loudly, fight with her siblings, or run away from home. She stays where she is and does not trespass borders. This systematic abstinence from following aggressive or exploratory impulses requires muscular effort. When such a person, later in childhood, experiences severe, emotionally threatening problems like the prospect of losing contact with a beloved relative, the emotional-muscular pattern becomes reactivated and firmly established. Later on, emotional expression, especially of aggressive feelings, and the desire to explore are linked to the threat of loss. This implies that anxiety is an underlying component of a personality structure that has become characterized by a control of emotions. The aggressive feelings represented by crying, biting, scolding, spitting, and beating during early childhood are dangerous feelings. They have to be kept in place or channeled indirectly. Most MPD patients do both. Partly, they restrain their aggression in the muscles of action (i.e., the masticatory muscles, the respiratory muscles, and the upper arm muscles); and they react with diffuse, anxiety-related phenomena like dizziness or nausea when this neuromuscular defense system becomes loosened by physiotherapy. They also channel their aggression through biting remarks about persons or events at a safe distance, simultaneously keeping a stiff upper lip.

They channel their perception of stress to conditions that are at a safe distance from their emotional life and present stress as being related to their nonfamily life (e.g., their working situation), or they do not report stress at all. They wait hopefully for a somatic diagnosis, which would represent an approvable pathway to relaxation and regression. Paradoxically, this represents regression from a response that by its repressive and overcontrolling manner is itself of a regressive nature.

Because of their personality structure and the sociocultural traditions, family problems are unmentionable to these patients. A psychiatrist may open up problems that are close to reality and cause emotional reactions. Although the case histories of Solveig and Ingrid may indicate that there is a substantial variation in the reaction pattern within the group of "typical MPD-patients," they have several personality, life-situation, and sociocultural factors in common.

The multiproblem patients, on the other hand, lack resources. They cannot afford a scratch in their facade and self-esteem. They need their pain as an admission ticket to continual regression and contact with the health system. Their more profound disturbance and lack of capacity for contact make them dependent on the health service system, which represents to them a set of limited and regulated possibilities for interpersonal contact. Dagmar is representative of the larger proportion of this group.

As can be seen from these three cases, the triggering mechanisms that make a person become an MPD patient are multifactorial, as is the etiology of the disorder.

The treatment should, in principle, be conservative. The dentist should realize that some patients need their symptoms for shorter or longer periods and should not feel a sense of failure and should not grow impatient when the patient does not immediately improve.

Function should be established by means of exercises for the jaw, biofeedback methods, or physiotherapy. The latter includes a chance for the patient to have the feeling of being taken care of and thus may constitute a guided regression weekly.

Soft occlusal splints that the patient may manage himself or herself are also approved remedies, which may neutralize the tension of masticatory muscles often manifested during sleep. Correction of occlusal conditions should be undertaken if they are severe.

First and foremost, however, the patient should be listened to.

REFERENCES

1. Lowental U, Pisanti S: The syndrome of oral complaints: Etiology and therapy, *Oral Surgery, Oral Medicine and Oral Pathology 40:2* 1978.
2. Laskin DM: Etiology of the pain-dysfunction syndrome, *Journal of the American Dental Association. 79*:147, 1969.
3. Schwartz L: The pain-dysfunction syndrome. In *Facial pain and mandibular dysfunction.* Edited by Schwartz L, Chayes CM. Philadelphia, Saunders, p. 140, 1968.
4. Kydd WL: Psychosomatic aspects of temporomandibular joint dysfunction, *Journal of the American Dental Association 59*:31, 1959.
5. Lupton DC: A preliminary investigation of the personality of female temporomandibular joint dysfunction patients, *Psychotherapy and Psychosomatics 14*:199, 1966.
6. McCall CM, Jr, Szmyd L, Ritter RM: Personality characteristics in patients with temporomandibular joint symptoms, *Journal of the American Dental Association 62*:694, 1961.
7. Shipman WG: Analysis of MMPI test results in women with MPD syndrome, *Journal of Dental Research.* (Special issue) Abstr. *82*:79, 1973.
8. Solberg WK, Flint RT, Brantner JP: Temporomandibular joint pain and dynsfunction: A clinical study of emotional and occlusal components, *Journal of Prosthetic Denistry 28*:412, 1972.
9. Fine EW: Psychological factors associated with nonorganic temporomandibular joint pain dysfunction syndrome, *British Dental Journal 131*:402, 1971.
10. Molin D, Edman G, Schalling D; Psychological studies of patients with mandibular pain dysfunction syndrome, *Svensk Tandlaekar-T. 66*:1,15, 1973.
11. Moulton R: Psychiatric considerations in maxillofacial pain. *Journal of the American Dental Association 51*:408, 1955.
12. Schwartz RA: Personality characteristics of unsuccessfully treated MPD-patients, *Journal of Dental Research 53* (Special Issue) Abstr. *291*:127, 1974.
13. Yemm R: Neurophysiologic studies of temporomandibular joint dysfunction, *Oral Sciences Review 7*:31, 1976.
14. Eggen S: Nevromuskulaer spenning som aarsak til kjeveleddslidelser, *Den norske tannlaegeforenings tidende 64*:123, 1954.
15. Helöe B, Helöe LA, Heiberg A: Relationship between sociomedical factors and TMJ-symptoms in Norwegians with myofascial pain-dysfunction syndrome, *Community Dentistry and Oral Epidemiology 5*:207, 1977.
16. Magnussor T, Carlsson GE: Comparison between two groups of patients in respect of headache and mandibular dysfunction, *Swedish Dental Journal 2*:73, 1978.
17. Berry DC: Mandibular dysfunction pain and chronic minor illness, *British Dental Journal 127*:170, 1969.

18. Franks AST: The social character of temporomandibular joint dysfunction, *Dental Practitioner. 15*:94, 1964.
19. Helöe B, Helöe LA: Characteristics of a group of patients with temporomandibular joint disorders, *Community Dentistry and Oral Epidemiology. 3*:72, 1975.
20. Agerberg G, Carlsson GE: Functional disorders of the masticatory system: I. Distribution of symptoms according to age and sex as judged from investigations by questionnaire, *Acta Odontol. Scand. 31*:335, 1973.
21. Helkimo J: Studies on function and dysfunction of the masticatory system, Dissertation, University of Gothenburg, 1974.
22. Agerberg G, Carlsson GE: Late results of treatment of functional disorders of the masticatory system, *Journal of Oral Rehabilitation. 1*:309, 1974.
23. Cohen SR: Follow-up evaluation of 105 patients with myofascial pain-dysfunction syndrome, *Journal of the American Dental Association 97*:825, 1978.
24. Laskin DM, Greene CS: Influence of the doctor-patient relationship on placebo therapy for patients with myofascial pain-dysfunction (MPD)-syndrome, *Journal of the American Dental Association 85*:892, 1972.
25. Thompson H: Temporomandibular joint problems, *British Dental Journal 3*:422, 1961.
26. Zarb GA, Thompson GW: Assessment of clinical treatment of patients with temporomandibular joint dysfunction; *Journal of the Canadian Dental Association 41*:410, 1975.
27. Lesse S: Atypical facial pain syndromes of psychogenic origin, *Journal of Nervous and Mental Disease 124*:346, 1956.
28. Lefer L: A psychoanalytic view of a dental phenomenon: Psychosomatics of the temporomandibular joint pain-dysfunction syndrome. *Comtemporary Psychoanalysis 2*:135, 1966.
29. Warner WL, Meeker M, Eells K: Social class in America: The evaluation of status. New York, Harper Torchbooks, The Academy Library, Harper & Row, pp. 72–84, 1960.

Chapter 14

Women and Alcohol Abuse

Barbara S. McCrady

Alcohol and drug abuse are becoming increasingly serious problems among American women. The most recent estimates suggest that there are from 1.5 million to 2.5 million adult American women with alcohol problems. The proportion of adult women who drink and the proportion of women among alcohol abusers have increased steadily over the last 10 years. Now, approximately one out of three alcohol abusers is a woman, as compared to one out of six women among alcohol abusers 10 years ago. Estimates of the number of women with other drug problems are equally alarming. Twice as many women as men use minor tranquilizers, 50% more women than men use barbiturates, three times as many women as men use amphetamines, and 30% more women than men use pills of various types to cope with stress. Although these numbers alone do not reflect abuse, the fact that so many women use so many potentially abused drugs increases the risk of abuse. The best estimates of the number of American women abusing any kind of prescription drug is 1 million to 2 million.

This chapter focuses primarily on alcohol abuse. Some information about other drugs is included because alcohol interacts with so many other drugs. This choice of focusing on alcohol abuse should not be seen as a statement that the abuse of other drugs is a minor problem. Rather, the problems of abuse are so vast that covering them all in one chapter would not be possible.

What is alcohol abuse? What are the indicators of abuse? What other drugs are most commonly abused, and how do they interact with alcohol abuse? What are the psychological issues that women face at different points in their development, and how do these issues inter-

Barbara S. McCrady, Ph.D. • Butler Hospital, Brown University, Providence, Rhode Island.

act with alcohol abuse? These are the questions that are addressed in this chapter.

DEFINITIONS AND PATTERNS OF ABUSE

A person is defined as experiencing problems in her use of alcohol or drugs if that use interferes with her functioning in any of the following areas: her physical health, her emotional well-being, her ability to function in her relationships with her family and friends, or her ability to fulfill her responsibilities in her job and/or in her home. *Functioning* is an admittedly subjective term, and *interference* may depend on the eyes of the beholder. For example, a woman may have a cocktail with her friends at lunch, or after work, and cook TV dinners that night or expect her husband to prepare the evening meal. Some husbands might conclude that the cocktails were "interfering," while others would see the same behavior as perfectly normal. Thus, defining "interfering with functioning" requires careful thought on the part of the woman, the people around her, and any professionals who may become involved with her. Another indicator of problems is seen when a person *requires* drugs or alcohol in order to function on a day-to-day basis. Again, *requires* is a very subjective criterion for abuse. However, the woman who experiences physical or emotional discomfort when she abstains from alcohol or drugs must be seen as "requiring" the drug.

Women who abuse alcohol and/or drugs vary widely in age, in occupation, in socioeconomic status, in education, and in their patterns of use, abuse, and problems. Several patterns of women's alcohol abuse have been described. One set of patterns, identified through factor-analytic studies of hundreds of women receiving treatment for alcohol problems, is described here.

1. *Classical-syndrome alcoholism.* Women with this pattern have the shakes after they drink, and they drink in the morning to get rid of them. They have frequent, long blackouts while drinking and are frightened by these. They feel unable to stop drinking once they have begun. (This is sometimes referred to as *loss-of-control drinking.*) They often miss work or lose jobs because of their drinking. While drinking, they don't sleep or eat and are afraid of what is happening to them. This pattern of abuse is similar to classical alcoholism in men.

2. *Physiological reactions.* Women with this pattern of alcoholism have blackouts, convulsions (seizures), and delirium tremens (severe reactions when stopping drinking, which include shaking, not knowing where they are, and seeing things that aren't there). They also tend to abuse other forms of drugs, such as tranquilizers. Although

this pattern overlaps with classical-syndrome alcoholism, the physical problems are predominant, more extensive, and more severe.

3. *Gregarious drinking*. Women who describe their drinking this way often drink for a few days and then stop. They do not drink alone or at home, and they feel that drinking helps them to socialize. This drinking pattern is more common in younger women.

4. *Steady, long-binge drinking*. These women drink every day, with severe binges lasting many days. They also tend to drink at a certain time every day.

5. *Psychosocial benefit*. Women who fit this pattern of drinking believe that drinking results in pleasant feelings of relaxation, alertness, and an improved ability to work. They also believe that alcohol enables them to make friends and feel superior.

6. *"Controlled" problem drinking*. Women who report this pattern often are employed full time, drink only on weekends, and began their serious drinking at an older age. Their drinking is described as "controlled" because the negative consequences of the drinking often do not pervade as many areas of these women's lives.

7. *Marital difficulties*. Women with this drinking pattern have husbands who are angry about their drinking, and they have marital problems. They drink daily and sleep a great deal. Their drinking appears to be getting worse, even when they seek treatment.

8. *Early-age drinking*. Women with this pattern began drinking and first became drunk at a young age. They began drinking at home and primarily drink beer.

9. *Anxiety–guilt–shame*. These women feel ashamed and guilty about their drinking but also feel that alcohol helps them relax and feel better about themselves. They tend to drink alone and resent it when others say anything about their drinking. This pattern is the one most stereotypically associated with female alcoholism.

The patterns described here illustrate that many different kinds of behavior are characteristic of alcoholism in women, and that no one stereotypical pattern can describe all women with alcohol problems. Clearly, these patterns overlap in some ways and are separated here to emphasize the diversity of alcohol problems among women, rather than to provide neat boxes to fit women into. It must also be emphasized that women may change their drinking patterns at different points in their drinking lives, although how, when, or why patterns change is unknown.

OTHER CHEMICALS OF ABUSE

The primary focus of this chapter is on alcohol and alcoholism. However, women frequently tend to abuse other drugs in addition to alcohol. Some of these drugs interact with alcohol in dangerous ways when taken in combination. Therefore, a brief description of the common drugs of abuse is included here.

There are eight major categories of drugs most commonly abused. These include:

1. *Alcohol*. Alcohol is one of the most commonly used depressant drugs. It is widely available without a prescription and is inexpensive. Used in moderate quantities, alcohol has no negative effects in most adults and has mild relaxant effects that are often accompanied by decreases in social inhibitions. Used in larger quantities, alcohol can cause damage to every part of the body: the brain, stomach, pancreas, liver, circulatory system, skin, teeth, and kidneys. Alcohol can be physically addictive as well. The signs of addiction include fear, tremulousness, nausea, vomiting and diarrhea the morning after drinking, daily drinking, and drinking in the morning. If a woman is addicted to alcohol, she may experience mild withdrawal symptoms when she stops drinking, such as tremulousness, fear, nausea, vomiting, and difficulty in sleeping. She may also experience severe symptoms during withdrawal, such as convulsions, hallucinations, and disorientation (not knowing where she is, what day it is, or the identities of the people around her). Severe withdrawal can be a fatal condition if not treated, but all withdrawals can be treated safely. About 90% of withdrawal symptoms resolve within five to seven days after cessation of drinking, but some symptoms, such as anxiety, difficulty sleeping, and strong cravings for alcohol, may last as long as 6–12 months.

2. *Amphetamines and other stimulants* (Benzedrine, Dexedrine, Methedrine, Desbutal, Desoxyn—uppers, thrusters, speed). Amphetamines have marked stimulant effects on the central nervous system. Psychologically, they tend to provide feelings of euphoria. Historically, amphetamines were prescribed to women as aids in dieting or for the treatment of depression. However, most physicians now consider them unnecessary for dieting, and the U.S. Food and Drug Administration has recently ruled that they can no longer be prescribed for dieting. Studies also show that amphetamines are not an effective treatment for depression. (However, other classes of drugs are safe and effective antidepressants for many people). Over time, tolerance for the euphoric effects of amphetamines occurs, which often leads patients to abuse their medication by taking larger and larger doses in order to achieve the same effects. While fatal overdoses are rare, prolonged use may result in psychosis. Amphetamines are not physically addictive, although psychological dependence is common.

3. *Barbiturates* (Verinal, Luminal, Amytal, Butisol, Nembutal, Seconal, Pentothal—downers, reds). Barbiturates depress the central nervous system. In small doses, they relieve tension and anxiety, but in

large doses, they cause drowsiness, sluggishness, and sleep. This property makes them effective anesthetics, and when appropriately prescribed, they can be effective anticonvulsants. In the past, it was thought that it was safe to use barbiturates as sleep-inducing medication (sleeping pills). It is now recognized, however, that after taking a barbiturate to sleep, it is easy to forget that you have done so and thus to take an accidental overdose. Again, it should be emphasized that there are other drugs that are relatively safe, effective sleeping medications.

Tolerance to the sedative effects of barbiturates occurs and can result in the user's taking increasing amounts. Barbiturates are physically addicting, and to suddenly stop taking them after prolonged or heavy use leads to withdrawal symptoms. These include weakness, severe tremors, anxiety, fever, rapid pulse, violent seizures, and sometimes vivid hallucinations. Untreated barbiturate withdrawal can be fatal, although medically supervised withdrawal is generally safe. Alcohol and barbiturates can potentiate the effects of each other; they can cause a severe depression of the central nervous system. That is, when taken in combination, this combination can be fatal, and the two drugs should not be taken together.

4. *Cannabis* (marijuana, hashish, THC—grass, pot). *Cannabis* is the general term for the various derivatives of the flowering or fruiting tops of the hemp plant. Cannabis is not a legal drug at this time, although its use in the treatment of glaucoma and in cancer patients is currently being studied. The physical effects of the drug include dizziness, buzzing sounds, dryness of the mouth and throat (when smoked), unsteady movements, loss of coordination, hunger (especially craving for sweets), sensations of warmth, burning of the eyes and blurred vision, and other occasional reactions. The psychological effects are quite varied, depending on the user's previous experience with the drug, the setting, and the user's preingestion mood. Reactions may include vague dreads, fears, or anxiety, and disoriented thinking, such as fragmented thoughts, memory problems, and interruptions in thoughts. Euphoria, giggling, body-image distortion, and disorientation in space and time are common. Heightened sensuousness and increased subjective sensitivity to colors, music, and pictures are common. Marijuana is not physically addicting, although psychological dependence can occur. It is not known to cause psychoses or deaths, and its use does not automatically lead to the use or abuse of other drugs.

5. *Cocaine* (coke). Cocaine acts as a stimulant on the central nervous system, with resultant euphoria and hallucinatory experiences. It is most commonly sniffed or injected. Tolerance and physical addiction do not occur. However, prolonged use can result in hyperstimulation; problems with nausea, appetite, and weight loss; insomnia;

delusions; and visual hallucinations. Chronic sniffing can also deteriorate the lining and bones of the nose.

6. *Hallucinogens* (DMT, LSD, mescaline, peyote, psilocybin, psilocin). This class of drugs generates hallucinations, which may become startlingly real, although the user usually knows that he or she is hallucinating. Hallucinations occasionally continue after the immediate effects of the drug have worn off. "Flashbacks," the recurrence of hallucinations weeks or months after the last use of the drug, have been reported.

7. *Heroin* (H). Heroin is a semisynthetic derivative of morphine. It is not legal to use heroin in medical practice today in the United States. In some countries, it is legal to prescribe heroin, either to legally maintain a patient's habit or to reduce pain in terminal disease. The primary effects of heroin are pain reduction, drowsiness, euphoria, constipation, vomiting, sedation, and relief of anxiety and tension. Heroin may be sniffed, injected subcutaneously ("skin popping"), or injected intravenously ("mainlining"). Repeated use of heroin leads to tolerance to the drug, so that increasingly larger doses are needed to achieve the same effect. With prolonged use, the euphoric effects of heroin are no longer achieved, but use continues because of physical addiction and the need to avoid withdrawal symptoms. Because heroin is both illegal and expensive, many women and men who are addicted become involved in such illegal activities as stealing and prostitution to support their drug habit.

8. *Minor tranquilizers* (Librium, Valium, Tranxene, Serax, Librax, Equanil, Miltown). Minor tranquilizers are usually used for the relief of moderate levels of anxiety and tension. Some are also used as muscle relaxants. They may cause drowsiness, uncoordination, dizziness, or stomach upset. Taken in large doses over long periods of time, they can be physically addicting. The dual use of tranquilizers and alcohol is a common and potentially deadly combination, because of the potentiating effects of the two drugs (i.e., the depressant effects multiply instead of merely being added together). Valium is the most commonly prescribed drug in the United States; Librium is third.

The first sections of this chapter have defined alcohol abuse and its symptoms, have described patterns of alcohol abuse, and have discussed other drugs that are commonly abused. We now turn our attention to the role of alcohol and alcohol abuse in the female life cycle.

OVERVIEW OF THE LIFE CYCLE

The development of any human being involves both physiological and psychological development and change. Our primary interest in this chapter is in psychological issues in development, and how alcohol use and abuse interact with various developmental tasks.

Psychological development alternates between periods of relative quiescence, equilibrium, or stability and periods of turmoil, upheaval, and disequilibrium. At each point of disequilibrium, certain important psychological changes occur. These changes may involve (1) cognitive capacities—the capacity to think, reason and comprehend; (2) emotional capacities—the capacity to react emotionally, to differentiate and label emotions, and to express feelings; (3) interpersonal capacities—the capacity to form relationships and to form different types of relationships with people; and (4) one's overall view of oneself as a person. Psychodynamic theorists dating back to Freud have written about these developmental changes; however, developmental changes have been extensively studied by researchers of many theoretical persuasions. It should be emphasized that all persons do not go through all the stages of psychological development in an identical fashion, but common issues and themes frequently emerge at certain points in people's lives. In this discussion of alcohol abuse and the life cycle, we focus on the effects of an alcoholic mother on the infant and the young child. Then, the focus shifts to factors in later childhood associated with the later development of alcohol problems. Then, we examine the emergence of alcohol problems in adolescence and young, middle, and late adulthood.

INFANCY AND EARLY CHILDHOOD

A child born to a mother who is an alcohol or drug addict may actually become addicted before birth to the drug that the mother has been abusing. The infant may consequently have to go through withdrawal from the drug. The withdrawal syndrome is a dangerous condition in adults, and it is even more dangerous for an infant. While the risk of being born addicted to alcohol is fairly low, children born to alcoholic mothers who are drinking heavily (an average of six or more drinks per day) during their pregnancy *are* at high risk for congenital malformations, low birth weight, irritability, and possible later learning disabilities. Data show that heavy drinking during pregnancy is strongly correlated with birth defects, but the same studies also indicate that heavily drinking women who stop drinking during their pregnancy have a very good chance of giving birth to healthy infants. The message is clear. Addicted women who become pregnant *need treatment for their addiction*. Such treatment, unfortunately, is complicated, since it is inadvisable to use drugs for the treatment of withdrawal in pregnant women, as these drug treatments may also cause birth defects.

In recent years, the fetal alcohol syndrome (FAS) has been studied professionally and discussed in the popular literature. The characteristics of the FAS include low birth weight, prenatal and postnatal growth deficiency, microcephaly (small head), shortened slits between the eyelids, joint abnormalities, altered crease patterns in the palms, heart problems, and problems in fine-motor coordination. The results of continued research have suggested that the incidence of the full fetal alcohol syndrome (including all the characteristics described) among children born to alcoholic mothers is not very high, but that the presence of some birth defects is very likely.[1]

In the postnatal period, children with birth defects are more likely to have abnormal sleep patterns and do not easily establish regular sleeping and waking cycles. Thus, even for a mother who is functioning well, children with irregular sleep–waking cycles are more difficult to care for, as they are more irritable, less predictable, and therefore more frustrating than children with regular cycles. When a mother is actively drinking, her irritability and unpredictable behavior interact with the child's unpredictable behavior, making it difficult to develop strong affectional bonds, to provide consistent parenting, and to establish basic trust between the child and the parent. The mother who is actively drinking is frequently sick, intoxicated, irritable, experiencing alcohol withdrawal, not caring for herself, having fights with her husband, and, in the midst of all this, trying to care for a difficult infant. It is a no-win situation that tends to exacerbate the alcoholism, and further impair the child's development.

To fully understand the relationship between a mother's alcoholism and early childhood development, it is necessary to consider the psychological tasks of early childhood. The primary psychological tasks of early childhood, according to Erikson,[5] involve three different areas. In the earliest months of a child's life, Erikson postulated that the most important psychological issue for a child to master is the development of a sense of basic trust in other people. The development of trust first occurs as a child learns that she or he is being cared for, and that someone will help alleviate the many physical discomforts of the infant. Feeling comfortable and associating special people with this feeling of comfort lead the infant to be able to let the parent out of sight without undue anxiety, because that parent has become "an inner certainty as well as an outer predictability."[5] Of course, for this sense of certainty and trust to develop, the parents have to be sensitive to the child's needs, as well as reliable and consistent. When the mother of an infant is drinking, it is difficult for her to be reliable and sensitive. It is also difficult for her husband, if he is there, to be caring, reliable, and consistent because he is also feeling stressed, angry, and disorganized by the dual stresses of having a young infant and a drinking wife.

As the child develops, Erikson postulated that the second basic psychological task is to develop a sense of autonomy. Autonomy is the feeling of being able to have control over things in one's world and being able to express oneself. Children enter this stage at about 18 months to 2 years of age. During this period, which lasts on the average until age 3, the child is frequently oppositional, saying no to the most gentle requests, throwing temper tantrums with little provocation, and generally showing the behavior that characterizes what has come to be known as "the terrible twos." The psychological danger to the child during this stage is that these expressions of autonomy and moves toward independence may be severely punished, leading the child to feel ashamed of his or her own impulses and, most fundamentally, to feel ashamed of his or her very existence. This is a difficult developmental stage for the parent. The need to be firm and set limits is clear, but the child often reacts against these limits in most unpleasant and trying ways. For a mother who is drinking, the tantrums and aggression of her young child may be extremely painful. She may feel guilty, fearing that her drinking is creating the child's behavior, and may respond to this guilt by trying to give the child whatever she or he may want. Giving in to the child's demands results in the child's ever escalating his or her demands, resulting in more frustration, anger, and guilt in the mother. Conversely, her own guilt and irritability may lead her to be unduly harsh and aggressive toward the child, so that the child may feel more and more ashamed of his or her very being.

In the next stage of early childhood development, the most important psychological task is the development of initiative. The child may become more relaxed, loving, and active. She or he continues to develop the sense of autonomy established earlier and enhances it by being able to begin activities and follow them through for the pure pleasure of doing so. The psychological danger of this stage is that the child may feel guilty about initiating acts or guilty about acts which she or he is considering. For the parent of a child at this stage, allowing the child and encouraging the child to develop initiative, begin activities, and follow them through, while at the same time maintaining firm limits and showing respect for the child, is a difficult task. Drinking makes the parent's tasks difficult, as the child's own identity and actions may often interfere with the drinking mother's plans for her drinking, or the mother's ability to handle the child's exuberance at this stage.

The above discussion of the relationship between early childhood development and maternal alcoholism is based almost completely on a theoretical analysis. To date, research studies do not exist on alcoholic-mother–child interactions during infancy and early childhood, or on the early and later adjustment of the children of alcoholic mothers. It is important to emphasize that many factors could exacerbate or attenuate the negative course of events postulated here. For example, the employment status of the mother, the presence or absence of the father, the relationship of the father and the child, the drinking patterns of the mother, the availability of other caretakers, or the presence of other family members in the home may affect the course of the early development of the child of an alcoholic mother.

CHILDHOOD

For the remainder of this developmental discussion, we will examine the factors associated with the development and emergence of alcoholism in the woman. Therefore, we will not focus on the effects of maternal alcoholism on children and adolescents; rather, we discuss the psychological patterns seen in children that appear to be related to the development of alcoholism in later life. Unfortunately, research studies in this area are scant. Throughout the remainder of the chapter, therefore, the reader should keep in mind that this discussion is based on incomplete information about alcohol abuse and the female life cycle.

In childhood, as a child enters school, he or she first learns to work. The concept of work—or "industry,"[5] in Erikson's term—means becoming productive and goal-directed, and experiencing a sense of completion and mastery through working, producing things, and accomplishing things. The danger for the child at this stage lies in the possibility of developing a sense of inferiority to others, rather than a sense of industry and accomplishment. At this developmental stage, traumatic events in the child's life and/or hostile, rejecting, or inconsistent relationships with the parents may seriously interfere with a child's ability to work productively. In such an emotionally disturbed family atmosphere, even if the child is able to be productive, she or he may not receive the kind of positive feedback and support from the parents that is so important in supporting a child's sense of accomplishment.

What are the childhood experiences of women who later become alcoholics? A caution is in order before attempting to answer this question. Data on the childhood of women who later develop alcohol problems have come primarily from studies of middle-class, white, married women, who have reported retrospectively on their childhood. Therefore, we know nothing about the childhood experiences of women of other racial backgrounds, marital or socioeconomic status, or homosexual or bisexual orientations. Keeping in mind the limitations of our information, we turn now to the available studies.

In one study,[6] loss of one or both parents at an early stage was frequently noted. Fathers were often unavailable because of death, divorce, alcoholism, or psychiatric problems. If both parents were present, the alcoholic woman described her mother as hostile, rejecting, cold, and harsh. The alcoholic women in this study stated that they were not closely attached to either parent, so that they did not turn to their parents for help in times of crisis. Of course, such a disturbed childhood does not cause alcoholism, as it can also occur in normal women and women with psychiatric problems, as well as in alcohol- or drug-addicted women. The retrospective nature of these studies also limits their use. We have no way of knowing whether, in fact, these women experienced their parents as rejecting and cold during childhood, or if their perceptions of their parents changed as a result of their current feelings of rejection, guilt, and shame because of their alcoholism. If, indeed, these women did experience such a rejecting childhood, this would certainly make it difficult to develop a sense of autonomy, productivity, and independence, and the rejection would reinforce feelings of shame, insecurity, and inadequacy. It should be pointed out, however, that such a childhood, although possibly contributing to the development of alcoholism, is not in itself a cause of alcoholism. If it were, then all women with such backgrounds would be alcoholics, which clearly is not the case.

ADOLESCENCE

Adolescence is a period characterized by intense physical and psychological growth. Puberty and the development of secondary sexual characteristics are the most obvious indications of the onset of the adolescent period. The development of a sense of unique identity is one of the most significant psychological tasks during this developmental period. The establishment of a unique identity often involves rebelling or fighting against many of the most important role figures in the adolescent's environment; such rebellion is a normal characteristic of this stage. If adolescence is successfully negotiated, the young woman emerging from adolescence has developed a sense of confidence in her meaning for others and also has begun to establish herself in a career or an occupational identity.

How does the use of alcohol fit into this adolescent period for the teenage girl? Recent reports show that the proportion of drinkers, heavy drinkers, and problem drinkers among youths increased steadily up to 1965.[1] Teenagers typically begin drinking alcohol at about the age of 13, with about the same proportions of boys and girls drinking alcohol during their adolescent years. Among junior- and senior-high students, approximately 4% of 7th-grade girls have problems in their use of alcohol, and this percentage increases to approximately 21% of teenage girls with alcohol problems in the 12th grade.

Some recent studies have attempted to identify the differences between teenage girls who drink and those who do not. These studies have also compared girls who are experiencing problems or who have potential problems with alcohol with teenage girls for whom drinking is not a problem. The data in this area are somewhat conflicting and sparse. The results of a national survey of drinking practices in adolescence[7,8] showed that young women who have problems with alcohol have different psychological characteristics, different perceptions of their environment, and different behavior patterns than girls who have no drinking problems. In general, teenage girls (and boys) who have alcohol problems tend to value academics less, to value their independence more than they value achieving, and to have lower expectations of their ability to achieve than do nonproblem drinkers. Problem-drinking teenagers tolerate deviance more, are less religious, and see more desirable aspects of drinking than do their counterparts who have no drinking problems. These problem-drinking girls also see conflict in their friends' relationships with their (the friends') parents, are more influenced by their friends than their parents, report that more of their friends use drugs and alcohol (compared with the nonproblem drinkers), and report that their friends do not disapprove of drugs and alcohol as strongly as do friends of nonproblem drinkers. Thus, these data suggest that girls with drinking problems hold different values, are in different peer groups, and behave differently from girls with no drinking problems.

Using the data from the same national survey, Wilsnack and Wilsnack[8] looked at the sex-role perceptions of these young women (including the nondrinkers, the drinkers, and the problem drinkers). These authors found that the girls as a group increased their desire for traditional femininity as they got older. Whether the girls in the study drank or not made no difference in their desire for traditionally feminine roles. The researchers found, in predicting drinking versus nondrinking, that the girls' grade in school, their religious affiliation, and

their attitudes about norms for women's drinking were stronger predictors of whether individual girls would be drinking than was sex-
role identification. However, the results also suggested that rejection
of the traditionally feminine role (on a six-item scale of traditional
femininity*) was more common among adolescent girls having problems with drinking than among those who drank but with no problems.

The above data suggest that teenage girls who are experiencing
problems with alcohol are not as accepting of traditionally feminine
sex-role behaviors as teenage girls who either drink without problems
or who do not drink. Their drinking appears to be associated with
different personality characteristics, with more deviant behavior, and
with a peer group that appears to support this drinking behavior, rather
than supporting nondrinking or nonproblem drinking. It appears that
such girls are struggling to develop a clear sense of identity, and that
their identity as young women and in the area of occupational functioning (as evidenced by poor school performance) is likely to be conflicted. Of course, rejecting traditional "femininity" can also lead to
high achievement. It appears that the combination of poor academic
achievement and a peer group that supports drinking intereacts with
nontraditional sex-role identification to contribute to the development
of drinking problems.

In contrast to these findings about teenagers with current drinking problems, a longitudinal study that followed girls from adolescence into adulthood showed that girls who became alcoholics as adults
were more likely to be described as submissive as youngsters rather
than as deviant and rebellious.[9] This study also concluded that adolescent girls who later have trouble with alcohol accept highly traditional
feminine sex-role stereotypes, but that in their midlife years (see below), they have more difficulty with accepting this stereotypical view.
It may be that extremes of rebelliousness contribute to teenage drinking problems. Submissiveness may contribute to low drinking as an
adolescent. However, as a submissive teenager matures, she may begin to experience conflict between her submissiveness and her role
functioning. A variety of life experiences, as described below, may
create further conflict between the maturing woman's submissive stance

---

*The authors used three data sources to measure sex-role orientation: (1) 12 adjective
phrases to describe the kind of person the girl would like to be, where, in previous
research, 6 were endorsed more often by men; 6 by women; (2) 6 Likert items on sex-
role performance; and (3) self-ratings of how much the respondents valued marriage,
children, and a career. From these data sources, a 6-item, face-valid scale of traditional
femininity was constructed, and this is the measure on which the authors' conclusions
were based.

and her life experiences. She may eventually turn to alcohol as a way to alleviate this conflict, and thus, she may develop drinking problems later in life.

In conclusion, it appears that girls who have problems with alcohol or who later develop problems with alcohol have an extremely difficult time shaping a clear identity, and that they are not highly successful in this psychological endeavor. Teenage girls who already have problems with alcohol are different from adolescent girls who develop problems with alcohol as adults. Both groups, though, seem to react at the extremes to the normal conflicts of adolescence. The limited data available suggest that girls who experience early problems with alcohol are more likely to reject traditional feminine stereotypes, whereas girls who initially are nonproblem drinkers but who develop problems with alcohol in their midlife years are more likely to try very hard to accept very traditional, highly feminine sex-role attitudes. It may be that when they reach midlife, they are no longer able to continue this passive acceptance of the "hyperfeminine" role.

Young Adulthood

In young adulthood, men and women are struggling to establish a firm sense of identity and to establish significant intimate relationships. At this stage, men and women are more eager and psychologically ready to form stable, committed relationships, even when these involve compromise and sacrifice. The psychological danger of this developmental period is in remaining distant, isolated, and aloof from opportunities for love and intimacy. Another important focus of young adulthood is for a woman (or a man) to attempt to master what she feels she is expected to do. For many women, these expectations are fully identified with the establishment of intimacy through marriage. (More and more women are developing their careers during this period; the issues of adult generativity through work are considered in the next section.) Until recently, a woman in her 20s was not expected to find an independent identity. She was expected to establish a relationship with a man who would be the stronger and protect her and care for her.

Because the issues of young adulthood revolve so much around intimacy and love relationships, this section focuses on traditional sex-role-related issues, including marriage, sexual functioning, and sex-role identity. Throughout the discussion of sex-role issues, the reader is cautioned to keep in mind that women in their twenties are an extremely heterogeneous group with regard to the use of alcohol. Among women in their twenties are (1) those who had alcohol problems in their teens but have outgrown them; (2) those who have not outgrown their drinking problems; (3) women who are showing alcohol problems now; (4) those who will develop problems anywhere from their 30s to their 70s; and (5) those women who didn't, don't, and won't have drinking problems. We know virtually nothing about how similar or different these five groups of women are.

Women who are or who become alcoholics get married at about the same rate as women without significant drinking problems. However, the rates of divorce and separation for alcoholic women are extremely high. In fact, the separation and divorce rates for alcoholic women are higher than the rates for alcoholic men, with some estimates suggesting that the husband of a female alcoholic is 10 times as likely to divorce his wife as is the wife to divorce a male alcoholic.

Extensive and detailed studies of men married to alcoholic women are sadly lacking. This lack of studies of husbands of alcoholics is due to several factors, including the lower rates of identification of alcoholic women, the less frequent study of alcoholic women, and an attitude of pity for rather than blame of men married to alcoholic women. This is in sharp contrast to the views of women married to alcoholic men, who have been viewed as being integrally involved in the cause and maintenance of their husbands' alcoholism. The research literature shows that such wives are in an acutely stressful environment, and that virtually all of the painful feelings and symptoms that they experience decrease or disappear if the alcoholic mate stops drinking for a while. In contrast to the studies attempting to find out what's "wrong" with the wife of an alcoholic male, one study of the husbands of alcoholic women stated that these men had become dominant in their marriages after the wives developed alcohol problems, and that this dominance was quite helpful to the women's recovery. The researchers suggested that the husbands' dominance allowed the women to function in their "feminine" roles, which, by implication, were seen to be important to good psychological health. The authors expressed no doubt that accepting traditional sex-role definitions was essential to recovery and did not even suggest that conflict about sex-role identity, or power–dominance conflicts between these alcoholic women and their mates could be issues in these marriages. They also did not explore at all the possibility that acceptance (by the women and their mates) of traditional sex-role identification could have contributed to the women's problems originally.

While few studies have actually looked at the marital relationships of alcoholic women, Gomberg[10] stated that women who become alcoholics have a significant need for love and reassurance because of the deprivations experienced in their childhood. She suggested that these women look to their husbands to fulfill these dependency needs, but that no marriage and no man can fulfill needs that are based on earlier difficulties or deprivations. The use of alcohol in such marriages allows the woman to escape a painful and unsatisfying relationship, enables her to express her anger at this man for not satisfying these unsatisfiable needs, and also provides her the sense of pleasure for which she so desperately wishes.

In addition to the psychological issues identified in the marriages of alcoholic women, statistical information suggests that a large proportion of female alcoholics are married to male alcoholics.[11] We do not know how many of these women became alcoholics before they met their husbands, how many developed problems before their husbands did, and how many developed drinking problems after their husbands did. We do know, however, that many women alcoholics drink along with their alcoholic husbands, and that recovery for such couples is extremely difficult. Each member of the couple has to deal with his or her own alcohol issues, and each lacks the support of the spouse, because that spouse is also looking for someone to help in his or her own recovery.

In addition to the early conflicts and disappointments that many alcoholic women experience in their marital relationships, alcoholic women also tend to have gynecological problems during their early adulthood. Of alcoholic women who have ever married, 78% have reported obstetrical or gynecological problems,[12] including difficulties in conception, repeated miscarriages, permanent sterility, and hysterectomies. Some research studies have found that these gynecological problems preceded the development of the alcoholism and therefore may have contributed to the alcoholism. However, other studies have found no time relationship between the gynecological and drinking problems. Therefore, we cannot conclude that gynecological problems contribute to the development of alcoholism, but it is clear that they are associated with alcoholism in women.

In looking at another physiological issue for women, some studies have shown that approximately half of menstruating women related the onset of drinking episodes to tension during the premenstrual phase.[13] However, premenstrual tension is extremely common among alcoholic and nonalcoholic women, and therefore cannot serve as an explanation for abusive drinking in women.

The effects of alcohol on sexual arousal and the variability of women's physiological responses to alcohol may also contribute to an understanding of female alcoholism. It is known that women reach higher blood-alcohol levels than men taking the same amount of alcohol, and that the level of alcohol in the bloodstream may vary greatly, in direct relationship to changing hormone levels during the menstrual cycle. It is also known that women on oral contraceptives metabolize alcohol more slowly than women who are not on such contraceptives;[14] therefore, such women become intoxicated more readily and stay intoxicated longer than they did when they were not on oral contraceptives. Thus, women find that they are more sensitive to the effects of alcohol, and that their responses are unpredictable from day to day, which makes it difficult to modulate and control their drinking. Also relevant is a recent study[15] that has shown that alcohol reduces sexual arousal in women, both physiologically and psychologically, which contradicts the stereotypical picture of alcohol's making a woman more sexually available and responsive (the "Candy is dandy, but liquor is quicker" notion). This marked discrepancy between a woman's actual experience and what society tells her she should feel may create further confusion about alcohol and its role in her life.

A picture of the alcoholic or potentially alcoholic woman begins to emerge in her twenties. The woman may enter marriage with a background of deprivation, and with high expectations that marriage will compensate for these earlier sadnesses in her life. She marries, but the marriage is characterized by a lack of emotional communication.[16] She may begin to drink, and to find that her response to alcohol is somewhat unpredictable and that the more she drinks the less she responds to her husband physically, which may lead him to become more withdrawn and distant. As she is married longer, the disappointments of her marital relationship become more evident to her, and she may also be experiencing gynecological problems. The disappointments of marriage, the developing sexual and marital problems, and the physical problems all contribute to and reinforce her confusion about her sex-role identity and her self-esteem.

A number of researchers and theoreticians have pointed to low self-esteem and confused sex-role identity as significant psychological factors among women with alcohol problems. Blane[17] has hypothesized that preoccupations with inadequacy, ineptness, and a sense of inability to cope successfully on one's own are central psychological features of alcoholic women. (Whether these psychological features precede or result from the alcoholism, however, is not known). Several studies have indicated that female alcoholics have a poor self-concept. The most recent studies[18] have found that self-esteem among women alcoholics is lower than that of male alcoholics and is also lower than the self-esteem of normal women, but is similar to the self-esteem of women in treatment for psychiatric problems not related to the use of alcohol.

Research and theories about sex-role identification and conflict in alcoholic women are both abundant and contradictory. Some researchers have postulated that women with alcohol problems have a "hyperfeminine" identification. In studies attempting to measure conscious and unconscious attitudes, some reports [19] suggest that alcoholic women do exhibit "overidentification" with traditional feminine sex-role stereotypes, but that measures tapping unconscious identifications and values find more "masculinity" and concern with power and assertiveness issues than in nonalcoholic women. This finding suggests that the alcoholic women studied experienced conflicts between their conscious desire to do what they were expected to do by experiencing themselves as traditionally feminine, and their less conscious desires to be "masculine." However, other studies [20] have come to the opposite conclusion, describing alcoholic women as having a conscious "masculine" identification and an unconscious feminine sex-role identification. Still other researchers [21] have postulated that the direction of sex-role conflict may vary with the individual woman. These researchers have postulated that drinking reduces sexual conflict, and an experimental evaluation lent support to their theoretical model. Unfortunately, they did not examine age variability in their study. It may be that younger and older women alcoholics experience sex-role conflict in quite different ways, as would be suggested by the studies showing markedly different sex-role issues among teenagers who have alcohol problems and those who develop them in later adulthood.

While most of the research on sex-role conflict has focused on the psychological aspects of sex-role conflict and sex-role identification, current research is beginning to examine sociological roles and role conflict. Conflicts may arise from a number of sources, such as (1) juggling a number of roles (e.g., among working mothers); (2) working in a traditionally male occupation after being socialized to function in traditionally "feminine" ways; or (3) the woman's experiencing a discrepancy between a woman's role and her evaluation of her competency in this role. These factors, currently being studied by Helen Metzner at the University of Michigan, may be more important aspects of sex-role conflict than the psychological conflicts considered separate from actual role functioning.

Some notes of caution in interpreting these studies on sex-role conflict in women alcoholics must be interjected at this point. Although these studies raise important issues, they may at the same time be perpetuating a subtle but powerful stereotype about women alcoholics that suggests that women's conflicts all revolve around sex-related issues, rather than a wide range of issues, some related to sex and some totally unrelated to sex. Also, the research on sex-role conflict has typically focused only on these variables, rather than attempting an analysis of multiple factors associated with women's alcoholism. Thus, while the sex-role conflict may indeed exist, it may not have been a major factor contributing to the development of alcoholism in many women.

While difficulties in marital relationships, confused sex-role identity, poor self-concept, marriage to an alcohol- or drug-abusing husband, and gynecological problems may set the stage for the later development of alcoholism, some women also develop problems with alcohol in their twenties. A recent study of almost 300 women admitted to a public detoxification facility [22] found that those who had drug-abuse problems and those with "antisocial personalities" showed an onset of alcohol problems in their twenties. The diagnosis of antisocial personality was established if the woman had had problems with her family, her school, the police, and her peers prior to the age of 16. The results of this study suggest that women who develop alcohol problems in their twenties may be similar to teenage girls with drinking problems, with an emphasis on social problems as well as particular personality and behavior patterns. As noted at the beginning of this section, we really do not know how different these women are from those whose alcoholism isn't apparent until their thirties and forties. Careful studies are sorely needed to compare alcoholic women in these different age groups on social variables, personality variables, and marital, sex-role identity, and self-concept variables.

THE THIRTIES

The transition from twenties to thirties, and the decade from the thirties to the early forties, has been described [23] as an "opening up" period, in which the individual begins to examine the choices she made in her twenties based on her perceptions of what she thought society expected her to do. Many a woman begins to examine these assumptions in light of a greater recognition of her current situation and her untapped capacities and capabilities. Such an examination may result in a growing realization that she may have the potential to succeed in many areas that have previously been unrecognized.

Erikson [5] has emphasized that one of the most significant psychological tasks of adulthood is to develop a sense of "generativity," a sense of productivity, creativity, and meaning in one's life as an adult. There are many routes to this sense of generativity, for example, parenthood or productive or creative work. Traditionally, women have achieved this feeling of generativity through their children, and through the creative work of reproduction, caring for and nurturing a child, and helping the child to develop emotionally, intellectually, morally, and spiritually. Some women also develop this sense of generativity through their involvement in volunteer work or through their employment and careers. For the woman who made the choice in her twenties to function primarily in wife, mother, and homemaker roles, a reexamination of her situation may result in considering her potential in the world of work, through beginning a job, developing a career, or returning to a career. For the woman who initially began to develop a career, a reexamination of her choices may involve reconsideration of her career or a yearning for marriage (if she is unmarried) or motherhood (if she is without children). The woman who is married may question her commitment to her marriage at this time, and if she remains married, the couple may go through a difficult but growth-producing examination of the spoken and unspoken agreements of their relationship during this period.

Although we have some general knowledge about the choices that women make in their 30s, we know very few specifics about which factors predict what patterns and choices women make in their 20s and 30s. We have no data on the incidence of these patterns among alcoholic women or on the problems that alcoholic women have in this transition from the 20s to the 30s. However, some review data[24] suggest that on the average, women develop alcohol problems in their early 30s. Therefore, examination of the 20s and 30s appears to be crucial to an understanding of some of the patterns in the adult development of female alcoholism.

As noted above, one of the common choices that women make in their 30s is to begin, develop, or expand their careers. Many women in their late 20s and early 30s find that they have to work outside the home, either because their intact family needs the money, or because they are single and need to support themselves, or because they are divorced or widowed and need to support themselves. What do we know about the employed woman alcoholic? Unfortunately, very little. As noted in the previous section of this chapter, reviews of the literature concerning women alcoholics pay great attention to sex-role identity issues, alcoholic women's relationships with men and children, fetal alcohol syndrome, and family histories (both psychologically and in terms of the incidence of alcoholism), but occupational status and occupational issues are most frequently not even noted. A notable exception to this omission is an early review by Lisansky.[25] She was one of the first and one of the few to discuss occupational classification in a study of the social histories of alcoholic women. Lisansky found that in her group of 46 subjects, 28 were employed. She attributed the high incidence (in 1957) of employed women to the large proportion of single, divorced, separated, and widowed women in her sample, and she also noted that many of the married women were holding part-time or full-time jobs. She observed that many of the women had high-status occupations, including nursing, teaching, social work, and writing, and that they appeared to be functioning efficiently in their jobs. Lisansky suggested that alcoholic women may show a degree of occupational integration that is similar to that of alcoholic men observed in outpatient settings. This picture contrasts with the stereotypical view of alcoholic women as either housewives or on skid row.

A recent, pioneering review[26] found that in 1977, a computerized search of major journals found no articles on the combined topics of employees, women, and alcoholism. This finding indicated that there were few, if any, studies of alcoholic women in the workplace. As a consequence, the author interviewed counselors working in various occupational programs in order to identify some of the unique problems of the employed alcoholic woman. The author noted (as is well known) that the employment rate among women has steadily increased, so that by 1975, 49% of the civilian work force was female. She also noted that among workers employed full time, women's median earnings were less than three-fifths of men's median earnings in 1973. Although data are not yet available, she and other workers in the field have hypothesized that women in employment settings feel that it is necessary for them to work harder and to be more competent than their male colleagues to prove that they are equal. The pressures to succeed in the job become overwhelming. In addition to the stresses of the employment situation, many of these women are heads of households and, when they return home, have to care for children, cook meals, and maintain their homes. They often have few job skills, are underpaid, and so are living at or below the poverty level. Surveys reveal that women (even if married and even if employed full time outside of the home) still do the vast majority of household chores. Thus, employed women experience stresses that are very different from those faced by employed men, because of the multiple responsibilities and pressures that women experience. It should be emphasized, however, that this combination of stresses cannot be considered the cause of female alcoholism, since most employed women are not alcoholics. However, these stresses certainly do not help women to remain nonalcoholic.

Women who are having trouble with alcohol behave differently on the job than do male alcoholics, and they also may be treated differently by supervisors and co-workers. Studies suggest[27] that alcoholic women drink on the job less than their male counterparts, which makes their problems harder to identify and to confront. Their supervisors often are males, and confrontation, reprimands for poor performance, and referrals for treatment are all tinged by the male–female relationship. Recent hypotheses suggest that women, when confronted with their alcoholism and the need to get treatment in order to maintain their jobs, often leave their jobs and move laterally to another position in another company. These kinds of moves are relatively easy to make for the many women employed in semiskilled positions. It is also felt that poor job performance is sometimes more difficult to recognize in women because of their lower job level, where the opportunities for mistakes are not as numerous, nor as obvious.

Thus, for the woman who works and has developed an alcohol problem, the problems are compounded. The stress of employment for a woman is different from the stress of employment for a man, the satisfaction is often less, and the stresses of combining home and job duties are difficult. Alcohol may appear to provide relief from these situations, but, of course, it only exacerbates problems, by adding to the woman's already poorly defined sense of identity, by increasing her level of guilt, and by decreasing her efficiency at her job and at home. Thus, the woman alcoholic is less able to perform competently; her incompetence, in turn, feeds her feelings of inadequacy about herself as a person and as a woman.

MIDLIFE

From her late 30s to her 50s, a woman begins to deal with the issues of midlife. Much has been written about "midlife crises," and they have become popular to talk about. In midlife, a woman realizes that she is halfway or more than halfway through her life and begins to examine what she has accomplished and what she has become. If she is married, she may again examine her relationship with her husband and look at it in comparison with the dreams and hopes that she had before she married. If, in addition, she has children, her children are beginning to leave home, and she is feeling the pain of their loss at the same time that she may be critically evaluating how her children, her creations, are turning out. If she has devoted herself to a career as a homemaker and mother, she begins to question what her functions in life are at this point, and what it is that will make her feel valuable now and in the future. If she has devoted herself to her occupation, she may question whether she has missed the satisfactions of parenthood. For single women, the choice or necessity of staying single may be examined once again.

This period in a person's life involves a serious examination of the issues described above and also often involves beginning to accept behavioral capacities not previously expressed. Thus, passivity may be questioned, and a woman may begin to become more assertive in expressing her own opinions, needs, and desires. At the same time, a man may become more expressive of emotional and affective dimensions.

Midlife is the time at which women are most likely to be identified as alcoholics, and the time at which they are most likely to come to treatment. Many women develop alcohol problems earlier, in their teens, 20s, and 30s. However, even if a woman develops a drinking problem prior to midlife, there are many factors that preclude women from seeking treatment and from even being identified as having alcohol problems prior to midlife. First, a woman with children who has an alcohol problem has a realistic concern that she may lose her children if she is labeled an alcoholic. If she is hospitalized and has few supports, she may have no way to have her children cared for other than by entrusting them to the state system, with foster care, and the resulting constant evaluation of her effectiveness and competency as a mother. Societal and family attitudes also militate against a woman's being identified as an alcoholic at an early age. Families often collude in protecting the woman from being identified as an alcoholic, by picking up her responsibilities for her, by ignoring obvious signs of her problem, and by making excuses for her when others notice that she is having difficulties. If an alcoholic woman is not employed, she is able to drink when there is nobody else home, can hide bottles more easily, and may actually be able to hide her drinking from her family for some time. As described above, because of women's employment status, and the feeling of many male supervisors that they wish to protect their women subordinates, women who are employed are often not confronted or urged to get early treatment. The drinking problem thus lingers on and on at home and on the job until finally it becomes impossible for employer, family, friends, or the woman herself to ignore it any longer.

Many professionals have suggested that women develop alcohol problems as a result of life stresses, and especially midlife stresses. Joan Curlee[28] studied 100 male and 100 female patients in an alcoholism treatment center. She concluded that alcoholism in women was more often related to specific life situations than was true for the men studied, and she believed that she had identified the specific stresses precipitating the alcoholism in 26% of the women she studied. Many of these cases were related to midlife issues, such as the "death of a husband, divorce, menopause, marriage of children, or other disruption of the role of wife and mother." Rosenbaum[29] found that when women were asked about the major causes of their alcoholic episodes, they reported marital conflict, anger, resentment, depression, problems with their children, and loneliness as likely to trigger alcoholic episodes. These two studies suggest that specific life stresses may be highly correlated with drinking in alcoholic women. What is not known is whether alcoholic women are more likely than men to have these specific life stresses as antecedents to their drinking, or whether, instead, alcoholic women feel more need to explain their drinking than do alcoholic men, since women's drinking is perceived as much less socially acceptable and much more shameful than men's drinking.

Not all studies support the hypothesis that life stresses contribute to the development of alcoholism in women. A recent study[30] found essentially no relationship between the experience of life stress events and the age of onset of alcohol problems. This study examined the relationship between alcoholism and gynecological events, the death of a member of the nuclear family or the family of origin, suicide attempts, separation or divorce, homosexual experiences, and drug problems and found no relationship between these events and the onset of alcohol problems. Thus, the results of this study raise serious questions about the contribution of midlife crises and other life crises to the development of female alcoholism.

The Sixties and Beyond

The later years in a woman's life can be ones of satisfaction and renewal, or of depression and disintegration. The woman who has successfully negotiated an integration of her sense of self, has achieved a sense of peace about the life that she has lived to this date, and has developed a sense of acceptance of the limitations of her life, her self, and her relationships may feel free in her later years to tap new sources of energy and interests for which she had not previously had the time. Thus, developing avocations and interests, deepening relationships, and developing a sense of peace about one's own life and one's aging are one form of resolution of one's psychological life work. At this point, many people begin to feel a greater need for involvement with friends and people whom they are close to, while others begin to feel the need to withdraw and develop a sense of peace with themselves in their own isolation.

Very little has been written about alcoholism among elderly women, and there are, in fact, few studies of alcoholism in the elderly in general. National surveys[1] reveal that 2%–10% of men over 65 and 2% of women in this age group have alcohol problems. These results reflect a number of factors. The number of persons who abstain from alcohol increases markedly above the age of 64 for both men and women. Also, since alcoholism reduces life expectancy, many alcoholics die before reaching this age, thus reducing the incidence of alcoholism among the elderly. In contrast to the survey data, a study of elderly patients receiving alcoholism treatment in England found that 60% of the population was female.[1] Also, Alcoholics Anonymous surveys show that fully 73% of women members, in contrast to 58% of men members report that their first AA contact occurred when they were age 50 or older. Taken as a whole, these results are somewhat contradictory. However, they do suggest that alcoholism programs for the elderly must fully address the issues of the large numbers of women in treatment.

Alcoholism in the elderly is a combination of the accumulation of numbers of women who developed alcoholism earlier in life and did not recover and women who first develop alcoholism in their later years. Often, the development of alcoholism in a woman's elder years may come after the death of her husband or retirement from her job, which may result in a sense of isolation, loneliness, and depression. Alcoholism in an elderly woman may also be an expression of the despair of aging, loss of abilities and faculties, and a lack of peace about the life that she has led.

Our preconceived notions about elderly women make it more difficult to identify alcoholism in this population (who can imagine an alcoholic grandmother?). The social isolation of many of these women also makes it harder for them to come to the attention of either their families or professional treatment personnel. Effective means of involving these women in treatment, developing treatment programs that address their unique needs, and helping them maintain the necessary changes in their drinking patterns are virtually unexplored areas at this point.

CONCLUSIONS AND COMMENTS

In this chapter, we have journeyed from birth to death in terms of women's use and abuse of alcohol. The pain that alcohol problems bring to the lives of women already living with pain, sadness, and stress is evident. However, what may be more evident than anything else from this journey is what we don't know, rather than what we do know. Few studies have looked at the issues involved in female alcoholism from a life cycle perspective. Therefore, the available data are often not broken down by age group, which makes it difficult to identify the unique issues associated with alcoholism at each age. Further, there are few studies of minority women who are abusing drugs and alcohol, few studies of lesbian women, few studies looking at varying socioeconomic status, and virtually no studies looking at different occupational groups among women with alcohol problems. For example, we know that there are nuns, nurses, physicians, teachers, clerical workers, and factory workers with alcohol problems. However, their identification, study, description, and treatment are rarely addressed. We know little about differences in rates and kinds of abuse among different ethnic groups (in women), or about how the families of different ethnic backgrounds react to women with alcohol or drug problems. How these families identify women in trouble, how they assist or impede the women in getting treatment, and how they respond to recovery are virtually unknown at this time.

Paradigms for treatment are just beginning to emerge. Controversies rage in this field, and the amount of hard data available is limited. Many feminist therapists believe that women should be treated in programs and in groups separate from men, and that they should primarily have women as therapists. There are no definitive studies that demonstrate either the effectiveness or ineffectiveness of such approaches. Whether women should be in group or individual therapy is not known. The differential effectiveness of Alcoholics Anonymous for women versus men is unknown. The need to address women's issues in treatment, such as sex roles and self-esteem, versus the degree to which traditional alcohol-focused issues need to be addressed, is also an important question for research. Women with alcohol problems who are seeking treatment are best advised at this point to seek treatment from an agency or a therapist who regularly works with women with alcohol problems, and who has a variety of services to offer. Then, if one approach is not effective, alternatives are available.

What we don't know and what we need to know about women alcoholics were the topics of a national effort in 1975 to study the needs and status of women with alcohol and drug problems, and a national report was issued.[2] What is needed in addition is the development of innovative programs, the effectiveness of which are studied in innovative but rigorous ways by means of criteria for success relevant to female populations. Additionally, basic research on many of the issues identified throughout this chapter is sorely needed. Any researchers studying female alcohol abusers should routinely consider their results for differences by age, socioeconomic status, ethnic background, racial background, drinking patterns, and occupational status. Such studies will help us to know more about the variability and uniqueness of patterns of alcoholism among women, so that we may move beyond simplistic, unifactor explanations of alcoholism to a real understanding of the multifactor etiology of substance abuse in women, and in men as well.

Acknowledgment

Special thanks to Toni Appel, Ph.D., and Carol Heckerman, Ph.D., for their helpful feedback on an early draft of the chapter. This chapter is dedicated to Andrew Blazer, M.D., for his sensitive understanding of women as patients.

References

1. Noble EP (Ed): *Third Special Report to the U.S. Congress on Alcohol and Health* (DHEW publication). Washington, D.C., U.S. Government Printing Office, June 1978.
2. *Drugs, Alcohol, and Women: Source Book*: Proceedings from the National Institute on Drug Abuse Program for Women's Concerns, Miami Beach, October 1975.
3. Horn JL, Wanbern KW: *Females are Different: On the Diagnosis of Alcoholism in Women*. Presented at the First Annual Alcoholism Conference of the National Institute on Alcohol Abuse and Alcoholism, 1972.
4. Kunnes R: Poly-drug abuse: Drug companies and doctors, *American Journal of Orthopsychiatry* 43:530–532, 1973.
5. Erikson EH: *Childhood and society*. New York, W. W. Norton, 1950.
6. DeLint JEE: Alcoholism, birth rank and parental deprivation, *American Journal of Psychiatry* 120:1062–1065, 1964.
7. Donovan JE, Jessor R: Adolescent problem drinking: Psychosocial correlates in a national sample study, *Journal of Studies on Alcohol* 39:1506–1524, 1978.
8. Wilsnack RW, Wilsnack SC: Sex roles and drinking among adolescent girls, *J Stud Alcohol* 39:1855–1874, 1978.
9. Jones MC: Personality antecedents and correlates of drinking patterns in women, *Journal of Consulting and Clinical Psychology* 36:61–69, 1971.
10. Gomberg ES: Women and alcoholism. In *Women in therapy*. Edited by Franks V, Burtle V. New York, Brunner/Mazel, 1974.
11. Miller WR, Hedrick KE, Taylor CA: *Relationship between alcohol consumption and related life problems before and after behavioral treatment of problem drinkers*. Paper presented at the Annual Meeting of the Association for the Advancement of Behavior Therapy, San Francisco, December 1979.
12. Wilsnack SC: *The needs of the female drinker: Dependency, power, or what?* Presented at the Second Annual Alcoholism Conference of the National Institute on Alcohol Abuse and Alcoholism, Washington, D.C., June 1972.
13. James JE: Symptoms of alcoholism in women, *Journal of Studies on Alcohol* 36:1564–1569, 1975.
14. Greenblatt DJ, Schuckit M (Eds): *Alcoholism problems in women and children*. New York, Grune & Stratton, 1976.
15. Wilson GT, Lawson DM: Expectancies, alcohol, and sexual arousal in Women, *Journal of Abnormal Psychology* 87:358–367, 1978.
16. Wood HP, Duffy EL: Psychological factors in alcoholic women, *American Journal of Psychiatry* 123:341–345, 1966.
17. Blane HT: *The personality of the alcoholic; Guises of dependency*. New York, Harper & Row, 1968.
18. Beckman LJ: Self-esteem of women alcoholics, *Journal of Studies on Alcohol* 39:491–498, 1978.

19. Wilsnack SC: Sex role identity in female alcoholism, *Journal of Abnormal Psychology* 82:253–261, 1973.
20. Parker FB: Sex-role adjustment in women alcoholics, *Quarterly Journal of Studies on Alcohol* 33:647–657, 1972.
21. Scida J, Vannicelli M: Sex-role conflict and women's drinking, *Journal of Studies on Alcohol* 40:28–44, 1979.
22. Schuckit MA, Morrissey ER: Psychiatric problems in women admitted to an alcoholic detoxification center, *American Journal of Psychiatry* 136:611–617, 1979.
23. Sheehy G: *Passages.* New York, Bantam Books, 1977.
24. Schuckit M: The alcoholic woman: A literature review, *Psychiatry in Medicine* 3:37–43, 1972.
25. Lisansky ES: Alcoholism in women: Social and psychological concomitants: I. Social history data, *Quarterly Journal of Studies on Alcohol* 18:588–623, 1957.
26. Masi FA: The employed woman alcoholic—Problems, solutions, and outreach strategies, *Labor-Management Alcoholism Journal* 6:38–44, 1977.
27. Bromet E, Moos R: Sex and marital status in relation to the characteristics of alcoholics, *Journal of Studies on Alcohol* 37:1302–1312, 1975.
28. Curlee, J: A Comparison of Male and Female Patients at an Alcoholism Treatment Center, *Journal of Psychology* 74:239–247, 1970.
29. Rosenbaum B: Married women alcoholics at the Washingtonian Hospital, *Quarterly Journal of Studies on Alcohol* 19:79–89, 1958.
30. Morrissey ER, Schuckit MA: Stressful life events and alcohol problems among women seen at a detoxification center, *Journal of Studies on Alcohol* 39:1559–1576, 1978.

PART III

Therapy

Chapter 15

The Therapeutic Alliance in Psychoanalytic Treatment

EARLE SILBER

Psychoanalysis is a special form of psychotherapy in which the relationship between the therapist and patient is the basic instrument of the treatment. This unique alliance between the patient and the analyst has been referred to as the *treatment alliance*, the *therapeutic alliance*, or the *work alliance*; all of these terms imply the importance of a cooperative and purposive goal shared by the two participants. As contrasted with other forms of therapy, the means by which analysis aims at assisting the patient is by involving the patient herself* in the process of the treatment and assisting her in pursuing and identifying her own goals in understanding her own unique feelings and attitudes by a process of investigation and understanding.

In contrast to the central role of investigation and interpretation in psychoanalysis, in other forms of psychotherapy different interventions by the therapist, such as suggestion, reassurance, and education, play a more prominent role. In addition, other types of psychotherapy are more limited in their goals than analysis. For example, goal-limited therapy would be indicated in helping someone face an acute crisis in relation to some external difficulty. Here, the focus of the work might be limited to assisting the patient in sorting out her feelings in order to gain some perspective in regard to a difficult life situation, to

---

*Since this volume is addressed to the issue of women as patients, patients are referred to in this chapter as women, and examples are drawn from women patients. I have therefore avoided using the grammatical form, "herself or himself," when referring to patients.

EARLE SILBER, M.D. ● Supervising and Training Analyst, Washington Psychoanalytic Institute, Washington, D.C.

consider alternatives, and to gain some emotional mastery of the issues involved in coping with this situation. Another possible goal of therapy is simply seeking the prompt relief of symptoms such as anxiety or depression with minimal consideration of the underlying issues in the patient's personality.

The analyst is also consulted by a patient who seeks help in order to alleviate some distress or painful symptoms. Ordinarily, analysis would be indicated for persons with symptoms of depression, anxiety, obsessive rumination, or personality problems about which the patient may feel in conflict and distress. A long-term exploration of the personality of the patient through analysis would be warranted when the emotional problems are repetitive, internal, and more related to enduring and long-standing personality characteristics than to immediate or difficult external situations.

While these distinctions between other forms of psychotherapy and analysis sometimes obviously overlap to some extent, the task of the participants differs, depending on the form of the treatment. In psychotherapy, the therapist is apt to be more active in encouraging the expression of feelings and in assisting the patient to sort them out in terms of their appropriateness to the present situation. The patient may be reminded of her past abilities and encouraged to use her personal resources in order to mobilize adaptive behavior. Sometimes, the therapist may enable the patient to lower her expectations of herself during a period of stress. At other times, the therapist is more actively reassuring and supportive. In analysis, the analyst helps the patient to look beyond her acute situation to a longer-term exploration of her personality. The goal is to make explicit the patient's personality difficulties and their origins so that the patient can face them consciously and deal with them in a better way. These difficulties are often related to some problem in resolving an earlier developmental task, such as achieving a sense of separateness from parents. This problem may repetitively block the patient's ability to deal effectively with her current life situation. Analysis helps to make the patient more aware of her own experience, with the goal of enabling her to be in charge of herself. Further, this insight is based on a compassionate awareness of those forces that have shaped the patient and influenced her in becoming the particular person that she is. The goal of this work is to enable the patient to develop the ability to see herself in some perspective and to understand the important influences in her development.

Insight plays a central role in the curative aspect of analysis. This insight, in order to be effective, is not restricted to the intellect—although the intellect does play a part—but is based on emotionally convincing experience in the analysis. The patient's defenses against her inner life are clarified and their functions understood so that the feelings that have been unconscious can be experienced, placed in the context of the patient's emotional development, and integrated in the personality. Insight also helps the patient to clarify her own psychological boundaries, that is to differentiate what is inside from what is outside, to be clear about what are her own thoughts and feelings, and to differentiate what belongs to the past from what belongs to the present.

What is therapeutic in this method of treatment? The process of collaboration itself is therapeutic insofar as it promotes the autonomy of the patient and enlists the patient's own skills and resources in dealing with herself. The means by which the treatment itself is conducted, and particularly the analyst's constancy in adhering to the task of understanding and compassionate inquiry, provide the patient with a model for collaboration. The patient internalizes the analyst's interest in analyzing rather than either condemning or indulging her neurotic difficulties. Through this process, the patient can come to view herself in a less critical and more compassionate way. The analyst's persistent attempt to put the patient's experience in some meaningful context enables her to organize her own experience in understandable human terms.

This method of treatment also helps by assisting the patient in differentiating herself clearly from the others around her. Analysis encourages realistic and appropriate forms of interdependence and autonomy, a capacity for clarity about the patient's psychological boundaries, and the real differences that define her as a unique person in her relationship with others. By helping the patient differentiate her past from the present, analysis enables her to be clear about how she may have perceived her present relationships in terms of important past relationships. All these factors facilitate the patient's psychological development and assist her in overcoming the internal handicaps that have interfered with her maturation as a full person. Thus, the long-range goal of analysis is to help persons face their problems and find new solutions for them through insight into the nature of the unconscious forces involved.

In addition, insight is a curative vehicle when there is sufficient time in the treatment for the patient to encounter her emotional problems in as wide a variety of contexts as possible, that is, to see how her internal difficulties interfere with her adaptation in her relationship to herself and to others, in her work, or wherever they occur. This process is referred to as *working through* and implies a need for the patient to confront and apply her understanding to her everyday life in order for the treatment to be effective. This is one of the principal reasons that analysis takes time. Enduring aspects of the personality are slow to change, and analysis requires this time for working through these issues in order to be effective. Intellectual insight alone cannot accomplish this.

Thus, the kind of learning that takes place in analysis is different from the learning associated with intellectual tasks. In analysis, feelings connected with important developmental experiences are relived in a new context. The safety of the analysis is also important in permitting the emergence of feelings previously excluded from consciousness and enables the patient to view them from the perspective of a more mature self.

Because of the particular goals and methods of the treatment, the psychoanalytic relationship is unique and in some ways peculiar. It differs from an ordinary social relationship in important respects. Since the purpose of the relationship is to assist the patient in exploring *herself* in the fullest possible way, the relationship tends to be unbalanced. It is the patient who does most of the talking and the work of self-exploration. The analyst's role is a facilitative and catalytic one aimed at assisting the patient in identifying and overcoming the barriers to her own self-understanding. Although the patient and the analyst share a similar goal, their tasks in the work are different.

In ordinary social relationships, persons reveal themselves to each other in a reciprocal way. This is not true in an analytic relationship. The analyst's principal communications to the patient are those of his understanding of her, and he or she helps the patient to say what she is thinking and feeling more clearly and explicitly. At times, the analyst may have little or nothing to add. Sometimes, he or she may raise questions or point out connections between certain aspects of the patient's remarks. On occasion, the analyst might identify for the patient some of his or her reactions for the purpose of assisting the patient to put her view of the analyst in some perspective. The patient is encouraged to talk about whatever is on her mind and to put as much of her experience into words as possible in whatever sequence her thoughts and feelings occur. Problems are explored by this method of "free association," which enables the patient to become aware of meanings, feelings, and memories that may be linked together in ways that do not follow ordinary, "logical" thinking. Free association permits the recognition of emotional connections that would otherwise remain outside awareness.

From what has been said, it can be seen that the therapeutic alliance offers a unique human situation in which the patient, with the analyst's help, has an opportunity to observe herself in a relationship, to identify her own responses, and to understand their origins. This is unique in human relationships. People ordinarily do not stop, step back, and say, "Let us look at what is going on between us. What are you feeling? Where is it coming from?" This is the position of the analyst with the patient. There are also some inherent frustrations in analysis because of the one-sided nature of the analytic relationship. The treatment is not for the purpose of the analyst's sharing his or her experiences with the patient; rather, it focuses on the patient. Issues that arise in the course of the treatment are looked at exclusively from the point of view of explicating the patient's experience. These and other constraints are necessary in order to preserve the unique characteristics of the relationship as a therapeutic one. They involve the analyst's maintaining an appropriate distance from the patient, and this, too, can be frustrating. The therapeutic alliance constitutes an enduring, dependable aspect of the relationship through all phases of the treatment.

From the very beginning, it is important for the patient and the analyst to understand why they are meeting and what the treatment is about. The analyst conducts the initial meetings with the patient in a style that is consistent with the goals of the analysis itself. That is, the analyst listens in a nonjudgmental way to assess where the patient is in her development, in which areas she is blocked in her growth as a person, and how he or she might be of help to the patient in relation to her psychological development. This approach means understanding how the patient's difficulties might reflect a developmental problem that repeats itself in a variety of forms. For example, difficulty in mastering fears related to competition with her mother may repeat itself over and over again without the patient's being conscious of this difficulty as an underlying problem.

In order to establish what type of treatment would be indicated, an initial consultation, which may extend over several sessions, precedes the onset of treatment. The analyst and the patient then clarify whether there is some work that the patient wishes to do in her psychological life with which the analyst might be of some assistance. This is the *means* of helping that the analyst proposes. Establishing a therapeutic alliance is ordinarily possible with persons who seek help voluntarily, who are able to identify an internal psychological problem, and who possess the capacities for self-observation and the psychological work that is involved in analysis. In addition, the patient must be interested in the long-term goals of self-understanding and must be able to manage the frustrations inherent in the analytic method. The following is a brief vignette of an initial consultation with a patient in which the basis of the collaboration was established:

A woman in her 30s had become very restricted in her life because her phobias had progressively limited her ability to move about, both literally and figuratively. An insightful and intelligent person, with a doctorate degree in mathematics, she was no longer able to travel because she was afraid of flying, driving in cars, and using public transportation. Finally, she was unable to leave her apartment unless she was accompanied by a friend.

In the consultation, several sessions were spent listening to her account of her difficulties and to some details of her personal life. The analyst told her that he would try to help her understand how her life had come to be where it was and the meaning of her phobias. She was interested in understanding herself, and they then began to discuss the arrangements about analysis in relation to this task. The definition of the work was not immediately focused on getting rid of the patient's symptoms. Since it was not possible to predict with certainty how long her phobic symptoms might persist, the analyst asked if she felt she could manage them and could make arrangements to come to the sessions in spite of her anxiety. She felt that she could and was willing to begin. The analyst explored directly with the patient whether she was interested in collaborating with him for the purpose of helping her to understand *herself* as a means of dealing with her problems, quite a different task than promising her immediate relief from her symptoms.

In this example, it was important that the analyst make clear that his principal task was to help the patient understand herself. Of course, the analyst hopes that the treatment may relieve the patient of her suffering, and if the patient does not feel the analyst's empathic interest and concern, this will also interfere with the development of an alliance. This is an unusual form of collaborative work between patient and analyst. The analyst is by no means simply a "paid friend" or an "agent of society," nor is the analytic relationship one between a superior and a subordinate. The therapeutic situation offers the patient an opportunity to talk and to explore rather than necessarily to be driven into action or to be endlessly inhibited from taking appropriate actions because of internal obstacles. The analyst is not peddling "happiness" or "adjustment"; rather, she or he offers an opportunity for psychological work.

Sometimes the patient comes to analysis not because of pressure from a symptom but because of something external that may also be a source of distress. The following is an example:

Ms. G had consulted other psychiatrists about her difficulty with her child and also about problems in her marriage. She described her unbearable relationship with her husband, who she felt was tyrannical and overbearing. She felt that the marriage had been a mistake. Another analyst, with whom she had consulted, had even advised her to divorce her husband. However, she was unable to do this. She was told by the present analyst that from her description, she was, indeed, in a very difficult life situation and that it was not clear what there was about this situation that might represent an internal problem belonging to her. An unhappy marriage is not necessarily a reason to enter analysis, but if there was something about herself that she wanted to understand better, it would be appropriate to meet again. She said that there was, and another appointment was arranged, to continue the consultation.

During the second appointment, she recognized that she was very vague about what she wanted to do with her own life and also that she tended to get caught up in fulfilling the expectations of others. This had been a chronic problem for her, and she felt that she did not know herself very well, that is, did not know what *she* really wanted. She had initially perceived her marital problems as if they existed outside herself and were unconnected to her as a person. The arrangements about analysis, which were made after several interviews, were based on the patient's interest in understanding her difficulty in defining her own interests rather than simply on her deciding what to do about her marriage.

In this example, the analyst made it clear that his task was not to relieve the patient of some external difficult reality. Rather, an effort was made to define a different task with the patient that both the analyst and the patient could agree on, that is, to assist the patient in some work of self-understanding. In these examples, the exploration of whether there is a mutually agreed-upon basis for the work constituted the beginning of the therapeutic alliance with the patient.

There are situations in which the patient's difficulties do not reflect her own internal problems. Unhappy marriages may result from a variety of causes, sometimes with a minimal contribution of the person who seeks psychiatric help. For example, obvious personality disorder or mental illness in the spouse, difficult external financial problems, and frustrating life situations may result in considerable psychological distress but are not indications for analysis. In such situations, other forms of psychotherapy or counseling might be indicated instead, with the aim of resolving pressing difficulties. In the consultative period, the analyst listens carefully to try to define whether the patient herself perceives that there is some *internal* problem for which treatment would make sense. In reality, of course, life is not always so clearly differentiated, and there may be a mixture of issues involved in any given situation. Some of the work of analysis consists of the clarification of those issues that are internal and those that are not. Analytic treatment offers a setting in which the patient can explore where her feelings are coming from, without necessarily assuming that every difficult situation involves an internal problem. Analysis strengthens the patient's sense of reality and her confidence in her own perceptions.

Sometimes a patient is uncertain about whether it would be preferable for her to work with a male or a female analyst. It is difficult to generalize about such an issue. Rather, since this choice is so dependent on the feelings of the particular patient, the question can best be explored in a consultation prior to beginning in treatment. If there is a strong preference for a male or a female analyst, the reasons need to be discussed so that some of the underlying assumptions can be brought to light, as in the following examples:

> In the consultation period prior to beginning in analysis, Ms. A felt very strongly that she wanted to work with a male analyst. Before seeing the male analyst, she had consulted a woman analyst but did not feel comfortable with her. The patient simply had a strong emotional conviction that a woman would not be able to help her. While she also recognized that this might not indeed be so, the assumption still influenced her feelings strongly enough so that she could not develop a therapeutic alliance with the woman analyst in question. She could, however, imagine working with a male analyst and felt more motivated to begin her analysis with him. As the work progressed, the deeper reasons for her preference came to light. Her emotional conviction that the woman analyst could not help her represented a projection of her own devalued view of herself as a woman onto the woman analyst. In addition, it represented a transference to the first analyst of her earlier depreciated view of her mother; similarly, her preference for a male analyst involved a transference of her earlier idealization of her father. These stereotypes were inextricably connected with the problems for which she sought treatment.

> Another patient felt uncomfortable about working with men. She tended to become overinvolved emotionally with men in ways that interfered with her own judgment about these relationships. Her compulsive addiction to the approval of men was part of the reason for her seeking treatment. She felt that she would be so preoccupied with having to seduce a male analyst that she would be unable to work realistically with him. In addition, her resentment of men was pronounced, and she did not feel that she could trust a male analyst. For this reason, she sought a woman therapist, with whom she established a good relationship and with whom she worked quite successfully in treatment. Her advancement in her career led to her move to another city. On the advice of her therapist, she considered now working with a male and sought a consultation. She had gained sufficient perspective about her relationships with men so that she now felt that she could profit from working with a man as well as with a woman. The reasons for her initial preference for a woman analyst were no longer as compelling, and she was freer to make a choice based on what might be more advantageous to her treatment.

Preferences for an analyst of one sex or the other obviously derive from many different sources and need to be explored as part of the treatment itself. Clearly, there is no point in a patient's forcing herself in one direction or another at the beginning of treatment if she doesn't feel a sense of trust in her ability to work with a particular analyst. It always remains uncertain how well a particular analyst and a particular patient will work together, no matter how competent the analyst or highly motivated the patient. Both the patient and the analyst need to evaluate this uncertainty together. The overriding issue is that the patient find the most competent analyst available with whom she feels she can work effectively.

The analyst's role as an expert has to do with his or her skill in establishing and delineating an analytic relationship with the patient and in safeguarding the conduct of analysis so that it has an optimal possibility of achieving its goals. Thus, the analyst helps the patient to define and work through her internal resistances to understanding herself. In this way, the analyst enables the patient to more clearly articulate and appreciate her inner feelings, psychological processes, and the way she functions as a person. The analyst is not an expert on the resolution of life's problems, nor does he or she have an omniscient awareness of how to best live one's life. The analyst's role, therefore, is not to advise the patient about her life decisions but to assist her as fully as possible to appreciate the range of her own interests represented in the choices that confront her. In this way, he or she protects and encourages, as much as possible, the autonomy of the patient. By clarifying how the patient sometimes confuses the present with the past, the patient can be helped to react to the present more appropriately. By better appreciating the sources of inhibition to action that have been unconscious, the patient can be helped to make choices free of old, repetitive dilemmas.

The analyst does not direct the patient's conversations; the patient is free to talk about whatever she wishes. For this reason, the analyst does not initiate the sessions but allows the patient to choose the topic for the day. In this way, the analyst keeps in touch with where the patient is and what is occupying her interest and attention on any particular day. It is not necessarily true that the analyst simply remains silent. The analyst may not answer certain questions but explore the patient's thoughts or feelings about them instead because the patient may learn more about herself in this way. On the other hand, certain questions might be answered because the answers could facilitate the patient's ability to explore something about her own feelings. This is a clinical judgment that the analyst makes. Much of the analyst's activity is concerned with listening and with promoting the patient's identification with the analyst's interest in understanding the meaning of her experience. The analyst listens quietly to assist the patient in learning to listen to herself, not to create a mystifying atmosphere.

Certain aspects of the arrangements of analysis are made in order to implement the goals of the work. For example, analysis is usually conducted with the patient reclining on a couch with the analyst out of sight. The use of the couch may assist the patient in expressing herself more freely and less self-consciously. Also, if the patient does not look at the analyst, the patient can more easily make free associations and note responses based on feelings that may also be less tied to reality. Thus, she may be able to explore issues in her emotional life that would otherwise remain out of awareness. The patient's inability to observe the analyst's expressions also helps her to articulate thoughts, feelings, and fantasies that might otherwise be censored. In addition, this arrangement puts less strain on the analyst and enables him or her to listen in a comfortable and freely attentive way.

Frequent appointments, four to five times a week, are necessary in analysis in order to provide sufficient time to explore the patient's feelings and attitudes in her day-to-day life. It is also necessary to meet this frequently to enable the patient to establish an important relationship with the analyst. The idiosyncratic elements of the patient's reactions to the analyst can then become an important vehicle for understanding the patient's inner life. Time is also required to provide continuity in the work and to explore the unconscious elements in the patient's reactions to life events as well as in the patient's relationship to the analyst. Other forms of psychotherapy with different goals do not require such frequent meetings. Sometimes, patients may be seen one or two times a week in a more goal-directed form of therapy or a therapy that is aimed at helping the patient contend with a more specific life situation. This difference in the arrangement reflects the difference in the tasks of the therapy.

Explicit fee arrangements are important not only in terms of meeting the analyst's requirements as a professional person, who earns his or her living from the analytic work, but also because these arrangements define important boundaries in the relationship. These involve reaching agreements about fees, schedules, cancellations, dates when payments are to be made, etc. Sometimes, during the course of the treatment, it may be necessary for the analyst to change these arrangements. Such a change requires discussion with the patient and an exploration of the patient's responses to such changes. Moreover, whenever the patient of the analyst changes the boundaries in the therapeutic alliance without discussion, it is a signal that something is occurring that needs to be talked about in order to be brought into the analysis for investigation.

The following is an example of how issues around money matters were explored as part of an analysis:

> After an initial consultation, arrangements were made with the patient
> to begin analysis. The patient and the analyst had discussed the fee and
> the analyst's preference that the fee be paid by a certain date each month.
> After the first month of treatment, however, the patient mentioned casually
> that she would be paying late that month since she was a little short of

funds. Rather than agreeing or disagreeing with her request, the analyst asked the patient if she might try to observe what was going on in order to understand something further about herself. The patient was able to do this and said that she often involved other people in her money problems. Although she was annoyed that the analyst simply hadn't gone along with her, she could see that she was passing the problem on to him. As she talked further, she also realized that she had been reluctant to discuss the matter with the analyst and had assumed that he would not be at all understanding about her difficulty and would be unwilling to consider any delay in payment, no matter what the reason. She began to see this feeling more and more as an example of her difficulty in cooperating with others. She felt that she had either to control things or to be helplessly controlled by the other partner in a relationship. Further associations led to recognizing that this feeling also had to do with a replication of expectations of her mother around similar issues.

In the beginning phase of analytic work, the particular style with which the patient begins the analysis becomes part of the subject matter to be investigated. While the patient is free to express whatever is in her mind without censorship, the analyst attempts to enlist the patient's cooperation in looking at her own behavior and verbal communications. He is interested not only in what the patient is saying but also in how she expresses herself.

The following example is an illustration:

Ms. J was a gifted person, quite bright, dedicated to her work as a teacher, and very skillful in working with children and counseling parents. She was familiar with analytic concepts and sensitive in applying her understanding of them in her work. She had been chronically depressed and felt that analysis might help her with this depression and also with certain aspects of her work. When she began in analysis, she plunged immediately into the work with some of the most difficult and painful recollections about her childhood. She pushed herself to talk about very painful material from the very beginning, and the analyst felt that she was really unable to integrate what she was dealing with. The analyst felt that she was quite anxious about beginning analysis and that she was overwhelmed with the material she was producing. Moreover, the analyst also felt that she was showing something about herself, namely, that she expected herself to undertake a great deal very quickly and that she had to master an uncertain situation immediately, beyond her real capacities to integrate the experience.

The analyst did not respond by trying to deal very much with the content of what she was talking about but tried to focus with her on her *style* of working and what this might be saying about herself. The analyst said that since he was just beginning to work with her, he could not yet appreciate the full significance of the kind of material that she was bringing into the analysis. He questioned whether she herself was really able to learn anything new from what she was forcing herself to recall and focused on her need to push herself so much. She explained that this approach was very much a part of her style of working and that she always tended to move into something new in this way. Rather than simply going on in this way, the analyst encouraged her to stand aside from her behavior and to try to understand it. This was an attempt to bring the patient's image of how she "ought" to be into focus for analytic inquiry. It was also an appeal to a more reasonable part of the patient's self, which could be enlisted to work in observing and understanding her struggles to fulfill an impossible ideal for her self. This problem was connected with the depression for which she had entered analysis. In these early hours of analysis, the nature of the real analytic relationship was clarified, and through interpretation, the therapeutic alliance was strengthened. The patient was encouraged to examine a recurrent part of her difficulties rather than simply to relive them.

As the work progresses, the patient may begin to experience certain feelings or attitudes toward the analyst that represent a reactivation of feelings derived from important early relationships in the patient's life. Sometimes, these attitudes and feelings reflect idealizations of the analyst. At other times, the patient may experience the analyst as representing a part of her own personality, such as her own conscience. These experiences, referred to as *transference*, can become a further opportunity for the patient to learn about her self. Such attitudes toward the analyst differ from the therapeutic alliance. The therapeutic alliance represents the patient's realistic and appropriate collaboration with the analyst, which tends to be more stable and more related to the goals of the treatment. The analyst does not base the work with the patient on her overestimation of her or him; instead, such distortions are identified and interpreted rather than being relied on as a basis for the analytic work.

Important and emotionally convincing experiences for the patient occur through a clarification of the roles that she assigns to the analyst. This enables the patient to put her past in some perspective. The differentiation of the actual role of the analyst, which remains constant, from the roles projected on him or her by the patient constitutes an important part of the work. Without being aware of it, patients begin to reenact in the analysis aspects of interpersonal difficulties from the past that they experience in other relationships. In this way, past interpersonal problems that the patient has carried around inside her are relived with the analyst and can be observed and understood firsthand in the analysis.

It is a common misconception that a woman patient inevitably "falls in love" with her analyst if the analyst is male. In fact, such reactions, particularly in the early part of treatment, may indicate a patient's difficulty in relating to the analyst *as an analyst*. Initial intense erotic feelings for the analyst may reflect the patient's resistance to entering into a more considered and realistic relationship with the analyst, as a basis for doing some psychological work.

Strong feelings between the patient and the analyst do develop during the work. These feelings include sexual feelings directed toward the male analyst by the female patient. When a good therapeutic alliance has been established, the patient and the analyst can cooperate in looking at the patient's feelings in order to understand their meaning and what they reflect about the patient. While it is also true that in any close relationship where such intense feelings are experienced, there is a potential for their enactment, the consistent adherence of the analyst to his role as analyst, dependably working with the patient by interpreting her transference, makes it possible for the patient to explore the full range of her feelings toward her analyst. The more the patient can depend on the analyst to remain in his role as analyst—that is, not to live out other roles with her as adviser, mother, father, etc.—the safer the patient can feel about expressing herself in the relationship. Often, the patient projects her own wishes onto the analyst and mistakenly interprets his interest in her psychological life as a sexual interest. If this projection can be viewed as an opportunity for emotional learning, it can be a useful and productive aspect of the work. There are times, as well, when it might serve the function of diverting the patient from her primary task, of achieving a fuller autonomy in her own right, and such eroticization of the relationship precludes the patient's capacity to work analytically.

The feelings that the patient transfers from the past or other ongoing relationships to the analyst are not obviated by a simple clarification at the beginning of the analysis about the nature of the real work between the analyst and the patient. Transference feelings persist and repeat themselves as the work progresses:

> One woman gradually presented herself in the analytic relationship in an increasingly helpless way. Her attention was drawn to her behavior, and she was encouraged to try to look at what was going on as an opportunity to learn something further about herself. Some of her complaints when she began analytic work had to do with her husband's tendency to dominate her and her own inability to assert herself in her marriage. This woman greatly valued her own potential for autonomy. At the same time, she seemed to be less aware of her own wish to be in a relationship with a man whom she could perceive as being very powerful and who would, in fact, dominate her. In reality, she and her husband lived out these complementary roles with each other. She had been unaware of the extent of her own feelings and perceived the danger to her autonomy as lying totally outside herself. She did not recognize her contribution to the pattern of this relationship, although her husband's behavior did, in fact, threaten her autonomy. Early in her life, she had internalized an image of herself as a person incapable of functioning in her own right without being directed by someone powerful. Since her husband lived out the complementary role to her helplessness by becoming more and more dominating, this progression made it impossible for her to appreciate her own contribution to the difficulty. However, in the analysis, her helplessness became more and more conspicuous as she invited the analyst over and over again to

rescue her from her distress and to enact with her her own internal image of herself. As she gained some understanding of her actions, she was able to look back at herself at the beginning of the analysis and say, "When I first came, it was because I was desperate. It was not to have the wish to really change anything, although it was what I wanted . . . but I didn't think about what I would do to try to make this happen. . . . I wanted to confess everything to you. . . . I wanted some kind of magic to happen. . . . I wanted there to be something you would work out for me."

A long period of work in analysis may be required even after the patient has gained some understanding of some of her principal internal psychological difficulties. This long period is necessary to strengthen the patient's self-understanding and to augment her capacity to make use of it in her day-to-day experience. Considerable time is required to examine the different aspects of the patient's life in which her problems are encountered. It is necessary to help the patient appreciate the full extent of these difficulties and to be able to identify the specific places in her life where such problems are lived out. This is also a period when the patient learns new patterns of behavior to supersede the old, as well as learning about the past. She must do so in order to minimize the likelihood of a recurrence of the previous patterns that stood in the way of her psychological development.

The notion that analysis focuses the patient only on the past is a misconception. The analyst is interested in the past insofar as it continues to be alive in the present. The analyst is also interested in helping the patient cope with her life with new forms of adaptation that have previously been inaccessible to her. When the analyst uses the word *adaptation*, he or she means the patient's dealing with external situations with a fuller consciousness of the different aspects of herself: her own feelings, values, standards of behavior, wishes, intentions, styles—all of the elements that make her the particular person that she is. *Adaptation* means dealing with the external world in a way that takes into account the fullest possible range of the patient's inner psychological world.

It is also a misconception of analytic work that the analyst can in any way make up for the patient's past. What is past is over. The analysis serves the function of helping the patient to mourn for the lost opportunities of the past. It is also a place for a gradual clarification of one's illusions about life. In this sense, the analysis seeks to enable the patient to become disillusioned in regard to fantasies about what life is supposed to be. It is to be hoped that this disillusionment will occur gradually and in a way that is manageable by the patient and enables her to see herself and others more realistically.

The aim of the work is toward sobriety, an appreciation of external difficulties as contrasted with those superimposed by the patient herself. The clarification and awareness of the self also includes a greater clarification of the patient's boundaries, that is, what is external to the self and what is not. These boundaries include the recognition of unhappy as well as potentially satisfying aspects of reality. It is therefore not a necessary requirement for the termination of treatment that the patient should reach some point where she has "resolved" all of her life problems. Rather, treatment is terminated when the origins of the patient's internal difficulties have been understood as fully as possible and there has been ample time to work through the major obstacles to the patient's emotional development. Further, termination is considered when the patient is in a position to continue the work of self-analysis by having internalized the analyst's interest in viewing her with nonjudgmental interest and curiosity. It always remains to be seen at the end of treatment what the effect of future life experiences will be and how favorably the patient's life situation will permit her to continue the process of self-development, which proceeds throughout the life cycle.

Certain problems recur in new forms with each phase of the life cycle. For example, conflicts about individuation and autonomy in relation to parents may be understood and successfully worked through by a young adult woman in analysis. These same conflicts will reemerge when the patient becomes a parent herself, and the same struggles may appear in yet a new form when her children have grown and are ready to separate themselves. For some persons, resumption of analysis for brief periods of work during these later developmental periods may therefore be quite useful in achieving further mastery of these issues. Just as the treatment begins with a collaborative agreement to undertake it, it is terminated collaboratively with an understanding that, of course, the analyst remains available to the patient if she should perceive the usefulness of returning for additional work in the future.

REFERENCES

Bibring E: Psychoanalysis and the dynamic psychotherapies, *J. Am. Psa. Assn.* 2:745–776.

Curtis HC: The concept of therapeutic alliance: Implications for the "widening scope." In *Psychoanalytic technique and theory of therapy*, Special Supplement, *Journal of the American Psychoanalytic Association* 27:159–193, 1979.

DeWald P: The process of change in psychoanalytic psychotherapy, *Archives of General Psychiatry* 35:535–542, May 1978.

Greenson RR: *The technique and practice of psychoanalysis*. New York, International Universities Press, 1967. Especially pp. 151–224.

Menninger KA, Hozman PS: *The theory of psychoanalytic technique* (2nd ed.). New York, Basic Books, 1973. Especially pp. 15–38.

Sandler J, *et al*: *The patient and the analyst*. New York, International Universities Press, 1973. Especially pp. 27–48.

Stone L: *The psychoanalytic situation*. New York, International Universities Press, 1961.

Zetzel ER: The concept of transference. In *The capacity for emotional growth*. New York, International Universities Press, 1970.

Chapter 16

Research on Gender and Psychotherapy

Lewis A. Kirshner, Stuart T. Hauser, and Abraham Genack

Although psychotherapists, at least since the time of Freud, have recognized and written about the importance of gender, until recently the sex of therapist and/or patient has not received much systematic attention in psychotherapy research. In their view of the literature on adult sex roles and mental illness, Gove and Tudor concluded that, "Sex acts as a master status, channeling one into particular roles and determining the quality of one's interaction with others."[1] At this point, however, the effects of these roles on the quantitative and qualitative aspects of psychotherapy remain poorly understood and to a degree controversial. In this chapter, we examine some of the relevant psychotherapy research, including our own work, and its implications for psychotherapy theory and practice.

In surveying the research on gender and psychotherapy, we will be looking primarily at empirical studies that have relied on methods ensuring systematic data collection (systematic sampling techniques, standard measures) and quantitative statistical analysis. But this review is not based exclusively on studies using these research designs. We also discuss several clinical papers, presentations based on detailed observation and the analysis of selected cases. Both types of investigation can contribute to refining concepts and generating hy-

Lewis A. Kirshner, M.D. • Department of Psychiatry, Harvard Medical School and Mount Auburn Hospital, Boston, Massachusetts. Stuart T. Hauser, M.D., Ph.D. • Department of Psychiatry, Harvard Medical School and Massachusetts Mental Health Center, Boston, Massachusetts. Abraham Genack, M.D. • Department of Psychiatry, Harvard Medical School and Mount Auburn Hospital, Boston, Massachusetts.

potheses in a field that deals with such a rich subject matter as psychotherapy. Still another aspect of these studies is that they include a wide range of therapists (using varied techniques and theories) from a variety of disciplines. For example, the therapists may be psychoanalyists, psychiatrists, social workers, clinical psychologists, nurses, or counselors. Despite this diversity of backgrounds, almost all of the studies we discuss here have investigated by means of therapies that use verbal discourse to explore the interpersonal and intrapsychic concerns of individuals who have sought help in resolving varied life problems. Consequently, we do not review the impact of gender on either behavior modification therapies or nonverbal, expressive group techniques.

EFFECTS OF SEX-ROLE STEREOTYPES

By *sex-role stereotypes,* we mean composite images or assemblages of personality traits that are generally believed by the population under discussion to characterize typical men or women. There is no doubt that questions raised by the women's movement of the 1960s about the influence of stereotypes on the lives and careers of women gave the major impetus to the study of gender effects in psychotherapy. One such study in particular has had a major impact: the work by Broverman, Broverman, Clarkson, Rosenkrantz and Vogel on the effects of stereotypes on clinicians' judgments of mental health.[2] Their research strategy was to ask a group of male and female psychotherapists to decide which of two polar descriptive words or phrases (e.g., "not at all independent–very independent," "very submissive–very dominant") applied specifically to "mature, healthy, socially competent" men or women. These therapists were then asked to use the same items to describe a "mature, healthy, socially competent person." They found that the male and female therapists were more likely to use the adjectives *unemotional, aggressive,* and *very independent* to describe men. In contrast, the therapists chose *gentle, expressive of tender feelings,* and *strong need for security* to describe women. Such a pattern clearly reflects the gender stereotypes held by a group of (male *and* female) psychotherapists. We do not know, though, to what extent these stereotypes are distributed across all groups in our society or vary along lines of professional discipline, social class, or ethnic or religious groupings.

Broverman and her colleagues also asked their sample of therapists to describe a "mentally healthy" person, using the same words and phrases. This new set of items was then systematically compared (using correlational analyses) with the gender-based constructions. The results of this second major component of the study revealed that both male and female clinicians held images of "psychological health" that were closely aligned with their pictures of "mature, healthy, socially competent" men. Do these results mean that clinicians' prejudices might work against the goals of female patients by conceiving of them as essentially less psychologically healthy, less "mature" than men? This important question—along with a second implication that clinicians might oppose, or at the very least, misunderstand the nonstereotypical aspirations of women—was certainly a major response to the Broverman research.

Another significant question that this research raises is whether this portrait of the "male chauvinist" therapist can be generalized beyond Broverman's sample. Do trained psychotherapists hold such clichéd views of gender roles—and, if so, do these stereotypes systematically influence therapists' work with their patients: We say *systematically influence* because, while no one doubts the existence of clinicians who act on this or that prejudice in their work, it is less clear whether the practice of all psychotherapists is significantly affected by gender stereotypes. To be more precise, is there a significant tendency for therapists to treat male and female patients differently? Research in this area is scanty, possibly because stereotypes are not easily detected or studied. To be sure, it is difficult to grasp what people "really believe" about anything. Moreover, it may be especially difficult to assess gender stereotyping on the part of therapists, as well as the impact of such stereotyping on actual clinical work, since psychotherapy involves many different features that are very likely interwoven with gender dimensions. In several of our later sections, we return to this important topic of the interplay between gender and other aspects of psychotherapy.

In terms of therapists' perceptions and expectations, several studies point out that therapists (and others) may not view masculinity and femininity as polar, "either/or" traits, but as independent dimensions that both form part of every individual.[3,4] From this perspective, mental health consists more of a mixture of "male" and "female" characteristics than of rigid adherence to the behaviors supposedly appropriate to one's own sex. In addition, other investigations in this area differ from Broverman *et al.* in finding that male therapists tend to have somewhat narrower conceptions of female roles than women themselves, and that female therapists are more likely to hold "androgynous," less sex-typed notions of psychological normality than males.[3,5,6]

When one turns from studying clinicians' beliefs or attitudes to their actual behavior, however, the picture becomes less clear. Put simply, it has not been possible to document any systematic, direct effects of gender stereotyping on the treatment process. Either therapists are able to keep their prejudices to themselves, or gender issues are not so visible in treatment that differences can be readily detected. For example, a study by Schwartz and Abramowitz[7] sought to uncover systematic effects of patients' race or gender on decision making by psychiatrists through the use of prepared case histories that differed only in these two variables. In the sample, the sex of the patient did not significantly influence the clinicians' judgments, either alone nor in interaction with other variables. Similar results emerged from an analogous study by Abramowitz et al.,[8] in which experienced group therapists were presented with a bogus patient history in which only the gender pronouns were varied. Although there were a few significant or near-significant statistical differences depending on the gender of the patient or the therapists in the choice of the therapeutic strategies employed, the overall conclusion was of a "surprisingly slight" impact of patient gender. Another measure of decision making by clinicians is reflected in length of treatment. Here, too, there is no clear-cut indication that women are kept in treatment longer than men or are recruited more avidly as patients.[9] This finding was confirmed in our own work. In general, then, the findings from a variety of studies suggest that the gender of the patient plays a limited role as a variable in psychotherapy. When patient gender is significant in influencing therapy outcome, it tends to be so in combination with other patient dimensions, such as age, marital status, and educational level.

"Real Differences" between Men and Women

Before embarking precipitously into treacherous currents, it is worth noting that a multitude of well-constructed research studies by developmental psychologists have been able to establish only a minimum of floatable conclusions about gender differences. One set of findings in this body of research describes females, in contrast to males, as showing "greater dependency, social conformity, and passivity," more interest in social activities, and "the gentler aspects of interpersonal relations."[10] Such personality attributes certainly might be expected to influence psychotherapy. But the controversial nature of these findings is amply demonstrated by the fact that Maccoby and Jacklin,[11] in their extensive review, concluded that related traits, such as attachment, affiliation, altruism, and nurturance, showed little gender differentiation. Given these conflicting findings, it becomes less evident how or whether patient and/or therapist gender influences psychotherapy. At most, we might anticipate that gender has a modest and complex impact on therapy.

In our own empirical work, we were interested in several implications that could be drawn from observations in the sex-difference literature. Since *some* of the studies, summarized by Mischel,[10] report a female advantage in emotional and interpersonal skills, we might expect to find a female patient effect and a female therapist effect. More specifically, we argued that female patients should be more responsive to the emotional strains of therapy and to the interpersonal exploration that forms its structure. Female therapists *pari passu* should be better at understanding and forming relationships with distressed patients.

These two hypotheses about a female advantage in psychotherapy formed the basis of a study of 189 patient–therapist pairs (in short-term psychotherapy) conducted by the authors at a large university health service.[12] The study used questionnaires to ask patients and their therapists to rate their psychotherapy experiences on several scales pertaining to satisfaction and improvement in different areas. These ratings were then used as outcome measures. Differences in outcome were analyzed statistically to determine effects of gender, age, social class, academic status, and therapist experience. As we had speculated, female gender (never male gender) turned up repeatedly in the significant or near-statistically significant category. In particular, we found two important patterns: (1) female patients reported greater improvement for themselves than male patients; and (2) female therapists were given higher satisfaction and improvement ratings than their male counterparts by the patients in our sample.

Our finding of a female patient advantage is supported by two other published studies, as compared with no reports in which males had superior outcomes.[13] One possible explanation for this gender effect may be that males are more difficult to treat. Phillips and Segal have elaborated an "expressivity hypothesis" that says that males in contemporary American culture are reluctant to express unpleasurable feelings because such behavior is considered "not masculine."[14] They believe that this unwillingness to acknowledge painful emotions may account for the preponderance of females as psychotherapy patients. If men are indeed more reluctant to admit emotional problems, one might hypothesize that they would have to experience more distress before entering therapy. Moreover, as Gove and Tudor[1] noted, men may be more likely to enter therapy in response to pressure from others when their behavior or level of performance does not correspond to social expectations. Thus, men may experience a greater element of coercion and less of inner motivation in seeking psychotherapy. Perhaps this possibility explains why the therapists in our study (especially the less-experienced therapists) were less satisfied with male patients.[12]

Our second set of findings concerns the female therapist effect. Patients were more satisfied with female therapists and reported more improvement with them. The studies of Light[15] and Cartwright[16] suggest one way that we can understand these findings. They observed a discrepancy between the men and the women who entered medical school. The female students combined "tough analytic" with "nurturant sensitive" traits much more than men. Similar findings were reported by Berzins[3] in a study of degree of adherence to narrowly defined gender roles among therapists and trainees, with women showing much more of a combination of traditionally male- and female-typed traits. A theoretical rationale for a female therapist advantage along similar lines was proposed by Carter.[17] These studies suggest obvious problems in the training of male psychiatrists. A paper by Alonso and Rutan,[18] which advocates opposite-gender supervision for psychiatric residents, speaks directly to this issue. Put somewhat differently, the results of our research point out that in a university-health-service setting using the modality of short-term psychotherapy, the patients are less satisfied with male (especially less-experienced male) therapists.

In sum, being female appears to be an advantage for both patient and therapist. This advantage may not reflect issues unique to the clinical situation as much as the effects of feminine socialization or differences in culturally sanctioned male and female roles *on* the process of psychotherapy.

Gender Matching of Patients and Therapists

Issues related to the choice of the sex of a therapist were discussed in depth by Thompson from a psychoanalytic perspective in a 1938 paper.[19] In her thoughtful review, she conceptualized a range of motives from realistic-conscious to fantasy-unconscious that operate in varying degrees when patients choose a therapist of a particular gender. Even at a wholly conscious level, patients' reasons for preferring like- or opposite-sex therapists are extremely diverse, as was recently documented by Davidson.[20] Clearly, patients have gender-related attitudes derived from past family and other relationships, from current relationships, from cultural stereotypes about what different sex therapists might be like; and from other feelings, facts, and fantasies. Because these attitudes are so individualized, it is exceedingly difficult, if not frankly impossible, to predict the effect of a particular gender match on a specific case. To take one common example, patients vary in their subjective comfort in talking to male or female therapists. In some cases, a strong sense of comfort may be essential to the development of a therapeutic relationship; in others, such comfort may represent an avoidance of important issues. Thompson advocated careful exploration of the meaning of a gender preference when it occurs, as well as attention to possible gender-related issues (for instance, the history of early relationships) in every patient. In this fashion, the importance of gender can be assessed for the individual, rather than calculated only on the basis of prevailing generalizations about who is good for whom.

Although many clinical beliefs are prevalent about the importance of gender matching for certain categories of patients (notably for adolescent and homosexual patients), meager empirical evidence can be found to support these positions. Most of the literature on gender matching—for example, the papers summarized by Ivey[21]—is anecdotal, if not political and exhortative.[23,23] However, when patients and therapists are observed from a research perspective, significant patterns of interaction by gender can be systematically investigated through objective measures and quantitative analysis. This area is of great interest because of the practical goal of making more rational matchings, as well as because of concerns about the real or imagined gender differences discussed above.

Since we found female-patient and female-therapist gender effects in our own study, it would seem plausible to predict that women working with women would have an advantage over the other possible pairings. There is some suggestive evidence in this direction. In their analysis of patient ratings in a study of trained undergraduate therapists, Persons, Persons, and Newmark[24] found that same-sex matches were advantageous, with women being especially responsive to female therapists. Reviewing their data from a sample of more experienced therapists, Orlinsky and Howard[25] concluded that while there was no overall effect of therapist gender, single women and depressed women felt more support and satisfaction with female therapists. Abramowitz et al.[8] reported that female therapists in their experimental design empathized more strongly with the (hypothetical) female patient. In our own study,[12] there were two significant findings concerning gender matching: (1) female patients paired with more experienced female therapists reported greater satisfaction and more improvement in self-acceptance and friendship when compared with other senior-therapist–patient pairs; and (2) female therapists treating female patients reported greater satisfaction with treatment.

Our research and that of others studying gender pairings show more strikingly, however, that gender per se has complicated interactions with other variables. For example, therapist experience in our study was an important variable, with "senior" therapists showing fewer gender effects than "juniors." Hill found that when female counselors were paired with female clients, the experienced therapists were more satisfied, empathic, and involved, while the inexperienced women were cautious and focused on technique.[26] This difference did not hold for male therapists. Similarly, whether female patients were undergraduate or graduate students in our study—or single, married, or divorced in Howard, Orlinsky, and Hill's study[27]—had significant effects on the psychotherapy. Patient expectancies, as Orlinsky and Howard[25] observed, are powerful factors in this context, perhaps overriding actual therapist characteristics. Boulware and Holmes reported in their review and experimental study that men and women tended to choose older therapists of the same sex for help with personal problems, although not for other types of counseling.[28] This result reached statistical significance only for women. These many observations of the interplay between gender and other characteristics suggest the conclusion that younger, unmarried, less-experienced patients and therapists are more vulnerable to gender-related feelings and stereotypes. On these grounds and from a clinical understanding of the impact of personal history, it follows that same-sex gender-matching should be strongly considered in those situations where these factors and a history of serious difficulty with the opposite-sex parent are present. Naturally, patients with a different preference of their own deserve to have the choice carefully respected. In such cases, it depends on the chosen therapist to bring to the treatment an informed sensitivity to gender issues.

Implications of Psychotherapy Research on Gender

Gender is a very broad kind of variable, and psychotherapy is a very individualized kind of procedure, which has the unique property of focusing on the response of a single person to his or her experience in seeming disregard of social forces. Psychotherapy research, however, can look for meaningful patterns within the universe of psychotherapy relationships and thereby document or draw attention to phenomena that might not otherwise be noticed. In general, as we have seen, the research on gender effects has not added much to the insights of earlier clinicians or of feminist critics of the past decade. Of the former, we may now say that the importance of gender as a significant variable in psychotherapy has been demonstrated. Its effects are modest, but meaningful, and must henceforth be taken into account in the teaching, practice, and scientific study of psychotherapy. Of the latter, we can confirm that therapists tend to share the stereotypes or biases of the culture, and that this is somewhat more true of men. These conclusions are echoed in two more recent reviews of the psychotherapy literature.[29,30]

Research on gender in psychotherapy also points up some neglected areas in theory and practice. These relate to the reluctance of men to seek help, to deficiencies in fledgling male therapists' appreciation of emotional issues, and to some discomfort for therapists in the treatment of men.

Our findings revealing female-patient and female-therapist effects suggest that the treatment of males—and the creation of productive therapeutic relationships by male therapists—may represent significant areas of weakness in psychotherapy. These observations have practical implications for the selection and training of therapists, particularly in those settings where academic achievement and intellectual skills are the major criteria of evaluation. Certainly, more considered explicit awareness of gender, gender roles, and gender stereotypes is a crucial response to these findings by mental health professionals engaged in training as well as treatment. In the individual psychotherapy case and in psychotherapy research, gender continues to deserve careful attention as a significant, often elusive, variable in the subtlety of therapeutic interaction.

REFERENCES

1. Gove WR, Tudor JF: Adult sex roles and mental illness. In *Changing women in a changing society*. Edited by Huber J. Chicago, University of Chicago Press, 1973.
2. Broverman IK, Broverman DM, Clarkson FE, *et al*; Sex role stereotypes and clinical judgments of mental health, *Journal of Consulting and Clinical Psychology 34*:1–7, 1970.
3. Berzins JI: Therapist-patient matching. In *Contribution to effective psychotherapy: An empirical assessment*. Edited by Gurmen AS, Razin AM. New York: Pergamon Press, 1979.
4. Bem SL: The measurement of psychological androgyny, *Journal of Consulting and Clinical Psychology 42:* 155–162, 1974.
5. Fabrikant B: The psychotherapist and the female patient: Perceptions, misconceptions, and change. In *Women in therapy*. Edited by Franks V, Burtle MA. New York, Brunner/Mazel, 1974.
6. Brown CR, Hellinger MC: Therapists' attitude toward women, *Social Work 20:* 266–270, 1975.
7. Schwartz J, Abramowitz S: Value-related effects in psychiatric judgment, *Archives of General Psychiatry 32:* 1525–1529, 1975.
8. Abramowitz S, Roback H, Schwartz J., *et al*: Sex bias in psychotherapy: A failure to confirm, *American Journal of Psychiatry 133:* 706–709, 1976.
9. Garfield SL, Affleck DC: An appraisal of duration of stay in outpatient psychotherapy, *Journal of Nervous and Mental Disorders 129*:492–498, 1959.
10. Mischel W: Sex-typing and socialization. In *Carmichael's manual of child psychology*. Edited by Mussen PH. New York, Wiley, 1970.
11. Maccoby EE, Jacklin CN: *The psychology of sex differences*. Stanford, Calif., Stanford University Press, 1974.

12. Kirshner LA, Hauser ST, Genack A: Effects of gender on short-term therapy, *Psychotherapy: Theory, Research, and Practice* 15:158–167, 1978.
13. Mintz J, Luborsky L, Auerbach A: Dimensions of psychotherapy: A factor analytic study of ratings of psychotherapy sessions, *Journal of Consultation and Clinical Psychology* 36:106–120, 1971.
14. Phillips D, Segal B: Sexual status and psychiatric symptoms, *American Sociology Review* 34:58–72, 1969.
15. Light DW: The impact of medical school on future psychiatrists, *American Journal of Psychiatry* 132:607–610, 1975.
16. Cartwright L: Personality differences in male and female medical students, *Psychiatry in Medicine* 3:213–219, 1972.
17. Carter C: Advantages of being a woman therapist, *Psychotherapy* 8:297–300, 1971.
18. Alonso A, Rutan JS: Cross-sex supervision for cross-sex therapy, *American Journal of Psychiatry* 135:928–931, 1978.
19. Thompson C: Notes on the psychoanalytic significance of the choice of analyst, *Psychiatry* 1:205–216, 1938.
20. Davidson V: Patient attitudes toward sex of therapist: implications for psychotherapy. In *Successful psychotherapy*. Edited by Claghorn JL. New York; Brunner/Mazel, 1976.
21. Ivey EP: Significance of the sex of the psychiatrist, *American Journal of Psychiatry* 2:607–610, 1960.
22. Chesler P: Patient and patriarch: Women in the psychotherapeutic relationship. In *Women in sexist society,* edited by Gornick V, Moran BK. New York, Basic Books, 1971.
23. Rice JK, Rice DG: Implications of the women's liberation movement for psychotherapy, *American Journal of Psychiatry* 130:191–199, 1973.
24. Persons RW, Persons MK, Newmark I: Perceived helpful therapist's characteristics, client improvements, and sex of therapist and client, *Psychotherapy: Theory, Research and Practice* 11:63–65, 1974.
25. Orlinsky DE, Howard KI: The effects of sex of therapist on the therapeutic experiences of women, *Psychotherapy: Theory, Research and Practice* 13:82–88, 1976.
26. Hill C: Sex of client and sex and experience level of counselor, *Journal of Consulting Psychology* 22:5–11, 1975.
27. Howard KI, Orlinsky DE, Hill JA: Patient's satisfactions in psychotherapy as a function of patient-therapist pairing, *Psychotherapy* 7:130–134, 1970.
28. Boulware DW, Holmes DS: Preferences for therapists and related expectancies, *Journal of Consulting and Clinical Psychology* 35:269–277, 1970.
29. Zeldow PB: Sex differences in psychiatric evaluation and treatment, *Archives of General Psychiatry* 35:89–96, 1978.
30. Mogul KM: Overview: the sex of the therapist, *American Journal of Psychiatry* 139:1–11, 1982.

Chapter 17

Special Issues for Women in Psychotherapy

Harriet E. Lerner

In recent years the practice of psychotherapy came under heavy fire from feminist critics, who turned in large numbers to women's rap groups or feminist therapy as alternatives to more established modes of treatment.[1] Concern about widespread sexist practices in the treatment of women was also voiced by mental health professionals from traditional training programs and work settings as well.[2,3,4] This chapter explores the nature and legitimacy of such complaints and identifies special issues of relevance to all women seeking psychotherapy.

Of the many criticisms leveled against traditional psychotherapies, a few may be summarized briefly. First, traditional psychotherapy—and in particular, psychoanalysis—tends to focus primarily, if not exclusively, on internal or intrapsychic conflicts rather than on the cultural context that has produced them. Such a therapeutic bias not only diverts energy away from potential social and political change but may also foster in the woman a sense of "uniqueness" regarding her "pathology" rather than helping her to recognize that her symptoms, which may be ubiquitous among women, stem naturally from patriarchal society's neglect and distortion of women's true intellectual, sexual, and social needs. Perhaps the most serious accusation against traditional psychotherapy is that in subtle but powerful ways, it may lead women to conform to male-defined notions of femininity and may discourage rebellion from the "feminine role" by interpreting such rebellion as pathological.

For many therapists, however, such accusations do not ring true.

Harriet E. Lerner, Ph.D. • Staff Psychologist, The Menninger Foundation, Topeka, Kansas.

As a staff psychologist in a traditional psychoanalytic institution, I can personally vouch for the good intentions of my colleagues. Well-trained psychoanalytic therapists do not strive to send their female patients back to the kitchen. Rather, the task of a good psychotherapy, psychoanalytic or otherwise, is to provide women with the opportunity to overcome the barriers that interfere with the full utilization of their capacities. This, in theory, is to be done in an atmosphere of therapeutic neutrality in which a woman is free to find a comfortable and honest definition of her femininity, based neither on predominant stereotypes about women nor on rancor and rebellion against them.

With such purity of intention, most therapists do not view sexism in treatment as a serious problem. Feminist concerns may be written off as naive, outdated, or simply misguided. It is indeed difficult for therapists to examine openly and critically how their own unconscious biases and perceptions adversely affect and limit their treatment of female patients. Yet, no longer can we close our eyes to the fact that every therapist has an implicit concept of "normality" for men and women that arises out of the cultural context in which she or he is embedded. As we will see in the pages following, a therapist's implicit (and often unconscious) absorption of cultural norms and values continuously affects the nature of the interventions that are made (or not made) in the course of the therapeutic process.

PSYCHOTHERAPY WITH WOMEN: DIFFERING IDEOLOGICAL PERSPECTIVES

Traditional therapists* tend to view women's symptoms and dissatisfactions as an expression of individual psychopathology, to be analyzed and understood in light of the patient's unique individual history. Even those therapists who are sympathetic toward feminist goals may not view "cultural factors" as the "real" or primary determinants that interfere with women's fulfillment. While cultural limitations on women may be superficially acknowledged, a patient's anger in response to these factors may be said to reflect an unhealthy sense of passive victimization that militates against constructive personal change. Thus, a patient's sensitivity to the social and cultural roots of her difficulties may not be legitimized by the therapist as an important focus for treatment. Rather, feminist concerns may be inter-

*By *traditional therapists,* I mean psychotherapists whose conceptualization of their patients' difficulties and their own therapeutic goals or clinical techniques has not been significantly altered or influenced by the past two decades of feminism. My experience with traditional therapists is largely with colleagues whose individual or group work is psychoanalytically based.

preted as the patient's defensive attempt to avoid painful inner conflict by placing the blame for her unhappiness outside herself.

In contrast, those who identify themselves as feminist therapists view the social and cultural context of the patient's problems as a legitimate and important focus of treatment. Indeed, to deny or minimize these sources of conflict is seen "as inappropriate as attempts to treat black persons while denying that racism is an ugly reality that affects us all."[5] The patient's capacity to identify and respond to ways in which women are depreciated, trivialized, scapegoated, or falsely defined in work and family is not viewed as peripheral to therapeutic work. Rather, the patient's expanded awareness of false and constricting values, myths, and pressures, which pervade the systems in which she operates, is seen as crucial to the process of self-definition and growth. It is when a therapist fails to legitimize the patient's realistic anger and protest that the patient becomes further inhibited in her capacity for creative and free-ranging thought and action.[5]

Most sophisticated therapists, whether feminist or traditional, do not maintain a narrow, single-minded focus on either intrapsychic or sociocultural realities, which would, in either case, be akin to listening for "the sound of one hand clapping." But therapists all differ, if not in conscious beliefs, then in the nature of their interventions and their approach to women's struggles during this period of social change. There still exists much controversy about whether women who angrily protest societal definitions of femininity and the feminine role are themselves expressing neurotic conflicts, or whether, on the other hand, it is our very definitions of femininity and the feminine role that are a pathogenic cause of female symptomatology. This is not simply a matter of theoretical interest, for a therapist's position regarding this controversy (whether conscious and explicit or unexamined and unconsciously held) determines the very course and process of treatment, despite that therapist's very best intentions to "help patients make their own choices" in an atmosphere that is "value-free."[6] To illustrate this point, let us consider the hypothetical case of Janet:

> Janet, a 34-year-old homemaker, has two healthy children and an ambitious, successful, and concerned husband. Janet tells herself that she "has everything"; yet she seeks psychotherapy because of feelings of depression and malaise as well as a growing anger and resentment toward her children and husband. From her own perspective, her dissatisfaction is entirely irrational, and she begins her first therapy hour by telling her psychotherapist, "I have nothing to be angry and depressed about." Her goal for treatment, as she initially states it, is to be a better and more satisfied wife and mother. Let us examine how two different therapists, Therapist A (traditional) and Therapist B (feminist), might conceptualize and work with Janet's problems.

Therapist A

Therapist A views Janet's anger and depression as a symptom reflecting unconscious conflicts that interfere with her capacity to nurture and care for others. Therapist A may explore with Janet deep-rooted feelings of neglect and deprivation from her own childhood, which now make it difficult for her to provide for her children without resentment and hostility. If Janet's anger at her husband is associated with the envious wish that she, too, would like to achieve and compete in the world outside the home, these "masculine strivings" may be interpreted in light of Janet's neurotic discomfort with her own feminine role.

Therapist A may also reassure Janet that a mother's job is a difficult one, particularly in her children's early years and may reassure Janet that to some degree her anger and ambivalence are a natural part of the difficult and challenging career of motherhood. In addition, Janet may be encouraged to find some time away from the children that is just hers alone, or perhaps to take up some independent hobby or activity. In a supportive and nonjudgmental context, therapist and patient may together explore a range of early conflicts and relationship paradigms with the goal (as Janet herself has stated it) of helping the patient to become a better and more satisfied wife and mother.

Therapist B

Therapist B may agree that Janet (like every human being) has neurotic conflicts that prevent her from parenting her children more competently and comfortably. However, these conflicts may not be viewed as a primary or even an important focus of treatment. Indeed, Therapist B may consider Janet's anger and depression healthy, legitimate, and realistic, despite Janet's own protests that it is "irrational." This therapist may first choose to explore with Janet the internal pressures and the external realities that caused her to lose sight of her own hopes, aspirations, and dreams for herself, and to choose instead to live vicariously through her husband and her children. Expressions of anger, competitiveness, or envy in regard to her husband, or men in general, may be interpreted as healthy strivings for mastery, success, and self-sufficiency, which are frightening for Janet to acknowledge. Historical and intrapsychic determinants may be explored at length,—however, not with the goal of making Janet "a better wife and mother," in the conventional sense. Rather, this therapist may use her or his skills to analyze the unconscious anxiety and guilt that prevent Janet from acknowledging and expressing more autonomous, self-seeking strivings for mastery and success.

In addition, Therapist B will help Janet to identify the familial and institutional realities that interfere with her potential fulfillment in both parenting and work pursuits. Therapist B may question Janet's assumption that the "good mother" (in singular contrast to the "good father") always puts the needs of her young children before her own growth and creative development. While Therapist B will recognize that Janet has her own private neurosis, it is not this neurosis that the therapist believes to be at the core of the problem. Rather, Janet's difficulties are seen as a symptom of the institution of motherhood and family (as it has been defined by male "experts"), which has excused the male sex from the real day-to-day task of child rearing, while demanding that a mother's growth and development be exchanged for the growth and development of the child she has borne.

The striking difference in focus between these two therapists illustrates the fact that we are living in a time of considerable controversy regarding our basic understanding of women's pleasures and problems. In the pages following I continue to demonstrate how psychotherapy invariably reflects the cultural context in which it is embedded. Every therapist, whether feminist or "Freudian," will express, in the course of treatment, her or his own values and visions for women. There is no "value-free" psychotherapy.

The Masculine–Feminine Dichotomy: Implications for Therapeutic Practice

Many therapists have absorbed culturally defined notions of masculinity and femininity and consciously or unconsciously view these concepts as reflecting what is healthy or "natural" for men and women. Therapists who explicitly label, or even privately conceptualize, certain of women's wishes, strivings, and behaviors as being "unfeminine" may unwittingly exacerbate their patients' inhibitions rather than increasing their options.[7] In certain cases, women may become further constricted in treatment as their aggressive strivings for dominance and power (which may indeed have certain pathological aspects) are labeled as *masculine* or *phallic* by the therapist, often without acknowledgment of the healthy and adaptive components of such behaviors. While purportedly providing insight, therapeutic interpretation may subtly be aimed at encouraging the patient to "stop" her aggressive, controlling, or competitive behaviors.[8] With men, however, the therapeutic goal would more typically be to help the patient achieve a healthier and more comfortable, conflict-free integration and expression of these same qualities or behaviors.

Failure to Analyze Conformity to Traditional Feminine Scripts. It is important to recognize that most good therapists do not consciously hold to narrow, stereotypical ideas about women; rather, they respect the patient's right to pursue treatment goals that may be out of keeping with the traditional feminine role. However, a subtle, serious, and more pervasive problem arises for the psychotherapy patient who does indeed fit the cultural stereotype, but for the wrong reasons (e.g., the traditional "feminine" woman who opts for full-time motherhood out of neurotic anxieties about competition, success, and intellectual achievement). In these cases, many therapists fail to analyze the conflicts and anxieties that keep the woman in her role and restrict her choices.[6,9] I have noted that unhealthy degrees of self-sac-rifice, dependency, and underachievement in women (except in their extreme and most conspicuous "masochistic" forms) are often not rec-ognized or questioned by the therapist since these may strike one as quite "natural" characteristics of the female sex. The failure of thera-pists to analyze sufficiently the defensive and maladaptive determi-nants underlying a patient's choice to conform to culturally prescribed notions of femininity is a common phenomenon in psychotherapy. The following clinical vignette offers an example of skillful therapeutic work, which unfortunately may be more the exception than the rule:

> Ms. B, a 28-year-old woman in intensive psychotherapy, announced to her therapist that she would be moving to a new city at the end of the year because of her husband's professional advancement. Although she was sad about leaving psychotherapy as well as her friends and her teach-ing job in a Montessori school, she expressed excitement about the chal-lenges that the move would bring and pride in her husband's success. Initial inquiry by the therapist as to any less enthusiastic feelings she might have met with a restatement of her positive reaction to the anticipated change. Certainly, it entailed losses for her, but these were well over-shadowed by the gains. Further, Ms. B was thinking about starting a fam-ily soon and thought she might stop work entirely for several years. She communicated clearly that she would like the issue dropped, and it was dropped for some time.
>
> Months later, when Ms. B was discussing some pains and pleasures of her work, the therapist once again commented that he was struck by how easily she had made her own job unimportant in regard to the planned move, and how adept she was at convincing him that this was the case. He also speculated as to why she might need to avoid taking her own professional life seriously and commented that it was difficult for her to be in competition with her husband or to ask him to make professional sac-rifices for her, although she had done so earlier for him. The therapist's questioning, which occurred in the face of her initial insistence that there were no further issues to discuss, led to her increased understanding of the neurotic anxieties that caused her to devalue her work, to treat it as less important than her husband's, and even to be ready to drop it entirely. The therapist's persistence in this line of questioning also had significant transference implications, since it communicated to the patient that he took her work seriously. The fact that he had dropped the issue, even though she had more than invited him to do so, had for her the unconscious meaning that he, like her mother, did not really want her to be a fulfilled individual. Ms. B and her husband did not move, and she has continued to advance professionally and now has a challenging position with consid-erably authority.*

In contrast to the therapeutic work presented above, many thera-pists fail to recognize, and thus to analyze, the patient's defensive or

*This vignette was previously published in the *American Journal of Psychiatry* 135(1):51, January 1978 (H. Lerner, "Adaptive and Pathogenic Aspects of Sex-role Stereotypes: Implications for Parenting and Psychotherapy").

neurotic conformity to the feminine role and to false and confining definitions of femininity. These errors of omission affect great numbers of female patients, for most women entering treatment are themselves unable to consciously acknowledge wishes or longings that are out of keeping with traditional feminine scripts. Indeed, many women who seemingly "choose" to relinquish self-seeking professional or autonomous strivings do so because they cannot freely, and without guilt and anxiety, fulfill themselves through personal achievement.[10] In my experience, it is not uncommon for a bored, exhausted, intellectually impoverished, and isolated mother of small children to begin treatment with the following goal, "Make me a better wife and mother to my husband and children." She may, quite literally, have no other vision for herself that feels acceptable, and the only form of protest she can voice is her symptoms, which frequently take the form of an unconscious wildcat strike against her "sacred calling"[11] (i.e., "I am too depressed/fatigued/confused to run the household and care for my children").

Traditional therapists, especially those who believe that small children need their mothers continually at home, often fail to skillfully explore with the patient other alternatives and options.[9] Further, they may not help her to clarify the nature of her legitimate anger and complaints against her "prescribed role," which the patient dare not herself express, except through her symptoms.

THE FEMALE-PATIENT–MALE-THERAPIST DYAD: REPLICATING PATRIARCHAL ARRANGEMENTS

Some feminist critics have warned that psychotherapy for women may entail a potential reenactment of male–female relationship paradigms as they exist in the culture at large.[1] It is indeed true that many women in psychotherapy become intensely dependent on an idealized male therapist, who may become the center of their fantasy life. If the relationship is eroticized, it may, much like an affair, dilute and eclipse other important relationships and pursuits in the patient's life and serve as a resistance to change. It may be so gratifying for a woman to receive support and empathic understanding from a warm, nurturant, male authority (and so gratifying for a male therapist to be able to comfortably express and be appreciated for these "maternal" qualities) that the therapeutic relationship itself may foster dependency without facilitating autonomous solutions.

Women have a long history of experiencing unegalitarian relationships with males as "natural" and of following leaders and "experts" compliantly. Cultural pressures on women to "please men" are so profound that the woman's desire to be attractive and admired by her therapist may override a more honest process of self-definition and self-determination. Women's attempt to fit themselves to definitions of femininity that are implicitly communicated by their therapist is often unconscious and subtle and may thus go unrecognized by both therapist and patient. I have spoken to a number of women who have participated in both individual treatment and feminist consciousness-raising groups, and who have stated in retrospect that the latter allowed them a greater opportunity to explore personal issues with real honesty and depth. Some of these women saw the limitations of their psychotherapy as stemming from their own deep-seated and often unconscious need to please the male therapist and to remain unthreatening. Others reported that their dependent, nonthreatening behaviors were induced, or at least unconsciously rewarded, by the therapist himself. Experienced supervisors do indeed report that male therapists may covertly and unwittingly encourage compliant behaviors and discourage a challenging, independent stance in female patients.[8]

While female therapists are hardly immune from adopting such attitudes, it is my observation that the problem occurs most intensely and with least conscious recognition in the male-therapist–female-patient dyad. Of significance is the fact that the feminine socialization process teaches females to protect the male ego at all costs by inhibiting any traits, qualities, and behaviors that may be threatening to men. Cultural pressures to "play dumb," "let the man win," or "pretend he's boss" are all crude, if not comic, expressions of a more subtle but powerful cultural injunction that states that in intimate male–female dyads, the man should be (or at least should feel like) the more capable, successful, and dominant partner. For the many couples who deviate from this arrangement, psychiatry has designed such terms as *role reversal, role confusion,* or *matriarchal family,* all of which are mildly pejorative terms suggesting that things are not in their natural place. Indeed, women who dare to compete openly with men on issues of competence and power may be labeled *castrating* or *unfeminine* and have their very attractiveness and love of humankind brought into question. As many authors have noted,[5,12,13,14] this patriarchal arrangement reflects, in part, men's persistent irrational anxieties about the dreadful effects of female aggression and dominance, as well as women's related irrational fears of their own destructive, "castrating" potential. These shared fears of female destructiveness date back to our long years of helpless dependency on women (i.e., our mothers and other female caretakers) and are rarely recognized consciously by either sex. Rather, these anxieties are contained and held in check by social arrangements that allow men to maintain power and control over

women, who are discouraged from expressing aggression and dominance except in indirect, covert, or manipulative ways.

Given such intrapsychic and cultural pressures, it is hardly surprising that male therapists, in particular, may encourage a patient to
be self-assertive and autonomous in her family and work life but may
subtly encourage her to have a "nice relationship" (e.g., to follow his
advice and to accept and value his interpretations) within the therapeutic hour. The paradox of therapeutic interpretations that are purportedly in the service of fostering the patient's independence, while
subtly patronizing her or undermining her autonomy within the therapeutic relationship, may go unnoticed by both therapist and super-
visor ("No matter how much I interpret, or try to push her, she still
won't be assertive with her husband!"). Further, the woman's healthy
expressions of anger, criticalness, or competitiveness directed toward
the therapist may be felt by him as an unhealthy display of aggression
or an attempt to control. If the woman is, in fact, hostile and controlling, he may interpret accurately the pathogenic components of such
behavior, but without recognizing the positive and adaptive aspects
of what the patient is attempting to communicate or accomplish.[8] Bernardez-Bonesatti[8] has commented on the especially strong feelings of
revulsion and disapproval that male therapists may feel when confronted with openly hostile and domineering behavior in their women
patients. Because women themselves have enormous unconscious fears
regarding their own destructiveness and the related fragility of the male
ego, both patient and therapist may fail to recognize the subtle ways
in which the woman is being "a good patient" at the expense of her
own autonomy and growth.

Bernardez-Bonesatti[8] has noted that women therapists may also
be prone to excessive disapproval of their female patient's anger or
competitiveness, especially if the target of the patient's hostility is a
male. Not only is a protectiveness for males aroused, but the female
therapist who unconsciously fears that her own unrestrained anger may
be hurtful to men is threatened by her identification with a female
patient whom she perceives as "destructive" or "castrating." I have
also been impressed by the need of female therapists to avoid identifying with women who are angry at men, even if they perceive them
as having a legitimate cause.

SEX OF THERAPIST

ADVANTAGES OF FEMALE THERAPIST. A significant number of factors go into the making of a good psychotherapist that far outweigh
the matter of one's sex. It is my opinion, however, that other things

being equal (level of skill, experience, quality of training, etc.), female patients may have much to gain in working with a woman therapist. At the risk of offering somewhat oversimplified generalizations, I would briefly outline certain advantages as follows:

1. Many women find it difficult to be open with a male therapist. For example, their frankness and specificity regarding sexual experiences may be limited. In general, a more honest exploration of self may be facilitated by work with a same-sex therapist. With a female therapist, the patient is less pulled to unconsciously fulfill stereotypical feminine behavior (e.g., "protectiveness" of the male therapist's ego and sense of importance, avoidance of direct confrontation and competition) that will block more creative, free-ranging work.

In intimate dyadic relationships, men have very little experience relating to women in a truly egalitarian manner, although many men may consider themselves exceptions to this rule. As noted earlier, men are more likely than women to overlook subtle aspects of female compliance, dependency, deskilling, etc., since these are the expectable and familiar ways that women relate to men in close dyadic relationships.

2. With a female therapist, sexualization of the relationship, which may serve as a major resistance against learning, is characteristically avoided. While homosexual feelings and fantasies may emerge with a same-sex therapist, these are usually not used defensively and seductively in the service of warding off anxiety and the threat of confrontation.

3. The opportunity to identify with a female therapist's professional skills and competence is extremely helpful for many women, particularly in instances where there is deep guilt and anxiety over issues of achievement and autonomous functioning. Some patients are better able to consciously acknowledge and express jealous and competitive feelings toward a therapist of their own sex, without having to feel "castrating" or unfeminine.

4. The firsthand experience of women therapists with specifically female emotional, physical, sexual, and spiritual experiences may facilitate a greater depth and intensity of clinical work. Women have incorporated a great number of male-defined myths regarding the "feminine experience," which can best be explored with a female therapist who has herself taken seriously the task of her own consciousness-raising.

5. Women's conflicts and inhibitions often have their roots in unresolved issues of autonomy and separation from the mother, although these conflicts may be masked by the girl–woman's transfer of dependency onto male authority figures and a premature flight into hetero-

sexual relationships.[15,16] A female therapist may allow for a richer and deeper exploration of the mother–daughter relationship and may facilitate an affective reexperiencing of the profoundly complex and ambivalent nature of this bond.

6. Affirmation by a same-sex therapist has especially significant meanings for certain women. To be accepted by another woman in the context of a close relationship characterized by trust and mutual respect may be more "validating" of one's worth and self-esteem than working with a cross-sex therapist. This, I have noted, is especially the case for narcissistic women with poor self-esteem who unconsciously experience male therapists (or men in general) as relatively more seducible, easily flattered, or fooled by appearances than are women.

7. A same-sex therapist offers greater opportunities for identification. While this is an advantage for all patients, it may be especially critical for the more disturbed individuals, who have not consolidated a stable and coherent sense of gender identity.

Paradoxically, the potential advantages of same-sex therapy, outlined above, are also associated with unconscious threats that may lead certain women to seek out male therapists. For example, a woman who is involved in an intense, unresolved struggle to separate from her own mother may experience considerable anxiety in anticipating dependency on the female therapist. Women who lack a stable and coherent sense of identity and fear themselves to be without substance and depth usually have consolidated a repertoire of cross-sex behaviors that make it easier to begin treatment with a male therapist, with whom these behaviors may help to control the anxieties inherent in beginning a therapy relationship. Women with unconscious conflicted wishes to achieve and succeed in the world outside the home may wish to avoid a relationship with a professional woman in which these conflicts will inevitably be stirred. In sum, many women consider a male therapist "safer" than a female therapist, although this feeling may not be their conscious experience. Rather, unconscious fears of women may be defensively masked by an experience of female professionals as less capable or authoritative than their male counterparts.

Prospective psychotherapy patients who voice a strong preference for male therapists may do so for adaptive, constructive reasons (e.g., a woman whose family life has included a psychologically or physically absent father may need to experience male nurturance). It is my clinical opinion that when a woman feels strongly that she wishes to see a therapist of a particular sex, male or female, her choice should be respected. While such preferences invariably include both adaptive and defensive components, the patient's anxieties should not be overriden or prematurely interpreted, and the wisdom of the patient's unconscious should not be ignored.

ADDITIONAL REMARKS. As is true of all generalizations, those stated here tell us nothing about the advantages or disadvantages of a particular therapist or the unique needs of an individual patient. Surely, being male does not condemn one to tunnel vision or to a rigid and unexamined adherence to patriarchal attitudes. Nor does being female guarantee one's freedom from unconscious biases and prejudices against women. As Alonso and Rutan[17] pointed out, there are female therapists who are male-identified, who look on their female patients with some measure of scorn, or who may lack empathy for women who have struggled less successfully than they have. Certainly, not all women therapists, by virtue of their femaleness, have their empathic understanding of women enhanced. Some, for example, may be vulnerable to greater distortion through overidentification and a reliance on projection, which may lead to a false assumption of "sameness" or understanding where it does not exist.

Similarly, a therapist's being a feminist tells us little about her professional expertise. While some feminist therapists have had excellent training, others have not, perhaps because they have avoided traditional, male-dominated institutions at a time when there are few alternative programs available that offer the opportunity for intensive, high-level clinical training. Certain feminist therapists, following an egalitarian treatment model that stresses demystification of the therapist's expertise, may engage in nontherapeutic openness and self-disclosure that blur the appropriate boundaries and fail to provide for the patient the optimal conditions for free-ranging fantasy and exploration. Feminist therapists, like traditional therapists, may be competent or not.

In light of the individual differences between psychotherapists and the many important factors that go into the making of a skilled professional other than his or her sex, it may be tempting to deny real differences between female and male therapists in the treatment of women. As Alonso and Rutan[17] noted, it is difficult for all of us to come to terms with the limitations of our own capacity to empathize and identify with patients whose experience we cannot enter. In discussing such limitations of empathy, these authors have reminded us of the painful experience that white liberals had during the racial tensions of the 1960s, and I recall vividly my own defensive reaction to being informed that blacks could not deal effectively with issues of power and self-definition in groups that included white members, and especially white "experts." Women, like blacks, have learned in the past decades of feminism that there is a certain development of consciousness and self-definition that can be achieved only in all-female groups. Along these lines, Bernardez-Bonesatti[16] has described the special advantages and benefits that an all-women's therapy group can provide for its members. Yet, perhaps because of unconscious fears about hurting or excluding men and incurring their anger and disapproval, even female mental-health professionals may deny or minimize the potentially powerful therapeutic benefits of same-sex therapy.

Conclusion

Psychotherapy can be a creative, expanding process of unfolding from the center, or it may reinforce conformity to constricted and externally defined notions of femininity. Similarly, the therapeutic process may free a woman to identify more clearly the sociocultural context of her difficulties, or it may "cool the mark" by encouraging her to cultivate her personal neurosis like a little flower garden, while minimizing the pathogenic effects of the system in which she is operating. To write off the more unhappy of these outcomes as isolated instances of "bad therapy" is tempting, for it allows therapists to avoid taking seriously the difficult task of critically evaluating their work with female patients. As I have tried to show here, good intentions and dedication to helping women become all they can be hardly ensure nonsexist work. It is only through a deeply felt commitment to one's own consciousness-raising that therapists can even begin to gain freedom from the unconscious biases and assumptions that adversely affect the treatment of women.

References

1. Chesler P: *Women and madness.* Garden City, N.Y., Doubleday, 1972.
2. Symonds A: Psychoanalysis and women's liberation. *Journal of the American Academy of Psychoanalysis* 6(4):429–431, 1978.
3. American Psychological Association: Report of the Task Force on Sex Bias and Sex-role Stereotyping in Psychotherapeutic Practice, *Am Psychol* 30:1169–1175, 1975.
4. American Psychological Association: Report of the Task Force on Sex Bias and Sex-Role Stereotyping in Psychotherapeutic Practice, Guidelines for Therapy with Women, *Am Psychol* 33:1122–1123, 1978.
5. Bernardez-Bonesatti T: Women and anger: Conflicts with aggression in contemporary women, *Journal of the American Medical Women's Association* 33(5):215–219, 1978.
6. Lerner H: Adaptive and pathogenic aspects of sex-role stereotypes: Implications for parenting and psychotherapy, *American Journal of Psychiatry* 135(1):48–52, 1978.
7. Kronsky B: Feminism and psychotherapy, *Journal of Contemporary Psychotherapy* 3(2):89–98, 1971.
8. Bernardez-Bonesatti T: Unconscious beliefs about women affecting psychotherapy, *North Carolina Journal of Mental Health* 7(5):63–66, 1976.

9. Group for the Advancement of Psychiatry, Committee on the College Student: *The educated woman: Prospects and problems,* GAP Report 92. New York, GAP, 1975.

10. Chasseguet-Smirgel J: Feminine guilt and the Oedipus complex. In Female sexuality: New psychoanalytic views. Edited by Chasseguet-Smirgel J. Ann Arbor, University of Michigan Press, 1970.

11. Rich A: *Of woman born.* New York, W. W. Norton, 1976.

12. Lerner HE: Early origins of envy and devaluation of women: Implications for sex-role stereotypes, *Bulletin of the Menninger Clinic 38*:538–553, 1974.

13. Lerner HE: Taboos against female anger, *Menninger Perspective 8*(4):4–11, 1977.

14. Dinnerstein D: *The mermaid and the minotaur: Sexual arrangements and human malaise.* New York, Harper & Row, 1976.

15. Lerner HE, On the comfort of patriarchal solutions: Some reflections on Brown's paper, *Journal of Personality and Social Systems 1*(3):47–50, 1978.

16. Bernardez-Bonesatti T: Women's groups: A feminist perspective on the treatment of women. In *Changing approaches to the psychotherapies.* Edited by Grayson H, Loew C. New York, Spectrum Publications, 1978.

17. Alonso A, Rutan JS: Cross-sex supervision for cross-sex therapy, *American Journal of Psychiatry 135*(8):929–931, 1978.

Chapter 18

Conflict and Psychological Development: Women in the Family

JEAN BAKER MILLER

Almost all family therapists have developed a concept that suggests that the family is "stuck" in one way or another. Most of their ideas revolve around the inability of families to move beyond a "pathological homeostasis,"[1] to disrupt a family myth,[2] to overcome a repetitive "double-bind" communication system,[3] to break out of a "pseudo-mutuality,"[4] to relinquish the recycling of "shared fantasies and projective identifications,"[5] and the like.

What these clinicians have not considered is that there may be an inherent factor that promotes stasis. This factor restricts the potential movement of the family, or, to put it more accurately, it restricts movement in the direction of growth. Despite the appearance of stasis, nothing truly stands still; this is certainly evident in families. It is a question of the direction of the movement, whether it is toward the enhancement of all family members or toward their constriction and distortion. This chapter considers the question of whether the family has been unable to encompass the experience of the woman; and whether this factor restricts the movement of the entire family.

In regard to intimacy, the necessity of encompassing change becomes particularly clear. An intimate relationship or system of relationships must be able to change with the changing needs and desires of the participants. If it does not, intimacy deteriorates.

It is commonly stated that when two people form a couple, they create a new "phenomenon," which is greater than the sum of the two individuals; and that this new combination has the potential to gen-

JEAN BAKER MILLER, M.D. ● Associate Clinical Professor of Psychiatry, School of Medicine, Boston University, Boston; Director, Stone Center for Developmental Studies and Services, Wellesley College, Wellesley, Massachusetts.

erate a greater level of adult creativity and growth than either individual has known before.[5] (For present purposes, other possible combi-
nations of adults will not be discussed.) For such growth to occur,
however, this new "community," this unit, must be responsive to the
experience of each partner, experience that is itself in flux.

Each child, in its attempt to grow, stimulates further disruptions
of the *status quo,* thereby forcing the parents to confront further change.
How have families met this repeated demand for change, and what
happens to the intimacy that the family members seek? One way to
explore the question is to consider the experience of one family, the
Ks. This family is described to illustrate the themes common in many
families. For brevity, only certain periods in the life of the family are
considered.

Many young people today state beliefs and goals that differ from
those of the Ks. These new values are making true differences in their
lives. For many people, however, the same forces continue to operate,
particularly on the psychological level. Past beliefs about the normative or "proper" family continue to exert a strong psychological effect,
not the least among members of the mental health professions. According to these traditional conceptions, the family is a unit in which
the man is the sole or major breadwinner and the woman is the non-
paid wife and mother. Today, only 16% of families conform to this
pattern, and 58% of mothers of school-age children are working, as
are over one-third of mothers of preschool children.[6] However, at a
major national convention, leading family therapists presented a major
survey of the field without mentioning either this change or the fact
that there has been a woman's movement that has produced a vast
literature on the family specifically, as well as on women in general.

An Example

The Ks had the appearance of an ideal American family, highly educated, devoted to their children, active in their community, helping neighbors, and desiring to direct their lives to the betterment of the larger world.
(The intent here is not to ignore families with fewer advantages but to
simplify for the sake of discussion. It is also, to suggest that poorer families
have problems that are similar in essence but are even more complex.)

Why in this ideal family did the wife, JK, come to a psychiatrist seven
years after marriage in a state of extreme distress? She was depressed and
immobilized and filled with feelings of inadequacy, hopelessness, and despair.

Her history revealed that the couple had met while each was attending
a prestigious college. They had decided that OK, the husband, would go
on to graduate training that would lead to an occupation in a field of social
reform. J shared an intense interest in this work. She hesitated about marriage because of her sense of lack of completion and the desire to test her

own abilities. However, she found a ready solution to her doubts by deciding that the more important course for her "as a woman" must surely be to marry this good man. The Ks believed that she would continue her pursuits—eventually. In the interim, she took "a boring job" to finance O's graduate training.

In 2½ years, the K's first child, a boy, was born, and 2½ years later, a girl was born. Both parents were delighted with the children at first, although J did almost all of the child care. O was finding, with much gratification, that he was becoming accomplished in his work, but the work was increasingly demanding. He arrived home tired and needy. J worked at trying to supply those needs. They involved bodily comforts in their concrete form: good feeding, comfortable surroundings, and the like. Much more importantly, they involved emotional and psychological accompaniment in his life and work.

Indeed, it emerged that while O was a very personable young man, he tended not to express, and often not to perceive, many of the issues that arose in his work. "After he talked things over with J," he found that he "always felt a lot better." He saw forces at work that he hadn't appreciated. Thus, J was providing for O's emotional and intellectual exchange and development. She was likewise supplying these same resources for the children.

By contrast, with the passage of time, J felt more alone with her part of life. She was increasingly unable to ask for O's participation because "It never seemed right. He was always pressured, needing to do some important thing for the world—or for his own deadlines."

The children learned to know J better than their father and to see her as the one who could "hear" their feelings and fulfill their needs and desires. As he later saw it, O gradually began to feel a mounting resentment toward his son. He felt that the boy lacked interest in him and turned to his mother more than he should. O was hurt by this tendency but did not define it as a problem. There were further problems with both children, but in the interests of brevity, they will not be detailed here.

Women's Needs

J seemed to go down an inexorable path of suppressing the examination and expression of a great many of her experiences, desires, and needs. Simultaneously, she developed many assets—and, in turn, a set of new and enlarged desires—but these were not clarified, nor could they emerge fully within the context in which the Ks lived.

J provided O with the sustained sense that someone was vitally interested in him; she was receptive to his emotional experiences and, more than that, was perceptive about emotions he could not express very fully. At a basic level, this provision created an overall "growth medium," as it were, the sustained environment of someone who took care of him and wanted to do so. Thus, for his remnants of unresolved problems, even on the most primitive level, O received enough reassurance so that he could function quite comfortably.

O loved J, but he did not think in terms of providing a comparable level of interest and involvement. Neither of the Ks had the concept that O should want to explore J's daily life or to accompany her in her emotional experiences.

In fact, J had many experiences that needed attention. Initially, she was left unsteady by the sense that she "wasn't certain about what she could do that was worthwhile in the world," and her unsatisfying job during early marriage added further to her doubts. O did not initiate thoroughgoing discussions about J's work as J did about O's. J's uncertainties in this realm contributed to her questions about her capacities and self-worth. These doubts further diminished her sense of her right to put forward her own needs in most areas of the marriage. O became defined as the worthy one and the one who had potential. J moved further in the direction of depending on his ability and his development. Everything had to go into aiding that development and anything that might distract from it or might trouble O had best be submerged. It is important to note the social congruence here. This position appeared "ego-syntonic" not only to O but to J as well.

The same basic factors reached out to affect realms beyond the family. The K's social life came to include primarily friends made through O's work. Finding herself excluded from much of the conversation and unable to follow a large part of it, J gradually gave up attempts to participate. Thus, in circles beyond the family, J felt increasingly alone—and increasingly inferior.

All of these events rendered J even less able to explain her feelings to O. They had notably few rows, and in those few, J soon retreated, feeling, as she later said in therapy, that "There were times when I thought I was right, especially about the children and I now see I was—even about matters other than the children. But when I kept hearing that O was such a promising 'thinker' and graduate student and I was mainly good at washing diapers, it became harder and harder not to think that he knew better about everything." Thus, J was encouraged systematically—if by no one's conscious intent—to limit the expression of her needs and her opinions even on matters intrinsic to the family, as well as on those beyond it. Her valuable perceptions and thoughts turned into sources of pain, rather than the assets and the basis of enhanced self-worth that they could have been.

By the time J sought therapy, all of these experiences had culminated in the feeling that she had "fallen out of love with O." She no longer felt "that deep sense of connection of souls" that was the way she described being in love. She had felt that "This connection was basic to everything, to our whole life together."

By this time, O was aware that J was depressed and troubled but had no clues about the reasons. He understood that she "had to get away from the house and kids sometimes." He tried to plan a romantic night out or an appealing gift. O had, in fact, begun "to rack his brain in attempts to try to be good to J and to make her happy." These attempts led only to more depression for J: "Here was O trying so hard and being so good to me. Another woman would be so happy to have such a husband, and there I was moaning and complaining," a self-image that she abhorred. O's attempts "didn't seem to be what I needed, and yet I couldn't tell him what it was I did need." To add to her self-contempt, she was now ungrateful. All of this served to confirm her feeling that there must be something terribly "wrong with me." Likewise, it convinced O that he "must have married a sick woman," a fate he had never envisioned.

Underlying Dynamics

In examining only a few points in the underlying dynamics, it is striking to note how similar the Ks were in several basic psychological configurations. Certain other factors, however, affected them differentially.

As do most people, both Ks had come to marriage with issues around what are often called *dependency needs*. It is perhaps more accurate to say that they had some problems about their continuing feelings of vulnerability and needs for other people. Both tended to deny these feelings. Instead, they gave to others and "did for others," a method that had been very effective in many ways. Each, in fact, could become quite angry when deprived, but both had problems with the recognition and the direct expression of anger.

Although both partners operated within this similar dynamic, there were important differential features. For one, O felt the right—and in his case, especially, the obligation—to develop himself so that he could serve others best. This conviction, plus a whole series of supports through high school, college, and graduate school, encouraged him. As a result, he did develop competence in the ways in which competence is usually rewarded—and the enhanced sense of self-worth that such competence can afford.

By contrast, the situation militated against J's development along these lines. She would have had to recognize her right and her need to think in terms of self-development and then to ask openly for consideration of her development. She would have had to ask her husband very directly, as things were made to appear—that is, ask O to take on much more of the provision for the family, including provision for her. She seemingly would have had "to ask" for consideration, also, from the children—that is, take time and attention from them, and thus confront the feeling of "depriving" them—again, as things were made to appear.

Asking for something was something that neither of the Ks "ever did." Demanding was even more threatening. O would have had a similar problem if he had had to do that. In fact, he did, at his work, but here, J provided continual encouragement. She could urge him to ask so long as it was for him, not herself. O was receiving many recognitions in his work, and these helped him further to ask for his due a bit more readily. Many of his rewards followed from the fact that he was such a kind and hard-working person. So was J—but she was feeling "more and more selfish and horrible." All of these factors converged to reinforce O's development, to enhance his sense of self-esteem, and, in turn, to make him more able to ask for what he wanted with an increased sense of safety about this whole area.

A second differential factor was the tacit acceptance by both partners that it was proper for J to serve and support O. It is quite common to find that, no matter what underlying dynamics exist, most men have been able to accept this kind of service. Indeed, even if the same type of dynamics is much more intense (i.e., denial of needs and simultaneous anger at their nonfulfillment), there is often a greater silent expectation and even violent demand that the woman serve the man. These factors are often prominent in instances of wife battering, alcoholism, and many other situations.

Both of the Ks had problems of a similar sort in other areas, for example, in the area of aggression. Both tended to deny their aggression. But, again, there were differential factors. O did not think openly of being aggressive in terms of extending himself and his influence to the world and to others in it, but his work pushed him along. He had to pass each test, meet each deadline, perform each task; and he did develop a sense of effectiveness. Here, too, he had J's encouragement. J would have had to consciously search out her desires in this area and therefore confront her problems about them more consciously; for example, she would have had to consider whether she wanted to be more aggressive; whether she could be so safely; what it meant when she was faced with opposition, disapproval, and the like—all of this in the face of the general cultural attitudes that assume that women should possess almost no need for assertion or aggression.[7]

J had to be assertive with the children and, at times, angry at them. These experiences added to her problems. They caused her to become upset and self-critical, since she held the common inner belief that the good mother has virtually no anger.

Worse problems arose for the Ks in regard to assertiveness with or anger at each other. They avoided overt anger whenever possible. Initially, this anger was suggested only by such hints as O's statement that he was "impatient" about J's failure "to get happy and carry on." Characteristically, he called this "self-indulgence." J called it self-indulgence, too, and condemned herself equally harshly, indeed more harshly.

As might be expected, because it involves pleasure for oneself, both K's had difficulty with sex. O, absorbing the common cultural influences, was able to overcome his restrictions on pleasure enough to allow himself to seek sex as his acceptable right. He tended to see it as a physical pressure that had to be relieved and that he had the right to have relieved, especially within the marital state.

Both partners shared the tacit sense that sex was something quite dirty and sinful and that their bodies were almost forbidden areas, not to be paid much attention and certainly not to be "indulged." It is clear that this shared belief was more consonant with O's notion of sexuality as relief. If he could relieve his sexual tension, then he had each time rid himself of the dirty, sinful thing; he could feel pure again and go on with his good work. J, however, was the recipient, left with the dirt and sin. O's " 'wham-bam' approach to sex," as she later termed it, and his lack of the ability to "indulge in sensuality" confirmed their shared fantasy and left J "carrying the bad and evil," as well as sexually frustrated. J eventually lost all interest in sex and felt "used" by O.

In addition to their shared notion, J, as a woman, had acquired much less sense of her right to sexual pleasure, and certainly not to "go out and seek it," as it seemed she'd have to do with O. She meant that the burden would have been on her to open up the whole area of sexuality, a sexuality that was limited for both of them. It emerged in therapy that J, like most women, had a concept of sex that differed from O's. She sought a more complete emotional and sexual experience. A change in the K's sexuality occurred as a result of therapy, but a description of it would require an extended discussion that can be summarized by saying that their total conception of sexuality was enlarged and transformed. This change occurred because J initiated it when she found ways of exploring and expressing her desires and needs.

GROWTH

If J had tried to define and pursue her desires and needs, she would have had, as she later stated it, "to make trouble," that is, to initiate conflict. It would have been conflict on many levels: with her husband, with his appointed role in life, with the usual family structure, with the larger institutions of society, and, most importantly, with her own internalized conception of herself as a woman.

At the same time, despite all of the above, J did develop many assets and, accordingly, other needs. Within the available conceptions and context, however, J's growth could not flourish nor even become recognizable in appropriate ways.

In order to discuss this lengthy topic, we may take one phase of the family's experience as illustrative, the phase of infancy. Children try to grow, and at each age, they inevitably evoke the caretakers' own emotions in relation to that phase. The adult reexperiencing of these issues offers a great opportunity for a creative reworking of them in a new context or for the opposite, the emergence of problems.

Thus, for example, in a child's infancy, the adult can learn that she or he can provide almost total care for another human being. This care requires complex qualities of perceptiveness and sensitivity that we are still attempting to understand.[8,9] For the adult, there are many reactions and gratifications of a kind never experienced before. However, the feelings generated in the direct care of another life are feelings of which the husband is usually deprived. Many husbands feel responsible for the care of the family, but it is in a more removed manner, not providing direct human emotion, but money and some of its equivalents. This can be a stressful burden without the intense emotional experience and enlarged emotional capacity that can follow from a close interaction with growth.

The man could participate more directly either by caring for the infant or by providing the complex emotional companionship that the mother needs at this time. In most families, neither of these is considered the man's major duty—or need.

If this were the case, both partners could become more aware of the existence of such feelings as neediness, helplessness, or vulnerability in themselves and could learn more about what tends to be fulfilling and what isn't and is, therefore, frightening and productive of anger, rage, envy and the like. Each could become more aware of the factors that make it difficult for her or him to provide for others; each could acquire a better sense of the scale and importance of these factors in her or his total personal makeup and could end in a better position to obtain fulfillment of them, for herself or himself.

Instead, it is most likely that the mother will inescapably have to confront a reawakening of these feelings. Whatever fear, rage, hate, shame, or guilt she herself has developed about them will be revived. The pressure of these reawakened feelings and the consequent shame, guilt, and other reactions often lead to self-blame and self-condemnation.

The man, for his part, is very likely not only to try to avoid but to react negatively to any reminder of these feelings.[7] Some men become particularly witholding from and/or attacking of the woman and child at this time. Clinically, it is very common to find a man embarking on extramarital affairs, becoming more alcoholic or more violent, or "acting out" in other ways at the time of pregnancy, childbirth, or the child's infancy, thus becoming particularly destructive precisely at the time when the woman needs his responsiveness most. This attack or withdrawal can serve to reinforce the condemnation that the woman is producing in herself by her own shame, guilt, or other self-reproaches. A period that could have been one of mutual creative reworking of a profound area of the personality for both partners can end in its opposite, a major source of problems for all.

This possibility is often augmented by the fact that these events occur at the time when the young man is at the height of trying to make his way in the world, garnering his resources to establish his "manliness" as manliness is currently defined. He is therefore often least able to allow himself to explore these realms. As it later emerged in therapy, this was true of O.

Examples of problems originating in this period are manifold; a few variations of the central theme may be mentioned. Some women never recover from their disappointment and resentment about the man's lack of responsiveness. A woman may feel that the man will not be there when she needs him most, especially if there is no change in the trend with time. The woman can conclude that the man does not love or value her, or the baby. Such feelings can combine with the woman's own reactivated conflicts to culminate in the resurrection of some version of archaic feelings that she will be not only condemned and deprived but abandoned by the man. (Some women are, in fact, abandoned.) That is, the feelings in this period can easily connect to more primitive feelings that she is needy, greedy, hateful, and dangerous. Her husband does not love the needy, hateful "baby" that she feels herself to be. He has become like a depriving, condemning parent. In turn, she hates him more. This process occurred in J, although both the Ks were totally unaware of it.

This same problem can be compounded. The man usually perceives a decrease in the care he has been receiving and resents this, rather than joining with the woman in a mutual attempt to increase their shared caretaking potential. O experienced this resentment, but he was not conscious of it. His resentment from this additional source was interpreted by J as further evidence of her unworthiness and unlovableness.

These forces obviously affect the children. As a result of her disappointment and anger with O, J tended to turn to her son for an increased sense that someone loved and cared about her. She, of course, provided for the child's care, but she moved toward the fantasy that this new "man" would bring her the love that she was beginning to believe her husband never would or could, the special connection that she could no longer feel with her husband. This was the close tie with her son that O envied and resented. Simultaneously, O's resentment was creating a block to his ability to fully love his son, a terrible deprivation for O, as well as for the child.

In another variation, some women come to resent the child as a

consequence of the man's anger and withdrawal. The woman's necessary attention to the child has made the husband less devoted to
her. In effect, the child has deprived her of her husband. At times,
there follows from this situation a dangerous focus on the child, which
combines great expectations and great anger. J had some tendency in
this direction, but this reverberating anger and expectation were not
carried to the extreme that they can sometimes reach.

We can see, however, that in a similar situation carried to a greater
intensity, we have a configuration leading to the problems in mother–
child "symbiosis" that have been described and also to many of the
other difficulties that are called problems in mother–child separation
and the like.

It is important to note again the asymmetry. J *did* develop in many
ways. She learned even more about the complex processes of so interacting with another human being as to foster the growth of that person, an accomplishment that could be seen as the most important of
all human endeavors. In addition, she did some reworking of her own
psychic forces, and this reworking changed her perceptions and attitudes. For example, her career goals were now more heavily influenced by a desire to participate in the growth of others and by the
belief that present occupational structures do not provide this opportunity. However, she did not have the confidence to put her perspective forward forcefully. Further, she was not accumulating the knowledge and credentials bestowed by education and work in the "real
world." Instead, she felt that she had fallen behind. Thus, she was left
with a common women's dilemma: How could she have a valid opinion if she was at the same time filled with such feelings of inadequacy
and conflict? (It may well be that some of men's "midlife crises" and
doubts about the value of their worldly accomplishments are a reflection of these same issues as they come round in another form.)

The complexities of just one stage of family life have been barely
suggested. Similar features, and their reverberating complications, occur through all of the phases of the life cycle, but they cannot be detailed here. The features mentioned, however, may offer some clues to
the underlying factors in families with greater difficulties.[3] Studies of
such families suggest that the needs of the parents, which are unresolved and of which the parents are unaware, are foisted onto the children. These needs come to be perceived (falsely) as the children's needs.
These studies have described, also, the indirect modes of communication that surround this process. Seen in today's perspective, it does
not seem too wild a conjecture to suggest that some of our most baf-
fling "disorders" may be the result of the family influences discussed
here, carried to a more intense level.

Another topic of major concern today is the dangerous effect of depression within the family. As illustrated by J, depression is a very likely outcome for the woman in the early child-rearing years. This assumption is borne out by current statistics.[10] There are many other matters that have gone under various clinical labels and that may bear reexamination in the light of recent understandings of the woman's situation, such as the mother–child separation issues mentioned above, phobias, and psychosomatic reactions.

For the Ks, specifically, the losses had been serious. In many clinical settings, J would have been diagnosed as "the patient." She may have been given various courses of antidepressants and/or tranquilizers; such prescriptions can convey confirmation of the message that the woman is the "sick" one. J would have lost the ability to love her husband; and he, her. Both loved their children, but the children's lives would have been marred by the covert conflicts in the family. Although the evidence has not been included here, it was clear that both children were on the path toward psychological difficulties.

COMMENT

O was pursuing the usual growth model—and certainly not consciously trying to oppress anyone. J, however, was carrying the seeds of conflict, and also the seeds of change, of movement toward a new integration. These seeds were being destroyed in *status nascendi,* and J herself was being destroyed.

Another way of putting the matter is to say that there had been a foreclosure on the possibility of engaging in growth based on the full interaction of two people; that is, there was a lack of a true encounter of differences. Men have been led to seek a continual renewal of male-defined goals and values, and women have been led to support this quest rather than to express their own experience in all of its depth and meaning. If women attempt to bring their *different* experiences into the interaction, they appear to be initiating conflict. Conflict, defined in a broad sense, does not mean a destructive process at all. Instead, the thesis here is that the suppression of this necessary conflict is the destructive factor. A situation that suppresses valid conflict between the sexes does not allow the full emergence of those aspects of life that women are supposed to embody. Conflict between the sexes does, at this time, imply engagement with those essentials that women have been made to "carry" for the total society, such as the part of life highlighted here, fostering the development of other people. (There are several other realms of life that women are supposed to carry for the total society, but they have not been discussed here.[11]) If change occurs, women will no longer be the sole "carriers" of these essentials, and the nature of the conflict will take on different configurations; it will be transformed.

Because adults have not learned how to engage in this conflict, most do not yet know how to go on to allow the full emergence of the next conflict, the generational conflict, that is, the conflict that children inevitably generate. There is a lack of psychological preparation for participation in the disruptions that children rightfully provoke, for example, in their intense demands and extreme opposition at various growth phases. Adults lack the background for the repeated psychological reorganizations that children's full growth demands. Likewise, adults are not impelled—forced—to learn the creativity that would emerge, I believe, when human beings attempt to truly engage in these conflicts. Instead, there has been a suppression of conflict and of the recognition that there is a *reason* for conflict. Without this recognition, we put obstacles in the path of family movement. We tend toward "pathological homeostasis," which becomes manifest in various forms. Only one common form, depression in the wife, is discussed here. In addition to the production of clinically defined problems, it is apparent that intimacy deteriorates: the "special connection" that J described is replaced by bitterness.

Many significant factors have not been covered, such as class, ethnic, and racial differences, as well as variations in individual personalities. In general, however, most families are heavily influenced by the general cultural forces suggested here. The main focus has been the exploration of some of the factors that become incorporated as psychological forces in families. I have not dealt with the question of large-scale social change nor with the basic question, raised by many people today, of whether marriage and the family as we have known them can or should continue to exist.

For the moment, a few immediate practical steps may be appropriate to suggest. It is certainly feasible to plan for both women and men to commit themselves to effective participation and leadership in all realms of life and to have children, if they so desire. Working hours, pay, excellent day care, and other necessaries could be devised. It is equally apparent that the attainment of such obvious rearrangements would require massive mobilization of the national will. Even then, a change in mentality will not ensue unless a constant struggle is conducted both on the larger social scene and in personal life. The very process of conducting a struggle for better practical arrangements can, however, simultaneously enlarge women's ability to believe in and establish their rights and needs.

Even as women have begun to campaign for changes in some of

the major institutions of society, they have recognized their need for immediate help at many (all) periods of life. Many women's groupings are now trying to provide these, for example, via pregnancy support groups and new models for childbirth.[12,13] While this help is crucial and while it may rest on women's readier ability to understand and respond to these needs at this time, I believe that the long-range goal must be a change in the major institutions of society and the cultural and economic forces impinging on both sexes. Until such change occurs, it is important that workers in the psychological fields recognize that conditions often labeled *external* are not solely external. They become internal and are part of the psychological forces acting on the formation of the mind within the most intimate of settings: the family.

REFERENCES

1. Jackson DD, Weakland JH: Conjoint family therapy: Some considerations on theory, technique and results, *Psychiatry* 24:30–45, 1961.
2. Jackson DD, Watzlawick P: The acute psychosis as a manifestation of growth experience, *American Medical Association Psychiatric Research Reports* 16:83–94, 1963.
3. Bateson G, et al.: Toward a theory of schizophrenia, *Behavioral Science* 1:251–264, 1956.
4. Wynne L, et al: Pseudo-mutuality in the family relations of schizophrenics, *Psychiatry* 21:20–220, 1958.
5. Pincus L: *Marriage: Studies in Emotional conflict and growth.* London, Tavistock Publications, 1973.
6. U.S. Bureau Labor Statistics: News release, March 8, 1977.
7. Miller JB, Notman M, Nadelson C, et al: Aggression in women: A reexamination. In *Changing concepts in psychoanalysis.* Edited by Klebanow S. New York, Gardner Press, 1979. (See also Nadelson C, Notman M, Zilbach J, and Miller JB, this volume.)
8. Mahler M: *On human symbiosis and the vicissitudes of individuation,* Vol 1. New York, International Universities Press, 1968.
9. Rich A: *Of woman born: Motherhood as experience and institution.* New York, W. W. Norton, 1976.
10. Weissman MM, Klerman GL: Sex differences and the etiology of depression, *Archives of General Psychiatry* 34:98–111, 1977.
11. Miller JB: *Toward a new psychology of women.* Boston, Beacon Press, 1976.
12. Seiden AM: The sense of mastery in the childbirth experience. In *The woman patient,* Vol. 1. Edited by Notman M, Nadelson C. New York, Plenum Press, 1978.
13. Turner MF, Izzi MH: The COPE story: A service to pregnant and postpartum women. In *The woman patient,* Vol. 1. Edited by Notman M, Nadelson C. New York, Plenum Press, 1978.

Glossary

These definitions pertain to usage in the text; they are not necessarily complete if used in another context.

Acting out: The tendency of some persons to unconsciously reproduce forgotten memories, attitudes, and conflicts by actions rather than by recognizing and verbalizing these issues.

Affect regulation: Ability to modulate expression of emotions.

Affective: Pertaining to feeling, emotion, or mood.

Affect regulation: The ability to modulate the expression of emotions.

Ambivalence: The simultaneous existence of opposite feelings, attitudes, and tendencies directed toward another person, thing, or situation.

Amenorrhea: The absence of menstrual periods. In *primary* amenorrhea, no menstruation has ever occurred; in *secondary* amenorrhea, menstruation has occurred, then ceased.

Anergic: Lacking energy, passive.

Anorgasmia: A condition in which the individual does not experience orgasm. Origin usually considered psychological.

Anticonvulsants: Drugs that prevent epileptic seizures.

Antisocial personality: This term is reserved for individuals who are basically unsocialized and whose behavior pattern brings them repeatedly into conflict with society.

Anxiety: Tension or uneasiness that stems from the anticipation of danger, the source of which is largely unknown or unrecognized. The accompanying physiological changes are similar to those in states of fear. May be regarded as pathologic when so extreme as to interfere with effectiveness in living or reasonable emotional comfort.

Atavistic: Refers to traits, dormant for one or more generations, which reappear in the offspring.

Behavioral psychotherapy: Therapeutic technique based in behavior theory, which postulates that symptoms are learned patterns of behavior that are unadaptive. Therapy is directed to the inhibition and/or extinction of the learned responses.

Blackouts: An alcoholic blackout is memory loss for events that occurred during a drinking episode. While in a blackout, a person is conscious and appears normal, although intoxicated. However, during that time, the individual is not learning and therefore, after the drinking episode, does not remember what occurred.

Borderline personality organization: A psychological diagnostic entity characterized by intense and fluctuating affective states: anger; perception of some people as all good and others as all bad; an inability to form stable, consistent, trusting relationships; the assignment of one's feelings to others.

Catharsis: A psychiatric term referring to the therapeutic release of conscious material

301

through talking, or to the release into awareness of repressed material from the unconscious.

Cathexis: The attachment, conscious or unconscious, of emotional feelings and significance to an idea or object, commonly a person.

Character disorder: A personality disorder manifested by a chronic and habitual pattern of reaction that is maladaptive in that it is relatively inflexible, limits the optimal use of potentialities, and often provokes the very counterreactions from the environment that the person seeks to avoid.

Corticoids: Any steroid that has certain chemical or biological properties characteristic of the hormones secreted by the adrenal cortex.

Countertransference: The effects of an analyst's or therapist's unconscious needs and conflicts on his or her understanding or technique. For example, a patient's personality or material may evoke some experience from the therapist's or analyst's past and this may color his/her relationship with the patient.

Defense mechanism: An unconscious psychic mechanism by which an individual handles excessive anxiety caused by conflictual issues.

Delusional: Refers to thinking characterized by delusions, or beliefs not based on realistic perceptions. Delusions arise from unconscious needs and are maintained against logical argument and despite objective contradictory evidence.

Dementia: Loss of intellectual function due to organic impairment.

Denial: A defense mechanism, operating unconsciously, used to resolve emotional conflict and to allay anxiety by disavowing thoughts, feelings, wishes, needs, or external realities that are consciously intolerable.

Depression: This term may refer either to a mood or an affect, or to a specific diagnostic classification. As a mood, it is characterized by feelings of sadness. In the diagnosis of depression are found individual experiences of lowered self-esteem, hopelessness, guilt, and diminished interest in activities. In addition, these mood disturbances may occur with objective signs, for example apathy, fatigue, loss of appetite, distrubances in sleep, constipation, and difficulty concentrating.

Displacement: A defense mechanism, operating unconsciously, in which an emotion is transferred or "displaced" from its original object to a more acceptable substitute.

Dissociation: A manifestation of confused thought processess and disorganized behavior in which the individual may be at different levels of organization and adaptiveness. We speak of dissociation of ego functions.

Double bind: A name for a type of interaction, noted frequently in schizophrenics' families, in which one member demands a response to a message containing mutually contradictory signals, and the other person is unable to comment on the incongruity or to escape from the situation.

DSM: Abbreviation for the *Diagnostic and Statistical Manual (of Mental Disorders)*, a guide to the nomenclature of psychological disorders.

Dysmenorrhea: The occurence of pain just before or during menstrual periods.

Dyspareunia: The occurrence of pain during sexual intercourse. The term is usually used in reference to women.

Dysphoric mood: A sense of dissatisfaction or unpleasantness.

Ego: one of the three functional dimensions of the mental apparatus as originally conceptualized by Freud. Ego is the integrative force that mediates between internal impulse or instinct and external reality.

Egocentric: Limited, in outlook or concern, to one's own activities or needs.

Ego functioning: A psychological theoretical construct; an individual's ability to integrate his or her perceptions and reactions derived from environmental stimuli and internal personal feelings.

Ego regression: A decrease in an individual's previous level of ego functioning.

Ego-syntonic: Describes aspects of an individual's behavior, thoughts or attitudes he or she views as acceptable and consistent with his or her total personality, as opposed to *ego-alien*. These aspects of behavior may be seen as acceptable or unacceptable by others.

Electroencephalogram (EEG): A graphic recording of the electrical activity of the brain.

Eysenck Personality Inventory: A psychological inventory that has scales for neuroticism and introversion–extroversion.

Grief: The normal, appropriate emotional response to an external and consciously recognized loss; it is usually self-limited and gradually subsides within a reasonable time. To be distinguished from depression.

Group delinquent reaction of adolescence: Individuals with this disorder have acquired the values, behavior, and skills of a delinquent peer group or gang to whom they are loyal and with whom they characteristically steal, skip school, and stay out late at night.

Hyperemesis Gravidarum: Pernicious vomiting in pregnancy.

Hysteria: A term used colloquially in a number of ways, sometimes to connote excessive emotionalism. Technically, it can designate a personality type or an individual who is dramatic, flamboyant, and labile, but not disturbed. Also, personality disorder characterized by excitability, emotional instability, overreactivity, and dramatization. Individuals with this disorder are often seen as immature, vain, and dependent.

Identification: An automatic, unconscious mental process whereby an individual becomes like another person in one or several aspects.

Id: In Freudian theory, that part of the personality structure harboring the unconscious instinctive desires and strivings of the individual.

Identification: The unconscious process by which an individual patterns himself or herself after another.

Impulse control: The ability to delay and regulate the discharge of sexual and aggressive drives.

Inadequate personality: This behavior pattern is characterized by ineffectual responses to emotional, social, intellectual, and physical demands.

Infantilization: The performance of activities or the imposition of rules that are immature or childish.

Introjection: An unconscious mechanism by which a loved or hated external object is symbolically taken into oneself.

Involutional: Refers to the changes or conditions occurring during late middle age in both sexes. The term is becoming outmoded.

Latency age: The period of childhood from ages 6 to 12, when sexual impulses were theoretically considered to be dormant.

Leukorrhea: A whitish discharge from the vagina resulting from inflammation or congestion of the mucous membrane.

Libido: Drive, energy; usually sexual.

Manic: Refers to a condition characterized by excessive elation, irritability, talkativeness, flight of ideas, and accelerated speech and motor activity. When there is a manic-depressive disturbance, manic episodes alternate with depressive episodes.

Masticatory: Refers to the parts of the jaw, including bones, teeth, joints, or ligaments.

Menarche: The onset of menstruation.

Metrorrhagia: Profuse bleeding from the uterus, especially between menstrual periods.

MMPI: The Minnesota Multiphasic Personality Inventory, a standardized, selfrating personality questionnaire consisting of 550 items concerning behavior, feelings, social attitudes, and symptoms of psychopathology.

Monism: The view that reality is one unitary organic whole with no independent parts.

Narcissism: The concentration of psychological interest on the self.

Neonatal: Relating to the newborn during approximately the first month after birth.

Neurasthenia: A term, rarely used in psychiatry today, that was taken literally to mean weakness or exhaustion of the nervous system characterized by chronic fatigue and lack of energy.

Neurosis: An emotional maladaptation characterized by anxiety and arising from unresolved emotional conflicts. This anxiety may be experienced directly or controlled by various psychological mechanisms that may cause other symptoms.

Obsessive-compulsive: A term characterizing the persistent intrusion of unwanted thoughts, urges, or actions that the individual is unable to stop, and that may become ritualistic or excessively concerned with conformity and adherence to standards. This term also described a personality state and character type of an individual who is rigid, conscientious (sometimes excessively so), perfectionistic, and who can also be indecisive.

Oedipal (complex, situation, conflict): A set of feelings arising within a family involving attachment of the child to the parent of the opposite sex accompanied by competitive, aggressive feelings toward the parent of the same sex. These feelings are largely repressed because of the fear of displeasure or punishment by the parent of the same sex. In its original use, the term applied only to the male child; it has since been extended to apply to both sexes. The term also represents a maturational development for the child, who is at this time able to relate to both parents in different ways at the same time, rather than to each one primarily as a need-satisfying figure.

Oligomenorrhea: Abnormally scant menstruation.

Oral fixation: An arrest in psychological development at an early period in life, when feeling was primary and attachments to people were dominated by these needs. In adult life, it manifests itself as intense wishes to have all needs gratified.

Paranoid: A disturbance in thinking in which delusions, generally persecutory or grandiose, are the essential abnormality.

Perinatal: Pertaining to the period of childbirth and shortly thereafter, usually beginning with the birth of a fetus of 20 weeks' or more gestation and ending 7–28 days later.

Personality disorder: A group of mental disorders characterized by ingrained maladaptive patterns of behavior, generally lifelong in duration and affecting the entire personality of the individual. When a personality trait becomes disabling or incapacitating, or leads to difficulty in relationships it is termed a *personality disorder.*

Phobia: An obsessive, persistent, unrealistically intense fear of an object or situation.

Pineal gland: A small, cone-shaped structure in the brain attached to the roof of the third ventricle between the superior colliculi. It produces melatonin, which has an unclear role in reproduction, and is also involved with indolamine metabolism.

Placenta previa: A condition in which the edge of the placenta overlies and partially or completely obstructs the opening of the cervix.

Potentiate: To increase the potential. When used in reference to drugs, the effect that one has on another to increase the potency of each.

Premenstrual tension (distress): Sometimes called *premenstrual syndrome.* The symptoms that sometimes occur just before the menstrual period, including headaches, nausea, psychological tension, and depression.

Projection: A defense mechanism based on the unconscious process of rejecting that which is emotionally unacceptable in the self and attributing those qualities to others.

Pseudocyesis: A condition in which a woman believes that she is pregnant and manifests some of the physical changes that accompany pregnancy when, in fact, she is not pregnant.

Psychoactive drug: When used in reference to psychopharmacological agents, this term refers to any drug (stimulant, depressant, or tranquilizer) with an effect on the mental processes.

Psychoanalytic psychotherapy: Psychotherapy based on psychoanalytic concepts and/or practices, in which association and dreams are traced and the unconscious is explored. The therapy seeks to eliminate or diminish unconscious conflict through conscious awareness and the regarding of old conflicts in terms of adult ego strengths.

Psychodynamics: The systematized knowledge and theory of human behavior and its maturation, the study of which depends largely on the functional significance of emotion. Psychodynamics recognizes the role of unconscious motivation.

Psychogenic: Due to psychological or emotional factors and not to detectable organic or somatic factors.

Psychopathic: Usually used to describe an antisocial personality disorder.

Psychosis: A major mental disorder in which the individual's ability to think, respond emotionally, remember, communicate, interpret reality, and behave appropriately may be so impaired that ordinary life demands cannot be met. It is often characterized by regressive behavior, inappropriate mood, diminished impulse control, and abnormal mental processes, such as delusions and hallucinations.

Psychotropic medication: Any drug with an effect on psychic function, behavior, or experience.

Rationalization: A defense mechanism, operating unconsciously, in which the individual attempts to justify or make consciously tolerable (by plausible means) feelings, behavior, and motives that would otherwise be intolerable.

Reality testing: The ability to appropriately understand, assess, and react to external and internal stimuli.

Regression: The partial or symbolic return to some earlier level of adaptation.

Repression: A defense mechanism, operating unconsciously, in which unacceptable ideas, affects, or impulses are banished from consciousness, or in which those that have never been conscious are kept from becoming conscious.

Schizoid: A personality disorder manifested by shyness, oversensitivity, seclusiveness, frequent daydreaming, avoidance of close or competitive relationships, and, often, eccentricity. Individuals with this condition often react to disturbing experiences and conflicts with apparent detachment and are often unable to express hostility and aggressive feelings.

Schizophrenia: A form of psychosis manifested by characteristic disturbances of thought, mood, and behavior. Thought disturbances are marked by alterations of concept formation that may lead to misinterpretation of reality and sometimes to delusions and hallucinations. Mood changes include flatness of affect, constriction, inappropriateness, and loss of empathy with others. *Schizophrenia* is sometimes used as a term for a group of related but not identical psychoses.

Separation–individuation: The process of separating from parents and differentiation into an individual, beginning in childhood.

Shakes: Shakes, or tremors, may be a sign that a person is addicted to alcohol. When an alcohol addict stops drinking, even for 5–12 hours, he or she begins to withdraw from the alcohol. Shaking in the morning after sleeping and not drinking for a few hours indicates addiction. A morning drink relieves the shakes by increasing the blood-alcohol level.

Somatization: The process of converting a mental disorder into physical symptomatology.

Splitting: The active process of keeping apart introjections and identifications of opposite quality, for example, good and bad self and object representations or images.

Stasis: In psychoanalytic theory, the accumulation of libidinous excitations or tensions because of the blockage of their motor discharge. When the free flow of libido has thus been dammed, stasis results, giving rise to the feeling of anxiety. This term is more frequently used in older psychoanalytic literature.

Superego: In psychoanalytic theory, that part of the personality associated with ethics, standards, and self-criticism. It is formed by the child's identification with important and esteemed persons in his or her early life, particularly parents. The supposed or actual wishes of these significant persons are taken over as part of the child's own personal standards to help form the "conscience."

Supportive psychotherapy: A technique of psychotherapy that aims to reinforce a patient's defenses and help him or her suppress disturbing psychological material. It utilizes such measures as reassurance, suggestion, inspiration, and education.

Temporal lobe: Part of the cerebral hemisphere which lies laterally and mediates the emotional aspects of behavior; integrates the visual, auditory, and cognitive functions.

Temporomandibular joint: The joint of the jaw.

Tolerance: Increasing resistance to the effects of a drug, so that higher doses are necessary for therapeutic effects.

Transference: In psychoanalytic therapy, the phenomenon of the projection of feelings, thoughts, and wishes from an important figure in the patient's past onto the analyst, who has come to be perceived as that person, transiently or in a more established fashion. The psychiatrist utilizes this phenomenon as a therapeutic tool to help the patient understand his or her emotional problems and their origins.

Unsocialized aggressive reaction of adolescence: This disorder is characterized by overt or covert hostile disobedience, quarrelsomeness, physical and verbal aggressiveness, vengefulness, and destructiveness.

Vaginismus: Involuntary spasm of the muscles surrounding the vaginal entrance, so that penetration in sexual intercourse is difficult or impossible.

Index

Femininity, concepts of (*cont.*)
  classical (*cont.*)
    penis envy, 23
  and drinking patterns
    adolescents, 228–229, 230
    young adults, 231, 234–235
  gender identity, 5, 25
  identity development, 7
  positive approach, 23–24
  reproductive function, 6–7
  (*See also* Sex roles)
Fetal alcohol syndrome (FAS), 224
Free association, 250
Freud, Sigmund, 19, 25, 152, 153, 154
  on incest, 69
  pleasure principle, 162
  suicidal attempt analyzed by, 123
  on superego, 31–32
"Frustration-leading-to-aggression"
    hypothesis, 97
Functional-organic controversy (*See* Dualism)

Gelles, R.J., 48
Gender identity, 5, 25
Gender roles (*See* Sex roles)
Generativity, concept of, 235–236
Genetic anomalies
  incest and, 70
  and violence, 38–39
Genetic transmission of depression, theory of, 193–194
Gift exchange and incest taboo, 68–69
Gilula, M.F., violence defined by, 36
Goal-limited therapy, 247–248
Gomberg, E.S., on alcoholic women, 231–232
Gove, W.R., 166, 195, 263, 267
Greek tragedy, violent women in, 29–30
Grief process, miscarriage and, 176–177, 179, 186
Group homes, adolescents in, 83–93
Guilt, miscarriage and, 177
Gynecological problems of alcoholic women, 232

Hallucinogens, 222
Hatching subphase in infant, 87
Heiser, J., violence defined by, 36
Heroin, 222
Homicide, 48
  women perpetrators, 36–38, 40–41
  case examples, 42

Homosexual incest, 79–80
Hospitalization
  and disorientation, 137–138
  miscarriage and, 183, 185
Hostility, depression and, 198
Hypochondriasis, diagnosis of, 159
  as depression/pain correlate, 161
Hysteria, 303
  neurasthenia vs., 143–144

Identification and aggression, 39–40
Illness vs. disease, 142, 148, 149
Incest, 65–81
  increased recognition, 66–67
  scope of concept, 65–66
  societal issues, 81
  taboo origins, theories of, 68–71
  types
    brother–sister, 79
    brother–daughter, 71–78
    homosexual, 79–80
    mother–son, 80–81
Infanticide, 42
Infants
  of addicted mothers, 223–225
  complaining, 150
  gender-based reactions to, 24–25
  from incestuous matings, 70
  psychological tasks, 224
  separation-individuation, 87, 88–90

Jacklin, E., 25, 26, 266
  quoted, 18
Jackson, D.A. and M., study by, 34, 36–37, 41
Jacobson, Edith, quoted, 83
Jealousy
  in abusive husbands, 52
  miscarriage and, 178
Jobs (*See* Careers)
Juvenile delinquency (*See* Delinquency)

Kaplan, E., 21
Kernberg, P., 123
Klein, D., quoted, 31
Klinefelter's syndrome, 38–39
Krout, B.M., 157, 158, 163, 164
Kumin, M., poem by, 155

Ladee, G.A., quoted, 160
Learned helplessness hypothesis of female depression, 195